Maternal and Perinatal Health
in Developing Countries

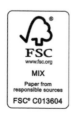

Maternal and Perinatal Health in Developing Countries

Edited by

Julia Hussein

University of Aberdeen, Scotland, UK

Affette McCaw-Binns

University of the West Indies, Kingston, Jamaica

and

Roger Webber

Argyll, Scotland, UK

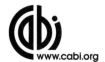
www.cabi.org

CABI is a trading name of CAB International

CABI	CABI
Nosworthy Way	875 Massachusetts Avenue
Wallingford	7th Floor
Oxfordshire OX10 8DE	Cambridge, MA 02139
UK	USA
Tel: +44 (0)1491 832111	Tel: +1 617 395 4056
Fax: +44 (0)1491 833508	Fax: +1 617 354 6875
E-mail: cabi@cabi.org	E-mail: cabi-nao@cabi.org
Website: www.cabi.org	

A catalogue record for this book is available from the British Library, London, UK.

Library of Congress Cataloging-in-Publication Data

Maternal and perinatal health in developing countries / edited by Julia Hussein, Affette McCaw-Binns, and Roger Webber.
    p. ; cm.
  Includes bibliographical references and index.
  ISBN 978-1-84593-745-4
I. Hussein, Julia. II. McCaw-Binns, Affette. III. Webber, Roger.
[DNLM: 1. Maternal Health Services. 2. Developing Countries.
3. Maternal Mortality. 4. Perinatal Care. 5. Perinatal Mortality. WA 310.1]

  362.198'32060091724--dc23

               2011049114

ISBN-13: 978 1 84593 745 4

Commissioning editor: Rachel Cutts
Editorial assistant: Gwenan Spearing
Production editor: Shankari Wilford

Typeset by SPi, Pondicherry, India
Printed and bound in the UK by CPI Group (UK) Ltd, Croydon, CR0 4YY.

Contents

—————————

The colour plate section can be found following p.126

Contributors

Endang L. Achadi is a medical doctor and public health practitioner. She is a senior teaching staff member and researcher at the Faculty of Public Health. Her main interests are in maternal and neonatal health and maternal nutrition. University of Indonesia, West Java, Indonesia; mcindo@indo.net.id

Kaosar Afsana is a public health practitioner with a medical and social science background. She is the Director of Health at BRAC and Professor at the BRAC School of Public Health. Her prime interests are in reproductive, maternal and child health and nutrition, community empowerment, gender and health system strengthening. BRAC, Dhaka, Bangladesh; afsana.k@brac.net

Iain Aitken is a public health physician. He is the Principal Technical Advisor at Management Sciences for Health. His main interests are in the integrated implementation of quality maternal, newborn and child health services. Management Sciences for Health, Cambridge, USA; iaitken@msh.org

Linda Bartlett is a family physician and maternal health epidemiologist. She is a senior faculty member at Johns Hopkins Bloomberg School of Public Health. Her main interests are in quality of care and expanding the evidence base for preventive and curative interventions at the community level to prevent maternal and perinatal mortality. Johns Hopkins Bloomberg School of Public Health, Baltimore, USA; lbartlet@jhsph.edu

Ann K. Blanc is a demographer. She is currently with the Population Council and previously Director of the Maternal Health Task Force. Her main interests are technical measurement issues, providing opportunities for knowledge sharing and consensus building, and identifying and supporting innovation in the maternal health field. Population Council, New York, USA; ablanc@popcouncil.org

Gilbert Burnham is Professor of International Health at the Johns Hopkins Bloomberg School of Public Health and heads the Center for Refugee and Disaster Response in the Department of International Health. He has a major interest in delivery of health services during conflict and post conflict situations, and in the needs of vulnerable populations affected by disasters. Johns Hopkins Bloomberg School of Public Health, Baltimore, USA; gburnham@jhsph.edu

Annabel Charnock is now a project officer at the Department for International Development and previously worked at the Nuffield Department of Obstetrics and Gynaecology at the University of Oxford. Department for International Development, London, UK; a-charnock@dfid.gov.uk

France Donnay is an obstetrician. She works at the Bill & Melinda Gates Foundation coordinating maternal, newborn and child health investments with a special expertise in maternal health. Her main interests are policy development and programme implementation in developing countries. Bill & Melinda Gates Foundation, Seattle, USA; France.Donnay@gatesfoundation.org

Tim Ensor is a health economist and health systems researcher. He is Professor of International Health Systems Research. He has a strong interest in health financing in low and middle income countries particularly in the areas of maternal health, costing and demand side financing. University of Leeds, Leeds, UK; t.r.a.ensor@leeds.ac.uk

Wendy. J. Graham is an obstetric epidemiologist and demographer. She is a professor at the University of Aberdeen and an evidence adviser at the UK Department for International Development. Her principal research interests are reducing and measuring the burden of maternal mortality and the translation of evidence into policy and practice. University of Aberdeen, Scotland, UK; w.graham@abdn.ac.uk

Sennen Hounton is a maternal health epidemiologist. He is Monitoring and Evaluation Adviser at the Technical Division of UNFPA. His main interests are surveillance of maternal and newborn deaths, design, implementation and cost-effectiveness evaluation of maternal and newborn interventions in developing countries. UNFPA, New York, USA; hounton@unfpa.org

Julia Hussein is a public health obstetrician and development practitioner. She is a senior researcher at Immpact, the College of Life Sciences and Medicine and Scientific Director of Ipact. Her main interests are in quality of care and strengthening research capacity in developing countries. University of Aberdeen, Scotland, UK; j.hussein@abdn.ac.uk

Gwendoline Quetoline Kandawasvika is a paediatrician. She is a lecturer in the department of paediatrics. Her main interests are in neonatal care audit and child development. University of Zimbabwe, Harare, Zimbabwe; gwenkandawasvika@gmail.com

Hannah Knight is a Research Associate at the Nuffield Department of Obstetrics and Gynaecology. Her main research interest is the use of evidence-based maternal health interventions in low and middle income countries. University of Oxford, England, UK; hannah.knight@obs-gyn.ox.ac.uk

Ana Langer is a physician specialized in paediatrics and neonatology, as well as a reproductive health expert, public health researcher and advocate for women's reproductive health and rights. She is Professor of the Practice of Public Health and the coordinator of the Dean's Special Initiative in Women and Health. Her main areas of expertise are women's health, maternal mortality, unsafe abortion and the quality of maternal health care. Harvard School of Public Health, Boston, USA; alanger@hsph.harvard.edu

Joy E. Lawn is an African born paediatrician and perinatal epidemiologist. She is Director of Evidence and Policy of Saving Newborn Lives. Her expertise includes national and global estimates for stillbirths, neonatal deaths and morbidity, and the design and evaluation of integrated maternal, newborn and child care services at scale, especially in sub-Saharan Africa. Save the Children, Cape Town, South Africa; joylawn@yahoo.co.uk

Adrienne Levay is a MSc in Global Health student at the School of Public Health. Her main interests are maternal health and nutrition in developing countries. University of Alberta, Edmonton, Canada; alevay@ualberta.ca

Tsitsi Mildred Magure is an obstetrician and gynaecologist. She is a lecturer at the department of obstetrics and gynaecology. Her main interests are in maternal and perinatal audit, the training of skilled attendants and cervical cancer screening. University of Zimbabwe, Harare, Zimbabwe; tmagure@uz.ucsf.co.zw

Dileep V. Mavalankar is a Public Health management expert. He is currently the Dean of the Indian Institute of Public Health, part of the Public Health Foundation of India and Government of Gujarat. His areas of interest include public health management, maternal health and reproductive health. Indian Institute of Public Health, Gandhinagar, India; dileep@iimahd.ernet.in

Affette McCaw-Binns is Professor of Reproductive Health and Epidemiology. In addition to teaching, research interests include improving quality of care for mothers and newborns through innovations in service delivery and measuring health outcomes, especially maternal mortality and quality of vital registration. University of the West Indies, Kingston, Jamaica; affette.mccawbinns@uwimona.edu.jm

Nicolas Meda is a medical epidemiologist. He is the Scientific Director of Centre MURAZ and Associate Professor of Public Health at the University of Ouagadougou. His main research interests are in HIV and maternal, neonatal and child health. Centre MURAZ, Bobo-Dioulasso, Burkina Faso; nmeda.muraz@fasonet.bf

Zubia Mumtaz is a physician and a public health specialist. She is an academic and researcher at the School of Public Health. Her main interests are in the social determinants of maternal health in developing countries. University of Alberta, Edmonton, Canada; zubia.mumtaz@ualberta.ca

Stephen Peter Munjanja is an obstetrician and gynaecologist. He is a professor of Obstetrics and Gynaecology. His main interests are the monitoring of levels of maternal mortality, audit of the quality of obstetric care and the provision of care by mid-level providers. University of Zimbabwe, Harare, Zimbabwe; spmunjanja@africaonline.co.zw

David Newlands is an international health economist. He is a Senior Lecturer in Economics. His main research interests are in the productivity costs of ill health and in equitable health care systems. University of Aberdeen, Scotland, UK; d.newlands@abdn.ac.uk

Ann Phoya is a public health nurse midwife and maternal and child health specialist. She is Director in the Department of Planning, Ministry of Health. Her main interests are in improving access to quality health services, especially for women and children, and midwifery education. Ministry of Health, Lilongwe, Malawi; phoyaann@yahoo.com

Emma Pitchforth is a health services researcher. She is Leader at RAND Europe Research. Her research interests include the application of social science methods and perspectives to study quality of care and users' experiences of health care. RAND Europe, Cambridge, UK; epitchfor@rand.org

Heather E. Rosen is a public health researcher. She is a senior research assistant in the Department of International Health. Her main interests are in strengthening community and facility based health services for mothers and newborns in developing countries. Johns Hopkins Bloomberg School of Public Health, Baltimore, USA; hrosen@jhsph.edu

Parvathy Sankara Raman is a demographer and researcher in public health. She is working at the Indian Institute of Public Health. Her main interests are in doing quantitative research in maternal and neonatal health. Indian Institute of Public Health, Public Health, Gandhinagar, India; parrathys@iiphg.org

Jeffrey Michael Smith is an obstetrician-gynecologist and public health practitioner. He is Maternal Health Team Leader at Jhpiego. His main interests are performance improvement and human resource development for maternal health in developing countries. Jhpiego, Baltimore, DC, USA; jsmith@jhpiego.net

Cynthia Stanton is trained in demography and epidemiology. She is an Associate Professor at the Johns Hopkins Bloomberg School of Public Health. Her work focuses on the measurement and evaluation of maternal and perinatal outcomes and processes. Johns Hopkins Bloomberg School of Public Health, Baltimore, USA; cstanton@jhsph.edu

Hannah Tappis is a humanitarian programming and research specialist. She is a doctoral candidate at Johns Hopkins Bloomberg School of Public Health. Her main interests are in strengthening health systems and quality of care in fragile, crisis affected states. Johns Hopkins Bloomberg School of Public Health, Baltimore, USA; htappis@jhsph.edu

Lisa J. Thomas is an obstetrician-gynaecologist with fellowship training in family planning. She is a Medical Officer in the Department of Reproductive Health and Research, where she serves as the focal point for sexual and reproductive health in humanitarian settings. World Health Organization, Geneva, Switzerland; thomasl@who.int

José Villar is an obstetrician and gynaecologist. He is professor of perinatal medicine at the Nuffield Department of Obstetrics and Gynaecology and the Women's Centre, John Radcliffe

Hospital. He is also Co-Director of the Oxford Maternal and Perinatal Health Institute and teaches obstetric research and perinatal epidemiology. University of Oxford, England, UK; jose.villar@obs-gyn.ox.ac.uk

Roger Webber is a specialist in communicable diseases. He was formerly Senior Lecturer in the London School of Hygiene and Tropical Medicine involved in teaching, research and consultancies. His interests include strengthening of health services in developing countries and preparation of teaching material, especially books. Argyll, Scotland, UK; r-webber@live. co.uk

Mary Nell Wegner is a maternal health programmer, with experience in reproductive health and gender issues in developing countries. She currently works as an independent consultant. Her main interests are in the quality of care in labour and delivery; obstetric fistula prevention and treatment and gender issues, especially as they apply to men's and women's roles in family planning and reproductive health choices. New York, USA; mnwegner@ comcast.net

Sophie Witter is a health economist and health systems researcher. She is senior research fellow in Immpact at the College of Life Sciences and Medicine, Reader at Queen Margaret University Edinburgh, and an Associate with Oxford Policy Management. Her main interests are health financing and financial barriers to care in low and middle income countries, health systems research, provider payments, complex evaluations, and maternal health care. University of Aberdeen, Scotland, UK; s.witter@abdn.ac.uk

Foreword

————————————

As Directors of the Maternal Health Task Force, we are often asked for recommendations from those looking for an introduction to and overview of the maternal health field. Until now, we have not been able to readily cite one source that is both comprehensive and practical. With the publication of this book, we will be able to point to an authoritative source.

The book fills a number of gaps, providing a history and overview of the field, summaries of the latest evidence and identification of critical gaps in knowledge. The individual chapters cover the gamut of key issues, including basic epidemiology, health systems and quality of care, financing and the demand for care. Readers will be able to assess both the progress that has been made in improving maternal health in developing countries and the many challenges that remain.

The editors have brought together a stellar group of international authors who bring both expertise and passion to the subject of maternal and perinatal health. As a group, they have both the research proficiency and the solid, on the ground, experience necessary to share important knowledge. We expect that the book will be a standard text for many years to come.

Ann K. Blanc, Ph.D. and Ana Langer, M.D.
Maternal Health Task Force Directors, phase 1 and 2

Acknowledgements

Acknowledgements are due to my co-editors and the authors for their contributions. Special thanks are due to Victor Ojodale Ogala, Katherine Ritchie and Ann Fitzmaurice for their assistance with referencing. The Kambia Appeal, Riders for Health, Paul Kwale, Lorney Kanguru and Navya Bezawada contributed to my search for photographs of transport modalities.

This book is a celebration – of what I've learned, and of the tireless efforts of the many, valued friends and colleagues I've learned from, who have dedicated their lives to improving maternal and perinatal health. May there be many others who feel the passion for joining our global 'community'.

Julia Hussein

Disclaimer

The authors alone are responsible for the views expressed in their chapters and they do not necessarily represent the decisions, policy or views of the organizations to which they belong.

List of Abbreviations

———————————————

AMTSL	Active Management of the Third Stage of Labour
CEE/CIS	Central and Eastern Europe/Commonwealth of Independent States
CI	Confidence Interval
EmOC	Emergency Obstetric Care
GNP	Gross National Product
HDP	Hypertensive disorders of pregnancy
HIV/AIDS	Human Immunodeficiency Virus/Acquired Immunodeficiency Syndrome
ICD 10	International Classification of Diseases version 10
IHME	Institute of Health Metrics and Evaluation
IV	Intravenous
MDGs	Millennium Development Goals
MHTF	Maternal Health Task Force
MNCH	Maternal, Neonatal and Child Health
OR	Odds Ratio
PMNCH	Partnership for Maternal, Newborn and Child Health
PMTCT	Prevention of Mother To Child Transmission
RAMOS	Reproductive Age Mortality Studies
RCT	Randomized Controlled Trial
RR	Risk Ratio
STI	Sexually Transmitted Infection
UK	United Kingdom
UN	United Nations
UNAIDS	Joint United Nations Programme on HIV/AIDS
UNFPA	United Nations Population Fund
UNICEF	United Nations Children's Fund
UNGA	United Nations General Assembly
UNSG	United Nations Secretary General
USA	United States of America
USAID	United States Agency for International Development
WHO	World Health Organization
WRA	White Ribbon Alliance

1 An Introduction to Maternal and Perinatal Health

Julia Hussein,[1] Ann K. Blanc,[2] France Donnay[3] and Affette McCaw-Binns[4]
[1]*University of Aberdeen, Scotland, UK;* [2]*Population Council, New York, USA;*
[3]*Bill & Melinda Gates Foundation, Seattle, USA;* [4]*University of the West Indies, Kingston, Jamaica*

Summary

- This chapter provides an overview of maternal and perinatal health in developing countries and presents a synopsis of the subsequent chapters in this book.
- Maternal deaths represent only a fraction of the burden of ill health and disability faced by millions of women and newborns as a consequence of complications during pregnancy and childbirth.
- Unnecessary maternal and perinatal deaths and ill health continue to occur in developing countries because of fundamental factors such as poverty and the lack of education and empowerment.
- Proximate determinants of maternal and perinatal mortality and morbidity are weak health systems, lack of access to health services and poor availability and quality of maternity care.
- Technical experts have agreed on core strategies to improve maternal and perinatal health, which include family planning, nutritional interventions, appropriate antenatal care, safe abortion care, skilled care especially during labour and delivery, emergency obstetric care and postnatal support.
- The global community has embarked on a united effort, with an expansion of interested groups which together can make a real difference in hastening the improvement of maternal and perinatal health.
- Some of the key challenges faced for the successful implementation of programmes at country level are to enhance the functionality of health systems as a vital foundation upon which to build programmes and to improve the integration of services. At global level, improved networking and clarity of mandates amongst the various partners will be fundamental to ensuring resources are directed effectively and efficiently.

The Burden of Ill Health

She had travelled for three days in the back of the cart, in labour, over stony desert terrain. On the second day, she delivered a dead child in the open desert. It was then that the bleeding started. She was unconscious and barely alive when she reached the hospital. I remember the sinking feeling I had when I saw her lying in the back of the cart, soaked in blood, as her husband looked to us for help, exhausted and covered in dust and dirt from the journey. The dead body of her baby lay swaddled and still beside her. We tried our best at the hospital, but she died minutes after she arrived. My enduring memory is of her husband leaving the hospital early the next morning, pulling his cart behind him, with two bodies wrapped in dirty rags, making a start to his long journey back home. To this day, I wonder what more I could have done to save her life.

J. Hussein, Jalalabad, Afghanistan, 1993

Each day, nearly a thousand women die as a result of the complications of pregnancy or childbirth. Over 98% of these deaths occur in developing countries. The precise numbers of deaths are not known as they are based on estimates with wide uncertainty intervals. The women who die are nearly all young, healthy and in the prime of their lives. These avoidable tragedies are difficult to make sense of in today's world, where information on health and disease is openly available, and drugs can be purchased at the touch of a button on the internet. Yet the spectre of death during pregnancy is the reality for many of the poorest and most disadvantaged women. The World Health Organization estimates that 358,000 maternal deaths occur annually (WHO, 2010) and that 88–98% of these are avoidable (WHO, 1986). Most maternal deaths in developing countries are from obstetric causes – bleeding, hypertensive disease, infection, obstructed labour and unsafe abortion (Khan *et al.*, 2006; see Stanton and McCaw-Binns, Chapter 4 this volume).

The full scale of the burden is not captured by the numbers of deaths alone. Much less is known about the scale of ill health resulting from pregnancy complications. Life-threatening complications are experienced in 15% of pregnant women, although some form of obstetric problem occurs in over 40% of pregnancies (WHO, 1994). It is estimated that over 300 million women suffer ill health as a consequence of pregnancy or childbirth, with 20 million new cases occurring annually (WHO, 2005). For example, 12% of women who survive severe bleeding will suffer severe anaemia (AbouZahr, 2003). Two million women are thought to live with obstetric fistula as a result of obstructed labour (Lewis and de Bernis, 2006). Depression is thought to appear during pregnancy in between 6% and 25% of women in developing countries (WHO and UNFPA, 2009). Infertility can result from infection, obstructed labour or unsafe abortion and affects an estimated 60–80 million people (Sharma *et al.*, 2009).

Pregnancy complications in the mother also result in death and illness in the fetus and newborn baby. Perinatal mortality is a term used to describe deaths of babies in the first week of life, plus the number of stillbirths.

The term is not favoured for measurement due to definitional difficulties (see Stanton and Lawn, Chapter 5 this volume) but remains a useful concept that serves to remind us of the obstetric origins of fetal and newborn wellbeing, and that poor maternity care or unsafe delivery has consequences before and after childbirth; as well as for the mother and newborn. Most perinatal deaths occur in developing countries and the poorest sectors of the population. Six million babies die each year, either as late fetal deaths or in the first month of life. Many of these deaths are preventable and the vast majority are associated with poor maternal health or mismanagement during childbirth (WHO, 2006). For instance, obstructed and prolonged labour can cause asphyxiation, occurring in 3% of babies and resulting in death or brain damage in half of them. Maternal infections and poor nutrition can result in newborn sepsis and low birth weight babies who are 30 times more likely to die in the first week of life. If the child survives these birth-related challenges, permanent neurological damage, seizures and severe learning disorders can result (Population Reference Bureau, 2002).

A maternal death can also result in a series of consequences that have profound effects on families and their livelihoods (de Kok *et al.*, 2010). A mother's death threatens her child's survival throughout infancy and beyond (Ronsmans *et al.*, 2010). Illness and the death of a mother can lead to loss of household earnings (Storeng *et al.*, 2008). Catastrophic debt is known to occur as a result of the costs incurred to seek care for complications in pregnancy. These circumstances can ultimately lead to disintegration of the family unit as a whole (Filippi *et al.*, 2006).

Why do Maternal and Perinatal Deaths still Occur?

The obstetric causes of maternal and perinatal death are well known and due to the complications outlined above. The time of highest risk for the mother is during the last 3 months of pregnancy and the first week post partum, peaking on the first day after childbirth (Ronsmans and Graham, 2006). In addition to the obstetric causes of death, as much as a third of maternal deaths are due to medical conditions including HIV, malaria, anaemia and heart conditions.

Understanding the reasons behind why maternal and perinatal deaths occur requires more than an appreciation of the medical and obstetric causes. Poverty, gender empowerment, rights and education underlie many of the problems leading to high maternal and perinatal mortality because they affect the demand for and access to appropriate care. Such factors affect people's preferences, knowledge and awareness of health care services. Cultural factors, costs, distance to health services, the availability and the quality of maternity services also influence demand. If facilities are not well supplied (with drugs and equipment) or are poorly distributed or inappropriately staffed, they may not be well used and may provide poor quality care. The attitudes of health workers, their motivation, knowledge and practices are other factors that affect the supply–demand dynamic of the health system that forms the all important foundation to improving maternal and perinatal health.

Taking Action

The good news is that recent estimates show a slow but significant decline in maternal mortality globally (see Stanton and McCaw-Binns, Chapter 4 this volume). This optimistic picture is supplemented by the successes of some developing countries such as Sri Lanka, Malaysia and Thailand and an upsurge of political will to support activities to accelerate progress globally (see Graham, Chapter 3 this volume). There is reason to believe that we now know more about how to reduce maternal and perinatal mortality, with improved technologies, clinical knowledge and ways to enhance efficiencies and learning in the health system (Hussein, 2007).

Yet improvements in maternal health, the fifth millennium development goal (MDG 5), have been identified as one of the hard to reach goals – maternal mortality is not falling sufficiently rapidly to meet the global targets set by the MDGs (Campbell and Graham, 2006). Although child mortality (MDG 4) is declining globally, it has only recently been recognized that the poor state of newborn health and the 'invisibility' of stillbirths are areas needing special attention. A concerted effort is required in a range of areas represented in the MDGs (see McCaw-Binns and Hussein, Chapter 2 this volume). This realization has brought a wide range of actors together – the challenge being that improving maternal and perinatal health is not only simply about preventing maternal deaths or treating complications in pregnancy – so multifaceted action is required, encompassing a range of different skills, outlooks and expertise.

Programme strategies

Making 'better' obstetric services available (see Phoya et al., Chapter 10 this volume) and accessible (see Munjanja et al., Chapter 11 this volume) are strategies on which much hope is being placed. Providing skilled attendance at delivery is now being recommended by the WHO as the single most important intervention to reduce the number of maternal deaths in developing countries (see Achadi et al., Chapter 14 this volume). Technical experts have come together to develop a core set of essential interventions, based on available evidence and categorized according to community, first and referral level care. For the promotion of maternal health the key strategies include family planning, nutrition, appropriate antenatal care, safe abortion care, skilled care especially during labour and delivery, emergency obstetric care and postnatal support (PMNCH and the University of Aberdeen, 2010). One of the key concepts underlying this essential package of interventions is the importance of providing services in an integrated way, to jointly address reproductive health needs more broadly (see McCaw-Binns and Hussein, Chapter 2 this volume).

The successful implementation of programme strategies requires a functioning health system (see Mavalankar and Sankara Raman, Chapter 6 this volume) and appropriate strategies to finance the provision of services (see Witter and Ensor, Chapter 7 this volume).

Implementing clinical and obstetric interventions that are safe and effective are at the heart of all maternal and perinatal health programmes. Evidence-based good practices to manage the obstetric causes of maternal death are known (see Langer *et al.*, Chapter 8 this volume), as are interventions for mothers affected by other medical conditions (see Webber *et al.*, Chapter 9 this volume). Apart from attention to providing high quality care, understanding the demand for care (see Mumtaz and Levay, Chapter 12 this volume) and ensuring that communities are empowered to act and actively participate in the health system (see Afsana, Chapter 13 this volume) are other areas of programme focus.

Underpinning every high quality programme is the need to monitor and evaluate the effects of the programme, as distinct from efforts to monitor progress at global level (see Hounton *et al.*, Chapter 15 this volume). Programmes that perform and achieve the intended results in one setting may not necessarily be successful in others, and adaptations may be needed when special situations arise, as in conflict and emergency situations (see Bartlett *et al.*, Chapter 16 this volume).

Who is involved? The maternal and perinatal health 'architecture'

The architecture – structure, institutions and networks that support maternal and perinatal health – has been characterized by a diverse array of groups working at international, national and local levels. Some of these institutions focus exclusively or primarily on maternal health while others have adopted a broader mandate that encompasses maternal health as well as other areas, such as child health, reproductive health, human rights, poverty reduction and women's empowerment. Unlike some related fields of public health, where the landscape is dominated by a few central institutions (HIV/AIDS, for example), the maternal health field is considerably more scattered. The fragmentation of the maternal health field is one of the possible reasons for its relative lack of policy attention and a factor impeding swifter progress on achieving improvements in maternal health (Shiffman and Smith, 2007). Shiffman and Smith's case study of the maternal health field characterizes its architecture as having 'weak guiding institutions' without an 'institutional home'. Some specific weaknesses include a lack of institutions to help engineer consensus around technical interventions and policy messages, weak and problematic links to other policy communities, such as newborn health, overlapping mandates, and competition between organizations for resources.

Over the last few years, however, as the slow progress in MDG 5 has become evident, the maternal health field has evolved rapidly with new vigour. Many new players as well as existing players in allied fields are now entering the arena. Some of these organizations are still defining their roles and their approach to maternal health. New leaders and champions are emerging. Coordination and technical consensus at the global level have improved (Family Care International, 2007).

Clearly, the delivery of maternal health services and programmes occurs at the country level. The majority of funding for health systems improvements comes from governments and individual families in high burden countries, while important regional, national and community-based organizations undertake roles of service delivery, coordination and advocacy. The focus of this section is at the global level, where much of the technical and policy guidance and support for external aid funds are generated. It is worth noting that, even at the global level, the boundaries of the maternal health architecture are indistinct. Since improving maternal health involves many aspects of overall health systems strengthening, there are many ways in which efforts at general strengthening of the health system are particularly beneficial for maternal health. Many organizations also have activities in a number of areas, for example, the WHO would provide policy guidance and participate in programme implementation as well as generating research evidence, so the categories identified below should be interpreted in that light.

Policy, advocacy and networks

Among the UN agencies, WHO takes the role of providing policy guidance and technical support and conducting research. UNFPA has enhanced its focus on maternal health with a broad spectrum of programmatic and advocacy activities. Four organizations – UNFPA, the World Bank, UNICEF and WHO – have recently formed a partnership called 'The UN Health 4', commonly abbreviated to 'H4', with the goal of accelerating progress on maternal and newborn health in the countries with the highest maternal mortality rates. It has been joined by UNAIDS to make the 'H4+'.

The Partnership for Maternal, Newborn and Child Health (PMNCH) was launched in 2005 by the merger of three existing alliances for maternal, newborn and child health. Hosted by WHO, PMNCH is comprised of over 250 national governments, UN and multilateral agencies, bilateral donors, non-government organizations, foundations and health professional associations. Its mandate is framed by a 'continuum of care' that emphasizes integrated services for mothers, newborns and children, and its activities centre around six priority actions: knowledge management, commodities, human resources, advocacy, core packages of interventions and monitoring of the MDGs.

The Countdown to 2015 Initiative is a collective effort of more than 20 institutions to track the coverage of interventions that reduce maternal, newborn and child mortality, such as antenatal care and skilled care at birth, at the country and global level, in an effort to increase government and other stakeholder accountability. It issues periodic reports that provide data for judging progress towards achieving MDGs 4 and 5 as well as supporting work that improves the use of such data.

Launched in late 2009 with a grant from the Bill & Melinda Gates Foundation, the Maternal Health Task Force (MHTF) aims to provide a neutral forum where researchers, programme implementers and advocates can collaborate to identify and fill knowledge gaps, build consensus, engage in dialogue and share lessons learned. The Task Force also provides support for new research and tools, an internship programme for young maternal health professionals and a new knowledge management system for maternal health.

A lead organization in grass roots advocacy is the White Ribbon Alliance for Safe Motherhood (WRA), a global coalition of individuals and organizations that promote public awareness of maternal and newborn health issues. WRA has attracted multiple high profile advocates in recent years in its work to bring increased attention to maternal health issues. Women Deliver is a global advocacy organization seeking to attract high level policy attention to a range of issues related to women's role in development, including a strong focus on MDG 5.

More recently, a number of organizations – including Amnesty International, Human Rights Watch and a partnership of organizations forming the International Initiative on Maternal Mortality and Human Rights – have undertaken work to place maternal health within a human rights framework.

Donors

The architecture of maternal and perinatal health is influenced by the overall aid architecture. Two seminal documents influencing aid practice are the 2005 Paris Declaration on Aid Effectiveness and the 2008 Accra Agenda for Action (OECD, 2005), which aims to improve the spending of aid funds. In accordance with the needs articulated in these declarations, official development assistance to maternal and newborn health has shown a rising trend since 2003, to US$1228 million in 2008 for 68 priority countries. This amount comprises about a third of total aid for maternal, newborn and child health (Pitt et al., 2010).

The USA and the UK stand out for two reasons – they are by far the largest bilateral donors to maternal, newborn and child health with a combined share of bilateral aid of 59% in 2008. Both countries have increased their focus on maternal and newborn health: UK aid rising by 249% and US aid by 637%, generating US$353 million additional funds for maternal and newborn health in 2008 (Kaiser Family Foundation, 2009; Pitt *et al.*, 2010). Norway is also a prominent donor to maternal health activities. The World Bank and other development banks are a key source of financial and technical assistance. UNFPA, the European Union and UNICEF are other important donors in the maternal and new-born health field.

Among large US-based private foundations, only the Bill & Melinda Gates Foundation and the John D. and Catherine T. MacArthur Foundation have explicit maternal health funding programmes, although there are several other foundations that support reproductive health internationally (Global Health Visions, 2011). The growing interest in eHealth and mHealth (the use of electronic and mobile communication devices for health services) in maternal health interventions in developing countries has given impetus for the global business communities to play an active role in supporting initiatives (Vital Wave Consulting, 2009).

Programme delivery

Numerous international organizations deliver services or provide technical assistance for maternal health programmes in developing countries. Many have already been mentioned. Family Care International was one of the earliest global organizations dedicated to maternal health and undertakes a range of activities including programme delivery, advocacy and evidence generation. Other examples include CARE, BRAC, Jhpiego, Save the Children, World Vision, Pathfinder International, EngenderHealth, Options and others. An example of a large global initiative is MCHIP (Maternal and Child Health Integrated Program), a USAID flagship implemented by a consortium of organizations and led by Jhpiego. Two leading initiatives specially relevant to perinatal health are: the Saving Newborn Lives Initiative led by Save the Children and the Global Alliance

to Prevent Prematurity and Stillbirth (GAPPS). These groups advance research and raise awareness about the causes of and interventions for preventing stillbirths and newborn mortality. Professional associations such as the International Federation of Gynecology and Obstetrics (FIGO, a confederation of national obstetric and gynaecological societies) and the International Confederation of Midwives are also involved in global programme delivery, provision of technical support and advocacy.

Evidence

Open access libraries with specific relevance to maternal and perinatal health in developing countries include the Reproductive Health Library, housed at WHO in Geneva, and the Cochrane Library, hosted by the Cochrane Collaboration. There are several universities that have played a leading role in setting research agendas and generating the evidence that is used for developing programmes and policies in maternal health. The Mailman School of Public Health at Columbia University implements the Averting Maternal Death and Disability (AMDD) programme comprising research, programme support and advocacy focused on improving health systems, especially emergency obstetric care and increasing equity in access to services. The University of Aberdeen, through the Initiative for Maternal Mortality Programme Assessment (IMMPACT), aims to assess the effectiveness of interventions and improve measurement in maternal health. In addition, the London School of Hygiene and Tropical Medicine, the Institute of Child Health at University College London, the Bixby Center at the University of California San Francisco, the Liverpool School of Tropical Medicine, the Institute of Tropical Medicine at Antwerp and Johns Hopkins University among others are leading research institutions in the field. The Health Metrics Network and the Institute for Health Metrics and Evaluation also address maternal health measurement.

Many non-governmental organizations working internationally contribute to generating evidence, testing new approaches and pushing innovation forward. Notable organizations in maternal health and family planning include PATH, Gynuity Health Projects, the Population Council, the Guttmacher Institute, the International Center for Research on Women, Pathfinder International, Family Health International, the Futures group and many others. A recent study by Management Sciences for Health commissioned by the Partnership for Maternal Newborn and Child Health revealed hundreds of 'knowledge producers' in the maternal and newborn health field. Readers are referred to the report for a more comprehensive review (Gill *et al.*, 2009).

Gaps and weaknesses

While many positive changes have occurred in the maternal health architecture recently, the field would benefit from several improvements that could be considered key elements of a cohesive and effective public health community.

- *Well-defined roles and clear mandates* – improved clarity on the roles and mandates of the institutions working on maternal health would strengthen the field. In other public health areas, donors have played a substantial role in this 'sorting' of institutions through close coordination, convening major players and making strategic funding decisions that provide long-term, adequate resources to strengthen selected institutions. A set of strong, well-funded institutions with defined roles could make the currently weak ties between evidence and policy more robust, attract more resources and link international and national efforts more effectively.
- *Centralized platforms for knowledge sharing and networking* – regular meetings that bring together researchers, advocates and programme managers for information sharing and debate have not been a feature of the field for a number of years, although the Maternal Health Task Force has already begun to address this need through holding global conferences and other networking activities. Another gap that has been identified by maternal health professionals is the creation of a Master's Diploma in maternal health (and/or

including perinatal and child health, to re-emphasize the continuum of care) or dedicated programmes in MPH curricula; as well as a major journal or small set of journals with a similar focus in which there is priority given to building the evidence base on effective interventions and their implementation. In addition, a system for tracking funding commitments and resource flows is not in place, although Countdown to 2015 is making an effort to improve this area. The creation of these platforms for knowledge sharing would strengthen the links between research and policy, nurture new leaders and fortify ties with other fields and between the international and national realms.

- *Stronger links with allied communities* – strengthening ties between institutions working in maternal health and those in allied communities, such as newborn health, malaria, HIV/AIDS, nutrition and heath financing, is likely to increase effective coordination and integration of programmes and use the limited resources available more effectively. Such links could possibly allow access for maternal health to tap into new resources. Closer ties with allied fields such as health promotion and environmental health could yield new resources for those working specifically on maternal health.

About This Book

This book takes a public health perspective, with its overarching aim being to improve the implementation of maternal and perinatal health programmes in developing countries. Maternal health is its primary focus, while recognizing that perinatal wellbeing will result from interventions which target the mother during pregnancy.

A practical approach is taken, providing the essential concepts, insights and guidance to development and public health practitioners, policy makers and programme officers to design, assess and improve the operationalization of their programmes. The book will also be useful for those unfamiliar with the topic who are seeking an orientation to the key issues in one volume.

The book is in two sections. The first five chapters provide a background on the global setting and concepts underlying international efforts to improve maternal and perinatal health. The second section brings together the main elements of maternal health programmes at a country level: the underlying health system and financial aspects; specific interventions to manage conditions that affect maternal and perinatal health; the means to improve availability, accessibility, demand for and quality of care; and the crucial foundation of monitoring, evaluation and research within programmes. The special circumstances of conflict and emergency situations are included. The intention of this book was to take a practical approach, so that the 'front line' realities of programme implementation are tackled. A number of the chapters are written by practitioners in sub-Saharan Africa and Asia and give a specific country perspective, including case studies and examples of good (and bad) practices to overcome implementation problems, drawn from the experience of the authors.

The landscape of maternal and perinatal health is fast moving and a constantly changing one, with new knowledge, insights and experiences emerging all the time. A book cannot aspire to remain abreast of these rapid fluxes and we have aimed to provide an overview of the broad parameters of the field. Readers are encouraged to use the material provided here as signposts and guides for further reading.

Conclusion

The rich developed nations have, thankfully, almost forgotten what a maternal death is. But, for the vast majority of women in the rest of the world, pregnancy and childbirth are still a dangerous journey from which there may be no return. We cannot allow this tragedy to be repeated over and over again. We know why deaths happen and what works to save the lives of women and their babies. The knowhow, technologies, safe contraceptives, powerful antibiotics and effective drugs are all widely available. What needs to be done is to ensure that these tools for survival can reach the right hands – the hands of women and their families, the health workers and the people at the front line of organizing and delivering services and programmes.

References

AbouZahr, C. (2003) Global burden of maternal death and disability. *British Medical Bulletin* 67, 1–11.

Campbell, O.M.R. and Graham, W.J. on behalf of The Lancet Maternal Survival Series Steering Group (2006) Strategies for reducing maternal mortality: Getting on with what works. *Lancet* 368, 1284–1299.

de Kok, B., Hussein, J. and Jeffery, P. (2010) Joining-up thinking: loss in childbearing from interdisciplinary perspectives. *Social Science and Medicine* 71, 1703–1710.

Family Care International (2007) *Safe Motherhood. A Review*. Family Care International, New York.

Filippi, V.D., Ronsmans, C., Campbell, O.M.R., Graham, W.J., Mills, A., Borghi, J., Koblinsky, M. and Osrin, D. (2006) Maternal health in poor countries: the broader context and a call for action. *Lancet* 368(9546), 1535–1541.

Gill, J.L., Aubuchon, J.W., Aitkin, I. and Silimperi, D. (2009) *Mapping Maternal, Newborn and Child Health Knowledge*. Report for the Partnership for Maternal, Newborn and Child Health at the World Health Organization. Management Sciences for Health, Cambridge, Massachusetts.

Global Health Visions (2011) US Maternal Health Donors: A Landscape Analysis. A report prepared for the Maternal Health Task Force. Available at: http://maternalhealthtaskforce.org/component/wpmu/2011/05/24/u-s-maternal-health-donors-a-landscape-analysis (accessed 10 October 2011).

Hussein, J. (2007) Celebrating progress toward safer pregnancy. *Reproductive Health Matters* 15(30), 216–218.

Kaiser Family Foundation (2009) *The US and Global Maternal and Child Health Fact Sheet*. KFF, Menlo Park, California.

Khan, K.S., Wojdyla, D., Say, L., Gülmezoglu, A.M. and Van Look, P.F.A. (2006) WHO analysis of causes of maternal death: a systematic review. *Lancet* 367, 1066–1074.

Lewis, G. and de Bernis, L. (2006) *Obstetric Fistula: Guiding principles for clinical management and programme development*. WHO Press, Geneva.

OECD (2005) Paris Declaration and Accra Agenda for action. Available at: http://www.oecd.org/document/18/0,3343,en_2649_3236398_35401554_1_1_1_1,00.html (accessed 2 August 2011).

Pitt, C., Greco, G., Powell-Jackson, T. and Mills, A. (2010) Countdown to 2015: assessment of official development assistance to maternal, newborn, and child health, 2003–08. *Lancet* 376(9751), 1485–1496.

PMNCH and the University of Aberdeen (2010) Sharing knowledge for action on maternal, newborn and child health. PMNCH knowledge summaries, PMNCH, Geneva. Available at: http://www.who.int/pmnch/topics/continuum/knowledge_summaries_introduction/en/index.html (accessed 2 August 2011).

Population Reference Bureau (2002) Hidden Suffering: Disabilities from Pregnancy and Childbirth in Less Developed Countries. Available at: http://www.prb.org/pdf/hiddensufferingeng.pdf 2002 (accessed 2 August 2011).

Ronsmans, C. and Graham, W.J. (2006) Maternal mortality: who, when, where and why. *Lancet* 368(9542), 1189–1200.

Ronsmans, C., Chowdhury, M.E., Dasgupta, S.K., Ahmed, A. and Koblinsky, M. (2010) Effect of parent's death on child survival in rural Bangladesh: a cohort study. *Lancet* 375, 2024–2031.

Sharma, S., Mittal, S. and Aggarwal, P. (2009) Management of infertility in low resource countries. *BJOG: An International Journal of Obstetrics and Gynaecology* 116, 77–83.

Shiffman, J. and Smith, S. (2007) Generation of political priority for global health initiatives: a framework and case study of maternal mortality. *Lancet* 370, 1370–1379.

Storeng, K.T., Baggaley, R.F., Ganaba, R., Ouattara, F., Akoum, M.S. and Filippi, V. (2008) Paying the price: the cost and consequences of emergency obstetric care in Burkina Faso. *Social Science and Medicine* 66, 545–557.

Vital Wave Consulting (2009) *mHealth for Development: The Opportunity of Mobile Technology for Healthcare in the Developing World*. UN Foundation and Vodafone Foundation Partnership, Washington, DC and Berkshire, UK.

WHO (1986) Maternal mortality: helping women off the road to death. *WHO Chronicle* 40, 175–183.

WHO (1994) *The Mother Baby Package. Implementing Safe Motherhood in Countries. A practical guide*. WHO, Geneva.

WHO (2005) *The World Health Report, 2005 – Make every mother and child count*. WHO, Geneva.

WHO (2006) *Neonatal and perinatal mortality: Country regional and global estimates*. WHO Press, Geneva.

WHO (2010) *Trends in maternal mortality: 1990-2008. Estimates developed by WHO, UNFPA, UNICEF and the World Bank*. WHO Press, Geneva.

WHO and UNFPA (2009) *Mental Health Aspects of Women's Reproductive Health: a global review of the literature*. WHO, Geneva.

2 The Millennium Development Goals

Affette McCaw-Binns[1] and Julia Hussein[2]
[1]*University of the West Indies, Kingston, Jamaica;*
[2]*University of Aberdeen, Scotland, UK*

Summary

- The MDGs are a contract between the developed and the developing world to improve the quality of life in developing countries, laying out the responsibilities of both groups of countries in working towards achieving these goals.
- Developed countries are expected to provide 0.7% of GNP in official development assistance to finance development programmes. Developing countries should provide an appropriate policy environment, while increasing their investment in these activities.
- Three of the eight goals are health related and aim to achieve between 1990 and 2015: a two-thirds reduction in child deaths (MDG 4); a three-quarters decline in maternal deaths (MDG 5); and reversal of the HIV/AIDS, malaria and tuberculosis epidemics (MDG 6).
- Doubling the proportion of girls with a secondary education from 19% to 38% could reduce fertility from 5.3 to 3.9 children per woman and lower infant mortality from 81 to 38 deaths per 1000 births.
- Other MDGs focus on public health (safe water, sanitation, environmental protection), alleviation of poverty and hunger, and the determinants of development (education, gender equity, fair trade, debt management).
- Income inequity exacerbates inequalities between the rich and the poor. Globally, only 36% of poor women have access to skilled care at birth compared to 85% among the wealthiest.
- In Africa and South-east Asia, the regions with highest maternal and child death rates, universal access to community, primary level and preventive interventions for newborns and mothers could reduce morbidity and mortality by half. Achieving the MDGs for maternal and child health would require universal access to clinical services as well.

Introduction

This chapter describes the Millennium Development Goals (MDGs), the 2015 targets and the interrelationships between the MDGs. Core global strategies to accelerate the pace towards the desired change are discussed, particularly in relation to the mother and newborn.

The world is divided into five major United Nations (UN) regions (Africa, the Americas, Asia, Europe and Oceania) and 21 sub-regions (Table 2.1). While Asia is the most populous, the small island states in the Caribbean and Micronesia are the most densely populated. Within the major regions, sub-regions classified as economically developed include Northern America (region of the Americas); Western, Southern and Northern Europe (European region); Japan (Asia) and Australia and New Zealand (Oceania); the

Table 2.1. United Nations regions and sub-regions, number of countries, population estimates and density per square kilometre (2008). Adapted from United Nations Statistics Division, 2011.

Regions	Sub-regions	Countries in sub-region	Population (millions)	Density (per square kilometre)
Africa	Subtotal	57	987.1	33
	Eastern Africa	19	310.6	49
	Middle Africa	9	122.5	19
	Northern Africa	7	205.8	24
	Southern Africa	5	56.9	21
	Western Africa	17	291.3	47
Americas	Subtotal	53	921.2	n/a
	Northern America[a]	5	345.1	16
	Latin America and the Caribbean	48	576.1	28
	Caribbean	26	41.6	178
	Central America	8	149.6	60
	South America	14	384.9	22
Asia	Subtotal	50	4075.3	128
	Eastern Asia (includes Japan[a])	7	1546.8	131
	South Central Asia	14	1728.5	160
	South Eastern Asia	11	575.6	128
	Western Asia	18	224.1	46
Europe	Subtotal	52	731.6	32
	Eastern Europe	10	293.5	16
	Northern Europe[a]	17	97.9	54
	Southern Europe[a]	16	152.3	116
	Western Europe[a]	9	187.8	170
Oceania	Subtotal	25	34.9	4
	Australia and New Zealand*	3	25.3	3
	Melanesia	5	8.4	16
	Micronesia	7	0.6	186
	Polynesia	10	0.7	83

[a]Developed sub-regions

remainder constitute the developing, or low and middle income economies, and are the target of the MDGs.

The Millennium Development Goals

In September 2000, the Millennium Declaration (UN, 2000) was adopted at one of the largest UN gatherings of 189 countries and 147 heads of state. The Declaration committed countries to work towards improving the quality of life for all people in the developing world. Subsequent negotiations between multilateral and bilateral agencies culminated in the 2001 development objectives known as MDGs. Poor and rich countries respectively accepted responsibility to provide an appropriate policy environment, good governance, transparency and openness in pursuit of these goals, with increased development assistance from the latter.

The eight MDGs and what their indicators measure is shown in Table 2.2. The three health MDGs include efforts to improve maternal (MDG 5) and child health (MDG 4) and reverse the impact of HIV/AIDS and other major communicable diseases (MDG 6).

Table 2.2. Millennium Development Goals, targets and factors measured by monitoring indicators (adapted from United Nations Statistics Division, 2008).

Goal and targets	What the indicators measure
Goal 1: Eradicate extreme poverty and hunger	
1A: Halve, between 1990 and 2015, the proportion of people whose income is less than US$1 a day	Extreme poverty; equitable access to resources
1B: Achieve full and productive employment and decent work for all, including women and young people	Employment opportunities; working poor
1C: Halve, between 1990 and 2015, the proportion of people who suffer from hunger	Malnutrition; access to food
Goal 2: Achieve universal primary education	
Ensure that, by 2015, boys and girls alike will be able to complete a full course of primary schooling	Access to primary education; literacy (young adults)
Goal 3: Promote gender equality and empower women	
Eliminate gender disparity in primary and secondary education, preferably by 2005, and in all levels of education no later than 2015	Gender discrimination in education, employment and state power
Goal 4: Reduce child mortality	
Reduce by two-thirds, between 1990 and 2015, the under-five mortality rate	Infant and under-five mortality Immunization coverage
Goal 5: Improve maternal health	
5A: Reduce by three-quarters, between 1990 and 2015, the maternal mortality ratio	Maternal mortality Access to skilled delivery care
5B: Achieve, by 2015, universal access to reproductive health	Access to family planning and antenatal care, including among adolescents
Goal 6: Combat HIV/AIDS, malaria and other diseases	
6A: Have halted by 2015 and begun to reverse the spread of HIV/AIDS	HIV prevalence; risk reduction knowledge and behaviour change; care of HIV/AIDS orphans
6B: Achieve, by 2010, universal access to treatment for HIV/AIDS for all those who need it	Access to antiretroviral drugs
6C: Have halted by 2015 and begun to reverse the incidence of malaria and other major diseases	Risk reduction/care for persons with malaria and tuberculosis
Goal 7: Ensure environmental sustainability	
7A: Integrate principles of sustainable development into country policies and programmes; reverse the loss of environmental resources	Deforestation; air and water quality
7B: Reduce biodiversity loss, achieving, by 2010, a significant reduction in the rate of loss	Protection of endangered species
7C: Halve, by 2015, proportion of people without sustainable access to safe drinking water and basic sanitation	Access to clean water and safe sanitation
7D: By 2020, achieve a significant improvement in the lives of at least 100 million slum dwellers	Quality of life for urban poor

Continued

Table 2.2. Continued.

Goal and targets	What the indicators measure
Goal 8: Develop global partnership for development	
8A: Develop an open, rule-based, predictable, non-discriminatory trading and financial system	Transfer skills/resources from developed to developing countries through increased development assistance; market access; debt sustainability
8B: Address special needs of least developed countries	
8C: Address special needs of landlocked countries and small island developing states	
8D: Comprehensively address debt problems of developing countries to make debt sustainable	Debt burden reduction
8E: In cooperation with pharmaceutical companies, provide access to affordable essential drugs in developing countries	Access to affordable essential drugs
8F: In cooperation with private sector, make available benefits of new technologies, especially information and communications	Access to communication technology

Education (MDG 2) empowers women (MDG 3) to make informed choices for themselves and their families. These goals are particularly relevant, as some of the slow progress in the health MDGs may be attributed to the social and economic issues women face. With 60% of the world's poor and two-thirds of the world's illiterate people female (Horton, 2010), and given their limited capacity to influence legislative decision making (fewer than one in five representatives worldwide are female), failure to address social and cultural barriers to gender equity will stymie achievement of the health MDGs (Shaw, 2009). Without health and education, efforts at poverty eradication (MDG 1) and environmental sustainability (MDG 7) cannot proceed at the pace needed to achieve the development (MDG 8) envisaged (UN, 2001).

The UN Secretary General at the time, Kofi Annan, described these goals as 'ambitious [but] technically feasible'. In 2002, the Monterrey Consensus committed developed countries to move towards the target of 0.7% of GNP as official development assistance to developing countries (UN, 2002). That commitment would increase donor aid from around US$70 billion to US$210 billion per year to support the scaling up of evidence-based interventions to achieve the MDGs.

The novelty of the MDGs, compared to earlier development initiatives, was the recognized interdependence of these basic goals to development, building on 20th-century experiences that, without addressing public health, hunger and education of the next generation, no true development can occur (Sachs, 2004). The other important element was the contract between developing and developed countries outlining their mutual responsibility for making this initiative happen, with clear criteria to monitor progress using a results-based approach.

The indicators for the three health MDGs have been subdivided into process and impact measures (Table 2.3). The use of these indicators highlights a number of key points. First, it shows that achieving the MDGs requires a complex set of activities that work together to achieve improved health outcomes. Second, the explicit inclusion of process and impact indicators emphasizes the value of monitoring at global level. The process indicators measure the provision, availability and use of services intended to achieve a particular outcome and can be monitored to ensure that programmes are on track to meeting the wider national and international goals. Programme officers can use some of these indicators for country-level monitoring (see Hounton *et al.*,

Table 2.3. Health MDGs and the related impact and process indicators (adapted from United Nations Statistics Division, 2008).

Goal	Process indicators	Impact indicators
MDG 4 Reduce child mortality	4.3 Proportion of 1-year-old children immunized against measles	4.1 Under-five mortality rate 4.2 Infant mortality rate
MDG 5 Improve maternal health	5.2 Proportion of births attended by skilled health personnel 5.4 Adolescent birth rate 5.5 Antenatal care coverage (at least one visit and at least four visits) 5.6 Unmet need for family planning	5.1 Maternal mortality ratio 5.3 Contraceptive prevalence rate
MDG 6 Combat HIV/AIDS, malaria and other diseases	6.2 Condom use at last high-risk sex 6.3 Proportion of population aged 15–24 years with comprehensive correct knowledge of HIV/AIDS 6.4 Ratio of school attendance of orphans to school attendance of non-orphans aged 10–14 years 6.5 Proportion of population with advanced HIV infection with access to antiretroviral drugs 6.7 Proportion of children under age 5 sleeping under insecticide-treated bed nets	6.1 HIV prevalence among population aged 15–24 years
	6.8 Proportion of children under age 5 with fever who are treated with appropriate anti-malarial drugs	6.6 Incidence and death rates associated with malaria
	6.10 Proportion of tuberculosis cases detected and cured under directly observed treatment short course	6.9 Incidence, prevalence and death rates associated with tuberculosis

Chapter 15 this volume) to ensure congruence of activities with global efforts. Third, the process indicators demonstrate that maternal mortality reduction is also affected by the key intervention of family planning through the inclusion of the indicators of unmet need and contraceptive prevalence. Finally, the indicators also highlight the concept of the continuum of care – which links the various stages across the reproductive life cycle, and the different places where care can be provided (see http://www.who.int/pmnch/about/continuum_of_care/en/index.html).

Maternal and child health (MDGs 4 and 5)

An estimated 15% of pregnant women experience pregnancy-related obstetric complications, half of whom will require care at referral centres – with 5% needing surgical intervention. The UN estimates that 358,000 women died during pregnancy or within 42 days of giving birth in 2008. The global maternal mortality ratio is falling, from 400 in 1990 to 260 in 2008, a decline of 34% over the period, far too slowly to reach the 2015 target reduction defined in Table 2.2 (Hogan *et al.*, 2010; WHO *et al.*, 2010; see Stanton and McCaw-Binns, Chapter 4 this volume). Four million babies also die within 1 month of birth, 75% in the first week of life (WHO, 2006) and many as a result of the complications experienced by the mother during pregnancy or childbirth. An additional 3.3 million babies are stillborn.

Total young child deaths are decreasing, from 12.6 million in 1990 to 8.8 million deaths in 2008 (UN, 2010). Black *et al.* (2010) estimated that, of the 8.8 million under-five deaths, Africa accounted for 48% of deaths and South/South-east Asia 27%. As efforts to prevent avoidable child deaths from infectious diseases succeed, the relative proportion of child deaths occurring in the neonatal period will increase, further emphasizing the importance of the maternal and perinatal continuum of care. Lawn *et al.* (2009a) indicate that, worldwide, 41% of under-five deaths occur in the first 28 days of life – the neonatal period. The higher the neonatal mortality rate, the more deaths that are preventable by interventions such as tetanus immunization in pregnancy, exclusive breastfeeding, neonatal resuscitation and, for preterm babies, attention to feeding, maintenance of warmth and early diagnosis and management of complications associated with early birth (e.g. respiratory problems, infection, jaundice) (Lawn *et al.*, 2009a). Although some of these interventions are amenable to care in the community, many require the same health system responses as those to prevent maternal mortality – antenatal care, skilled care and emergency care at birth and in the postnatal period.

The interrelationship of maternal and infant mortality risks and availability of skilled care from pregnancy into the neonatal period is demonstrated in Plate 1, where 193 countries were organized in five neonatal mortality rate categories as markers of health system performance. An ecological association between neonatal mortality and skilled attendance was demonstrated, but cannot be assumed to be causal (Lawn *et al.*, 2009b).

Maternal ill health or death also negatively impacts household survival and function, especially affecting the youngest children, who need the food, care and emotional support mothers are most relied on to provide. Ronsmans *et al.* (2010) documented what we instinctively know – that a mother's death compromises children's chances of survival, with risks greatest in the first year of life. Mothers are also more likely to support children's educational development, important for achieving their full potential and realizing a pathway out of poverty; demonstrated by lower school attendance rates among AIDs orphans (UNICEF, 2009). No similar effect was noted if the father died.

Reducing unwanted pregnancies

A reduction of maternal mortality levels can be achieved by a focus on prevention and treatment of the causes of death and also through prevention of pregnancy itself. This underscores a fundamental principle underlying the measurement of maternal mortality, where two distinct components should be differentiated – the risk of being pregnant (related to the number of times a woman might become pregnant, hence the role of family planning) and the risk of dying once pregnant, called the obstetric risk (see Stanton and McCaw-Binns, Chapter 4 this volume). Family planning can reduce pregnancy rates in adolescents and in older women, and also decrease the numbers of high parity births, all of which contribute to higher risks of maternal mortality (Campbell and Graham, 2006). Birth spacing has also been shown to have effects on improved perinatal outcomes (Conde-Agudelo *et al.*, 2006).

The association between contraceptive use and mortality is demonstrated in Table 2.4. When indicators of universal access to reproductive health care are presented alongside the mortality risk, regions with low contraceptive prevalence and high total fertility rates (South Asia and sub-Saharan Africa) can be seen to have the lowest access to skilled care and the highest maternal mortality. Clearly, the need for investment in family planning will vary, with the greatest benefit to be realized in countries where fertility rates, including adolescent fertility, are still high. Adolescent fertility rates are much higher in sub-Saharan Africa than South Asia (Fig. 2.1), which may explain the added risks of early and frequent childbearing and higher lifetime fertility.

Abortion accounts for one in eight maternal deaths worldwide. In 2003, 48% of all abortions worldwide were unsafe and more than 97% (19 million) were in developing countries. The induced abortion rate (abortions per 1000 women 15–44 years) was 29 per 1000 in 2003 (Sedgh *et al.*, 2007). Legal restriction of abortion does not appear to affect incidence, with an estimated abortion rate of 28 in Europe where abortion is usually legal and 29 in Africa where, in many countries, abortion

Table 2.4. Universal access to reproductive health care, fertility and maternal mortality, 2005–2009 (adapted from UNICEF, 2011).

| | Contraceptive prevalence | Total fertility rate | Antenatal care | | Delivery care | | Maternal mortality ratio 2008 |
			1+ visits	3+ visits	With skilled provider	In facility	
West and Central Africa	17	5.2	72	46	51	48	720
Eastern and Southern Africa	29	4.8	72	39	37	35	550
South Asia	51	2.8	70	45	48	42	290
Middle East and North Africa	54	2.8	78	–	77	65	170
Latin America and Caribbean	75	2.2	95	86	89	87	85
East Asia and Pacific	77	1.9	90	76	90	78	88
CEE/CIS	69	1.7	95	–	97	93	34
Global summaries							
Africa	28	4.5	72	45	48	43	590
Asia	66	2.3	79	51	66	58	200
Least developed countries	31	4.3	68	37	41	35	590
Developing countries	61	2.7	79	53	64	58	290
Industrialized countries	–	1.7	–	–	–	–	14
World	61	2.5	79	53	65	58	260

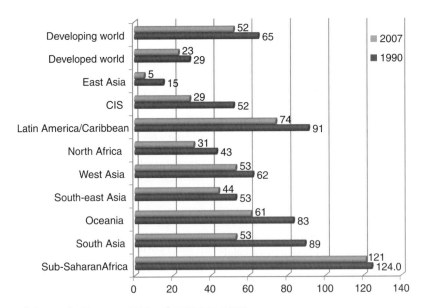

Fig. 2.1. Adolescent fertility rates, 1990 and 2007 (UN, 2010).

is not legal (Myers and Seif, 2010). The leading causes of death from unsafe abortion are haemorrhage, infection and poisoning from substances used to induce abortion (Grimes *et al.*, 2006).

Eliminating or liberalizing restrictive abortion laws requires prolonged and coordinated efforts from lawyers, health researchers and activists. In Nepal, this process involved 20 years of research and legal activism. Strategies employed by successful advocates included demonstrating the conflict between existing laws and international agreements, building coalitions of advocates, providing evidence on the scale of unsafe abortion and the poor health, social and economic consequences of restrictive abortion laws and involving the media. Once legal hurdles are cleared, the next stages involve establishing facilities, training staff (including modifying curricula in medical and midwifery schools) and overcoming cultural barriers and the more subtle stigma associated with use of these services (Myers and Seif, 2010). Scaling up the safe delivery of abortion services will require training of mid-level clinicians, midwives and nurse practitioners, especially those who work in rural or remote areas where physicians are scarce and few surgical facilities and little equipment exist (Yarnall *et al.*, 2009; Kishen and Yvonne, 2010). Creative mechanisms to deliver safe abortion services (Gomperts *et al.*, 2008) to women where access is not legal have been employed by the group 'Women on the Waves' (http://www.womenonwaves.org), who offer a telemedicine consultation, medication by mail and follow-up over the internet (http://www.womenonweb.org). The accessibility of these services to the poorest women who are most in need is likely to pose difficulties due to its reliance on the internet.

Effectiveness of core strategies

Hu *et al.* (2007) compared the cost-effectiveness of alternative maternal morbidity and mortality reduction strategies in Mexico by simulating the natural history of pregnancy (planned and unintended) and pregnancy-related complications in a cohort of 15-year-old women followed over their lifetime. They compared the health outcomes and costs of the current maternal health standard of care or current practice with strategies to achieve coverage levels recommended by WHO. Increasing family planning coverage by 15% and access to safe abortion for women desiring elective termination of pregnancy resulted in a reduction of maternal mortality by 43% and was cost saving compared to current practice. The most effective strategy added a third component, enhanced access to comprehensive emergency obstetric care for at least 90% of women requiring referral. This strategy reduced mortality by 75% and cost less than current practice. They concluded that increasing provision of family planning and assuring access to safe abortion are feasible cost-effective strategies that would provide the greatest benefit within a short time-frame. Incremental improvements in access to high-quality intrapartum and emergency obstetric care would further reduce maternal deaths and disability consistent with MDG 5 expectations.

Similar studies done for sub-Saharan Africa and South-east Asia identified a similar mix of strategies for those regions. These included: antenatal care (tetanus toxoid, screening for pre-eclampsia, screening and treatment of asymptomatic bacteriuria and syphilis); skilled attendance at birth, first-level maternal and neonatal care around childbirth; and emergency obstetric and neonatal care, including the community based newborn care package. Scaling up the interventions to 95% coverage would halve neonatal and maternal deaths. Providing community-based primary care preventive interventions for newborns and mothers were cost-effective strategies to reduce morbidity and mortality; however, to achieve the MDGs for maternal and child health would require universal access to clinical services as well (Adam *et al.*, 2005).

HIV/AIDS and the health of women and children (MDG 6)

HIV prevalence ranges from under 1% in Asia up to 28% in southern Africa (UNAIDS, 2008).

Improvement in maternal mortality has been slow at a global level (see Stanton and McCaw-Binns, Chapter 4 this volume) and the contribution of HIV infection to maternal mortality is considerable. Hogan *et al.* (2010) estimate that there were 61,400 extra maternal deaths due to HIV in 2008. While maternal mortality had been declining at a rate of 2.2% in 1980, the onset of the HIV epidemic in the early 1990s saw the rate of decline dropping to 1.8% between 1980 and 1990 and 1.4% from 1990 to 2008. Southern Africa bore the greatest burden with maternal mortality rates increasing in 2008 compared to 1980 in Botswana, Lesotho, Malawi, Mozambique, Namibia, South Africa, Swaziland, Zambia and Zimbabwe. In South Africa, 54% of maternal deaths due to tuberculosis were attributable to HIV infection, demonstrating the increased susceptibility to tuberculosis among HIV-positive women during pregnancy (Khan *et al.*, 2001).

Globally over 15 million women live with HIV disease (Table 2.5), more than 2 million of whom become pregnant each year. HIV infection has been associated with decreased fertility and increased risk of spontaneous abortion, stillbirths and child deaths (McIntyre, 2005). With improving access to antiretroviral therapy, AIDs-related maternal deaths should decline; however, women living with HIV/AIDS may be more susceptible to direct or obstetric causes of maternal mortality, such as postpartum haemorrhage, puerperal sepsis and complications of Caesarean section, in part due to concurrent AIDS-related anaemia or immune deficiency.

Tracking the number of women living with HIV is important to control perinatal infection through mother to child

Table 2.5. HIV disease burden, 2009 (UNICEF, 2011).

Summary HIV indicators	Estimated adult HIV prevalence rate (aged 15–49)	Estimated number of women (aged 15+) living with HIV (thousands)	HIV prevalence among young people (aged 15–24)		Orphan school attendance ratio
			Male	Female	
Sub-Saharan Africa	4.7	12,300	1.1	3.3	93
Eastern and Southern Africa	7.2	8,800	1.9	4.8	92
West and Central Africa	2.7	3,300	0.8	2.0	94
Middle East and North Africa	0.2	190	0.1	0.2	–
South Asia	0.3	930	0.1	0.1	73
East Asia and Pacific	0.2	750	<0.1	<0.1	–
Latin America and Caribbean	0.5	660	0.2	0.2	–
CEE/CIS	0.5	690	0.1	0.1	–
Global summaries					
Industrialized countries	0.3	570	0.2	0.1	–
Developing countries	0.9	14,700	0.3	0.6	81
Least developed countries	2.0	5,000	0.7	1.5	85
World	0.8	15,900	0.3	0.6	–

transmission and to monitor the unique risks to women associated with their vulnerability to sexual coercion, lack of power and child marriage. Table 2.5 shows that, in the industrialized world, males record higher rates of HIV disease than females. In Africa, however, prevalence rates are two to three times higher among young women. The increased risk among young women is associated with having multiple sexual partners, having sex with older men, abuse or working in the sex trade (Day, 2009). Orphans are less likely to have the opportunity to attend school compared to non-orphan children of the same age.

The UN strategic approach to prevention of mother to child transmission (PMTCT) includes: (i) primary prevention of HIV infection; (ii) prevention of unintended pregnancies among HIV-infected women; (iii) prevention of HIV transmission from infected women to their infants; and (iv) provision of care and support to HIV-infected women, their infants and families (Luo et al., 2007). Pregnancy provides an opportunity to reach women and men with HIV prevention and care interventions and may be the only time women that age interact with the health services. The motivation to protect their offspring often provides an incentive for the required behaviour change to occur (McIntyre, 2005). Box 2.1 shows the potential but also the challenges of implementing PMTCT programmes in the real world, where, despite understanding the importance of prophylaxis during pregnancy and labour and the risk of HIV transmission posed by breastfeeding, women were reluctant to disclose their HIV

Box 2.1. PMTCT Pilot Study – Jamaica (Harvey and Thame, 2004)

Background

Prior to the introduction of antiretrovirals, Jamaica was home to an estimated 24,000 HIV-positive individuals, many of whom were unaware of their status. Each year, women gave birth to 150 to 300 HIV-positive children. Mother to child transmission accounted for 7% of all reported HIV/AIDS cases in Jamaica up to the year 2000.

Pilot study

A pilot intervention was undertaken in 15 antenatal clinics across the four health regions of Jamaica between January 2001 and December 2002. The programme was intended to: offer HIV testing; antiretrovirals for HIV-positive women in labour and their newborns; and offer these women counselling that recommended against breastfeeding.

Results

Of 8116 participating women (12% of births at the 15 facilities), 1.4% tested positive in 2001 and 1.6% in 2002, yielding 176 cases (123 new, 53 previously diagnosed). Of 143 mothers (81%) on whom data on antiretroviral therapy were available, 77% (110) received therapy; 58% took antiretrovirals before delivery and 77% at the onset of labour. Of 136 babies, 83% (113) received antiretroviral prophylaxis. The majority of women (95%) knew that both antiretroviral therapy at birth and not breastfeeding could prevent HIV transmission. While 69% of mothers received replacement feeds, 25% breastfed at some point, reluctant for various reasons to not breastfeed.

Children were followed for a mean of 22.6±5.4 months (range 9–33 months); 51 of 59 infants had an HIV test, 8 (16%) of whom tested positive; 10.3% among those who received antiretrovirals, 23.8% among those who did not. Breastfed infants were significantly more likely to test positive (50%; 6 of 12) than non-breastfed (6%; 2 of 34) babies. Nearly 30% of the participants reported feeling victimized because of their HIV status; most reported being victimized by health-care workers (35%) or neighbours (29%).

Conclusions

Antiretroviral prophylaxis, supported by advice and the means to not breastfeed, can reduce MTCT; however, stigma and discrimination remain a serious barrier for persons living with HIV/AIDS accessing services within the health sector. Possible victimization by health workers may contribute to women's failure to disclose their HIV status to hospital providers at the time of delivery.

status to hospital staff at delivery or expose themselves to questions from community members regarding why they were not breastfeeding their infants; thus they increased the risk of transmitting HIV to their infants.

Other MDGs and their links with maternal and perinatal health

Poverty alleviation and the poverty trap (MDG 1)

Resource constraints are the biggest barrier to achieving the MDGs. While Africa bears 24% of the global disease burden, it has only 3% of the world's health workforce and 1% of the financial resources at its disposal (WHO, 2005). Even in middle income developing countries, the poor are too under-resourced to overcome hunger, disease and their inadequate housing to equip themselves and society for economic growth. Their impoverished state limits the disposable income needed to create savings and resources for private investment. Persons earning below the tax threshold do not contribute to tax revenues that finance public investment and day to day public sector operations, further restricting access of the poor to resources for development such as physical infrastructure (roads, water, sanitation, hospitals, schools) and the related health services and education.

Women make a significant contribution to social and economic progress at household, community and national level. During pregnancy, they are exposed to life-threatening risks, which may endanger their ability to become productive members of society. Indeed, maternal ill-health has been shown to throw families into debt and profound poverty as a result of loss of the earning potential of a woman and also from the costs of accessing care (see Witter and Ensor, Chapter 7 this volume).

It is generally well known that the coverage of all types of health care is worse in poor compared to richer households, but skilled care at delivery shows the widest poor–rich gap. Worldwide, only 48% of women in the poorest quintiles make three or more antenatal visits compared to 82% in the wealthiest quintile. The gaps are even wider for skilled

care at birth, ranging between 36% and 85%, respectively, with eight-fold differences in access in South Asia and three-fold differences in sub-Saharan Africa (Gwatkin et al., 2007). Such gaps are in contrast to child-related interventions; for example, 57% of the poorest households have access to oral rehydration therapy compared to 71% in richer sectors of the population.

The burden of maternal mortality is clustered disproportionately amongst the poor with as much as six-fold differences between the poorest and richest sectors of the population in some countries like Peru (Ronsmans and Graham, 2006). Improved and equitable access to and use of maternal health services will reduce the economic impact of death and disability in the poor and vulnerable, so contributing to poverty reduction overall.

Educating girls, empowering women and gender equity (MDGs 2 and 3)

Educating girls and women is critical to achieving improved health for women, children, families and society (Malhotra et al., 2003). MDG 2 targets access of boys and girls to primary education while the related MDG 3 on gender parity in primary and secondary education contributes to achieving this objective. Post-primary education helps enable women to reject gender-biased norms and access alternative opportunities and social roles, especially where girls and women face substantial discrimination. Subbarao and Rainey (1995) estimated that doubling the proportion of girls with a secondary education from 19 to 38% would reduce the total fertility rate from 5.3 to 3.9 children per woman and lower infant mortality from 81 to 38 deaths per 1000 births. Smaller families free household resources for qualitative investment in the more manageable family unit, reducing malnutrition and other morbidity, improving infant and young child survival.

The two regions with the highest maternal mortality burden, sub-Saharan Africa and South Asia, are also hobbled by lack of skilled staff (Filippi et al., 2006). With most skilled care delivered by female providers, a more educated female population is a prerequisite to achieving the rapid coverage that is needed through training, deployment and retention of midwives.

By the late 20th century, women's life expectancy exceeded males in most regions of the world. Modern family planning methods enable women to reduce the risks associated with excessive child bearing and limit the burdens of child rearing. Global growth in tertiary education for women has created a pool of technicians, managers, advocates and decision makers sensitive to the challenges women face, motivated to work towards addressing their needs in a gender sensitive way.

Social inequities increase the risk of poor health outcomes. HIV/AIDS is a case in point, where more women 15–24 years old are infected than their male counterparts (Grown et al., 2005). Gender inequities can be expressed in many different ways, not least through the problem of selective feticide (Box 2.2).

Environmental sustainability and women's health (MDG 7)

A safe environment (clean water, safe waste disposal) reduces transmission of communicable diseases that disproportionately affect children. Use of solid fuel for cooking is most prevalent in the poorest regions and among impoverished households, with three of four such households dependent on this form of fuel. As women usually prepare the families' meals, they are more often exposed to the negative health effects of indoor air pollution. Women exposed to indoor smoke are 3.2 times (95% CI, 2.3–4.8) more likely to suffer from chronic obstructive pulmonary disorders, such as bronchitis and emphysema, than women who use electricity, gas or other cleaner fuels. Exposure to indoor air pollution is also associated with risk of preterm birth (Smith et al., 2004) and low birth weight (Pope et al., 2010). Preterm infants contribute disproportionately to under-five deaths or survive with disabilities (Arpino et al., 2010) with further likelihood of depleting family resources to meet immediate and long-term health care needs (Miljeteig et al., 2009).

The links between population growth and environmental sustainability are varied, although there is agreement that, while large families heighten degradation of natural resources, they are also more vulnerable to the effects of extreme climate change. Without

---

Box 2.2 Selective feticide – the absent females of Asia

One downside to better reproductive technology and opportunities to terminate unintended pregnancies is the capacity for abuse. In India technologies such as chorionic villus sampling in early pregnancy or amniocentesis and ultrasonography later in pregnancy are being used to identify the sex of offspring and abort, more often than not, female fetuses. This practice has grown such that the 2001 census documented the lowest ever sex ratio, with 927 girls to 1000 boys aged 0–6 years (Registrar General of India, 2001). This trend continues with the sex ratio at the 2011 census even lower, at 914 girls to 1000 boys (Jha et al., 2011). The ratio is most skewed in wealthier regions. While fetal sex determination and medical termination of pregnancy due to fetal sex have been illegal since 1994, there is persistent evidence of sex determination and female feticide, taking older customs of female infanticide and neglect to a new level, especially in urban areas by the more educated.

In many Indian and Chinese (Zeng et al., 1992) communities characterized by strong patriarchal values, couples prefer sons to continue the family name and bloodline, earn money, look after the family and care for parents in their old age. Daughters are often regarded as a liability, especially where the custom of dowry prevails, with families sometimes forced to borrow money to fund them. An unmarried, uneducated daughter is a burden to parents if unable to work (Sheth, 2006). These preferences are manifested in a variety of ways, from differential expenditure on male and female children, including educational opportunities, to neglect of female children to selective infanticide and feticide. Solutions include education of women and opportunities for their integration into the labour force. Developing social security systems are long term strategies to provide a secure retirement income. As social customs run deep they will take a long time to modify; public education is essential to change the attitudes of families about the sex of their children.

primary care services such as family planning, poor couples continue to have larger
families, contributing to rapid population
growth and environmental degradation
(Rehfuess *et al.*, 2006) as forests are cut down
for shelter and fuel (Sachs and McArthur,
2005). Women and children are often responsible for fuel collection and fetching water,
activities which are time consuming depending on proximity of local fuel wood and water
resources to the household. Alleviating the
drudgery of these chores, reducing cooking
time and clean-up through more efficient
devices, can free women for productive
endeavours (MDG 1), access to education
(MDGs 2 and 3) and child care, and will
reduce the risk of assault and injury for
women and girls (Rehfuess *et al.*, 2006).

Global partnerships for development (MDG 8)

The Millennium Project recognizes the need
for a new partnership between rich and poor
countries based on good governance,
expanded trade, aid and debt relief to help
finance the infrastructure and human capital
needed to attract private investment and
stimulate growth and development (Sachs
and McArthur, 2005). While scholars such as
Adam *et al.* (2005) and Stover *et al.* (2006) have
estimated the cost and value of scaling up
interventions to achieve the MDGs, investments have been slow.

The UN Secretary General, Ban Ki-Moon,
embraced the concept of global partnerships
in the 'Global Strategy for Women's and
Children's Health' (http://www.who.int/
pmnch/activities/jointactionplan/en/index.
html). The document clearly sets out the importance of partnerships to improve the lives of
women and children. Complementary roles of
the various partners – governments, donor
countries, multilateral organizations, global
philanthropic groups, civil society, the business
community and academics – are clearly set out.
In particular, this encouragement to enhance
partnerships for development has spurred
involvement of the business community to
develop partnerships with others for the use
and application of technologies for achievement of the MDGs.

Conclusion

The eight MDGs form a framework to catalyse global development and stimulate action
to meet the needs of the world's poor. The
interlinkages that exist between the MDGs
serve to emphasize the complex nature of
health and development. Progress towards
MDGs 4 and 5 is dependent upon as well as
likely to contribute to the other MDGs.
Evidence for what programmes are needed
to improve maternal and perinatal health
outcomes exists; however, the challenge is in
their equitable and consistent provision. For
the achievement of all MDGs, high-income
countries need to jump-start the investment
cycle and enable developing countries to
invest in health, education and basic infrastructure; otherwise some communities will
remain trapped in the cycle of poverty (Sachs
et al., 2004).

References

Adam, T., Lim, S.S., Mehta, S., Bhutta, Z.A., Fogstad, H., Mathai, M., Zupan, J. and Darmstadt, G.L. (2005)
    Cost effectiveness analysis of strategies for maternal and neonatal health in developing countries. *British
    Medical Journal* 331, 1107.
Arpino, C., Compagnone, E., Montanaro, M.L., Cacciatore, D., De Luca, A., Cerulli, A., Di Girolamo, S. and
    Curatolo, P. (2010) Preterm birth and neurodevelopmental outcome: a review. *Childrens Nervous System*
    26(9), 1139–1149.
Black, R.E., Cousens, S., Johnson, H.L., Lawn, J.E., Rudan, I., Bassani, D.G., Jha, P., Campbell, H., Fischer
    Walker, C., Cibulskis, R., Eisele, T., Liu, L. and Mathers, C. for the Child Health Epidemiology Reference
    Group of WHO and UNICEF (2010) Global, regional, and national causes of child mortality in 2008: a
    systematic analysis. *Lancet* 375(9730), 1969–1987.

Campbell, O.M. and Graham, W.J. (2006) Strategies for reducing maternal mortality: getting on with what works. *Lancet* 368(9543), 1284–1299.

Conde-Agudelo, A., Rosas-Bermúdez, A. and Kafury-Goeta, A.C. (2006) Birth spacing and risk of adverse perinatal outcomes: a meta-analysis. *Journal of the American Medical Association* 295(15), 1809–1823.

Day, M. (2009) Young women are at more risk of HIV infection than young men. *British Medical Journal* 338, 883.

Filippi, V., Ronsmans, C., Campbell, O.M.R., Graham, W.J., Mills, A., Borghi, J., Koblinsky, M. and Osrin, D. (2006) Maternal health in poor countries: the broader context and a call for action. *Lancet* 368(9546), 1535–1541.

Gomperts, R.J., Jelinska, K., Davies, S., Gemzell-Danielsson, K. and Kleiverda, G. (2008) Using telemedicine for termination of pregnancy with mifepristone and misoprostol in settings where there is no access to safe services. *BJOG: An International Journal of Obstetrics and Gynaecology* 115(9), 1171–1175.

Grimes, D.A., Benson, J., Singh, S., Romero, M., Ganatra, B., Okonofua, F.E. and Shah, I.H. (2006) Unsafe abortion: the preventable pandemic. *Lancet* 368, 1908–1919.

Grown, C., Rao Gupta, G. and Pande, R. (2005) Taking action to improve women's health through gender equality and women's empowerment. *Lancet* 365, 541–543.

Gwatkin, D.R., Rutstein, S., Johnson, K., Suliman, E., Wagstaff, A. and Amozou, A. (2007) *Socio-economic Differences in Health, Nutrition and Population.* World Bank, Washington, DC.

Harvey, K. and Thame, I. (2004) The impact of a programme to prevent mother-to-child transmission of HIV: disease transmission and health-seeking behaviour among HIV-positive mother-child pairs in Jamaica. Operations research results. Quality Assurance Project for USAID, Bethesda, Maryland. Available at: http://www.hciproject.org/node/698 (accessed 8 June 2010).

Hogan, M.C., Foreman, K.J., Naghavi, M., Ahn, S.Y., Wang, M., Makela, S.M., Lopez, A.D., Lozano, R. and Murray, C.J.L. (2010) Maternal mortality for 181 countries, 1980-2008: a systematic analysis of progress towards Millennium Development Goal 5. *Lancet* 375(9726), 1609–1623.

Horton, R. (2010) Gender equity is the key to maternal and child health. *Lancet* 375(9730), 1939.

Hu, D., Bertozzi, S.M., Gakidou, E., Sweet, S. and Goldie, S.J. (2007) The costs, benefits and cost-effectiveness of interventions to reduce maternal morbidity and mortality in Mexico. *PLoS One* 2(1), e750.

Jha, P., Kesler, M.A., Kumar, R., Ram, F., Ram, U., Aleksandrowicz, L., Bassani, D.G., Chandra, S. and Banthia, J.K. (2011) Trends in selective abortions of girls in India: analysis of nationally representative birth histories from 1990 to 2005 and census data from 1991 to 2011. *Lancet* 377(9781), 1921–1928.

Khan, M., Pillay, T., Moodley, J.M. and Connolly, C.A. for the Durban Perinatal TB HIV-1 Study Group (2001) Maternal mortality associated with tuberculosis–HIV-1 co-infection in Durban, South Africa. *AIDS* 15(14), 1857–1863.

Kishen, M. and Yvonne, S. (2010) The role of advanced nurse practitioners in the availability of abortion services. *Best Practice and Research Clinical Obstetrics and Gynaecology*, doi:10.1016/j.bpobgyn.2010.02.014.

Lawn, J., Kerber, K., Enweronu-Laryea, C., Massee, D. and Bateman, O. (2009a) Newborn survival in low resource settings – are we delivering? *British Journal of Obstetrics and Gynaecology* 116(Suppl. 1), 49–59.

Lawn, J.E., Kinney, M., Lee, A.C., Chopra, M., Donnay, F., Paul, V.K., Bhutta, Z.A., Bateman, M. and Darmstadt, G.L. (2009b) Reducing intrapartum-related deaths and disability: can the health system deliver? *International Journal of Gynaecology and Obstetrics* 107(Suppl. 1), S123–S142.

Luo, C., Akwara, P., Ngongo, N., Doughty, P., Gass, R., Ekpini, R., Crowley, S. and Hayashi, C. (2007) Global Progress in PMTCT and Paediatric HIV Care and Treatment in Low- and Middle-Income Countries in 2004–2005. *Reproductive Health Matters* 15(3), 179–189.

Malhotra, A., Pande, R. and Grown, C. (2003) *Impact of Investment in Female Education on Gender Equality.* International Centre for Research on Women, Washington, DC.

McIntyre, J. (2005) Maternal health and HIV. *Reproductive Health Matters* 13(25), 129–135.

Miljeteig, I., Sayeed, S.A., Jesani, A., Johansson, K.A. and Norheim, O.F. (2009) Impact of ethics and economics on end-of-life decisions in an Indian neonatal unit. *Pediatrics* 124(2), e322–e328.

Myers, J.E. and Seif, M.W. (2010) Global perspective of legal abortion – Trends analysis and accessibility. *Best Practice and Research Clinical Obstetrics and Gynaecology*, doi:10.1016/j.bpobgyn.010.04.002.

Pope, D.P., Mishra, V., Thompson, L., Siddiqui, A.R., Rehfuess, E.A., Weber, M. and Bruce, N.G. (2010) Risk of low birth weight and stillbirth associated with indoor air pollution from solid fuel use in developing countries. *Epidemiology Reviews* 32(1), 70–81.

Registrar General of India (2001) *Census of India, Provisional Population Totals – Series I, Paper I.* Office of the Registrar General, New Delhi.

Rehfuess, E., Mehta, S. and Prüss-Ustün, A. (2006) Assessing household solid fuel use: multiple implications for the Millennium Development Goals. *Environmental Health Perspective* 114(3), 373–378.

Ronsmans, C. and Graham, W.J. (2006) Maternal mortality: who, when, where and when (2006). *Lancet* 368(9542), 1189–1200.

Ronsmans, C., Chowdhury, M.E., Dasgupta, S.K., Ahmed, A. and Koblinsky, M. (2010) Effect of parent's death on child survival in rural Bangladesh: a cohort study. *Lancet* 375, 2024–2031.

Sachs, J.D. (2004) Health in the developing world: achieving the Millennium Development Goals. *Bulletin of the World Health Organization* 82(12), 947–949.

Sachs, J.D. and McArthur, J.W. (2005) The Millennium Project: a plan for meeting the Millennium Development Goals. *Lancet* 365(9456), 347–353.

Sachs, J.D., McArthur, J.W., Schmidt-Traub, G., Kruk, M., Bahadur, C., Faye, A. and McCord, M. (2004) Ending Africa's poverty trap. In: Brainard, W.C. and Perry, G.L. (eds) *Brookings Papers on Economic Activity* 1. Brookings Institution Press, Washington, DC, pp. 117–240.

Sedgh, G., Henshaw, S., Singh, S., Åhman, E. and Shah, I.H. (2007) Induced abortion: estimated rates and trends worldwide. *Lancet* 370, 1338–1345.

Shaw, D. (2009) Access to sexual and reproductive health for young people: Bridging the disconnect between rights and reality. *International Journal of Gynaecology and Obstetrics* 106, 132–136.

Sheth, S.S. (2006) Missing female births in India. *Lancet* 367(9506), 185–186.

Smith, K.R., Mehta, S. and Maeusezahl-Feuz, M. (2004) Indoor air pollution from household use of solid fuels. In: Ezzati, M., Lopez, A.D., Rodgers, A. and Murray, C.J.L. (eds) *Comparative Quantification of Health Risks: Global and Regional Burden of Disease Attributable to Selected Major Risk Factors*. WHO, Geneva, pp. 1435–1493. Available at: http://www.who.int/publications/cra/chapters/volume2/1435-1494.pdf (accessed 27 May 2010).

Stover, J., Bertozzi, S.L., Gutierrez, J., Walker, N., Stanecki, K.A., Greener, R., Gouws, E., Hankins, C., Garnett, G.P., Salomon, J.A., Boerma, J.T., De Lay, P. and Ghys, P.D. (2006) The Global Impact of Scaling Up HIV/AIDS Prevention Programs in Low- and Middle-Income Countries. *Science* 311, 1474–1610.

Subbarao, K. and Rainey, L. (1995) Social gains from female education. *Economic Development and Cultural Change* 44, 105–128.

UN (2000) The Millennium Declaration. UN General Assembly document A/RES/55/2, 8 September 2000. Available at: http://www.un.org/en/development/devagenda/millennium.shtml (accessed 2 August 2011).

UN (2001) *Road map towards the implementation of the United Nations Millennium Declaration*. General Assembly document A/56/326, 6 September 2001. United Nations, New York. Available at: http://www.un.org/documents/ga/docs/56/a56326.pdf (accessed 2 August 2011).

UN (2002) Report of the International Conference on Financing for Development. Monterrey, Mexico, 18–22 March 2002. Available at: http://www.un.org/esa/ffd/monterrey/MonterreyConsensus.pdf (accessed 2 August 2011).

UN (2010) Millennium Development Goals Report, 2010. Available at: http://www.un.org/millenniumgoals/reports.shtml (accessed 2 August 2011).

UN Statistics Division (2008) Official list of MDG indicators. Available at: http://unstats.un.org/unsd/mdg/Host.aspx?Content=Indicators/OfficialList.htm (accessed 28 July 2011).

UN Statistics Division (2011) Population, rate of increase, birth and death rates, surface area and density for the world, major areas and regions. Available at: http://unstats.un.org/unsd/demographic/products/dyb/dyb2008/Table01.pdf (accessed 22 July 2011).

UNAIDS (2008) *Report on the Global AIDS Epidemic, 2008*. UNAIDS, Geneva.

UNICEF (2009) *Progress Report for Children Affected by HIV/AIDS*. UNICEF, New York.

UNICEF (2011) State of the World's Children. Available at: http://www.unicef.org/sowc2011 (accessed 22 July 2011).

WHO (2005) *The World Health Report 2005: make every mother and child count*. WHO, Geneva.

WHO (2006) *Neonatal and Perinatal Mortality: Country, regional and global estimates*. WHO, Geneva.

WHO, UNICEF, UNFPA and the World Bank (2010) *Trends in Maternal Mortality: 1990 to 2008*. WHO, Geneva.

Yarnall, J., Swica, Y. and Winikoff, B. (2009) Non-physician clinicians can safely provide first trimester medical abortion. *Reproductive Health Matters* 17(33), 61–69.

Zeng, Y., Tu, P., Gu, B., Xu, Y., Li, B. and Li, Y. (1992) Sex ratio of China's population deserves attention. *China Population Today* 9, 3–5.

3 The Politics of Progress: The Story of Maternal Mortality

Wendy J. Graham

University of Aberdeen, Scotland, UK

Summary

- The history of measuring maternal mortality reflects the evolution of two broader strategic priorities: maternal health (safe motherhood) and health information systems.
- Three main periods can be distinguished: mid-1980s to 2000, 2000–2010, and 2010 to the present day, which broadly coincide with the phases of 'awareness', 'acknowledgement and enquiry' and 'commitment' used to describe the evolution of safe motherhood.
- Over the last 12–18 months, there has been an unprecedented level of political support and activity to accelerate progress towards achieving MDGs 4 and 5, reflecting stronger harmonization and alignment among major global actors, national governments, civil society organizations and other constituencies.
- Under the auspices of the United Nations Secretary General's Global Strategy for Women's and Children's Health, the WHO-led Commission on Information and Accountability has highlighted the need not only to generate reliable and powerful evidence but also to ensure its effective **use** in informing remedial actions at national and international levels.
- The Commission's recommendations include the maternal mortality ratio as one of 11 core indicators for judging progress within a framework for results and accountability, and ensure the continuing political prominence of this outcome in global health.
- The renewed attention to women's and children's health provides an opportunity to strengthen the information systems *within* countries. Although models and modelling will continue to play a useful part in estimating maternal mortality, particularly at a global and world region level, this should not be at the expense of investment in or attention to strengthening country-owned information systems and capacity.

Introduction

The imperative to demonstrate progress in reducing maternal mortality has a long history. From the early parish registers of Sweden (Högberg and Wall, 1986) to the strengthening of vital registration across Europe (Loudon, 1992) and on to the use of confidential enquiries into maternal deaths (Drife, 2011), the story in the global North is one of 'progress driving progress'. Identification of maternal deaths provided the basis for the virtuous cycle of calling for action, demonstrating reductions and sustaining commitment – a clear demonstration of 'what you count is what you do'. This well-documented history reveals the driving role of political necessity to show progress along with technical innovation in health information systems. The significant reduction in the level of maternal mortality in high income countries now presents other challenges in terms of demonstrating progress, with numbers of deaths often too small to produce stable trends (Macfarlane, 2001). There remains, however, a high burden of maternal deaths in low income countries – accounting for an estimated 98% of the annual global total. Here the desire to achieve and show progress is receiving heightened national and international attention as the 2015 deadline for the MDGs approaches – with MDG 5 on maternal health still regarded as the most 'off-target' (World Bank and International Monetary Fund, 2011).

The purpose of this chapter is to describe the evolution of the politics of progress in maternal mortality over the last 30 years, primarily from an international rather than individual country perspective. Maternal mortality provides a lens which amplifies the inevitable tensions from balancing the political power of advocacy with the technical realities of monitoring health outcomes in developing countries – tensions found in several other areas of public health (Setel *et al.*, 2007). The chapter ends by considering recent shifts in the international landscape around women's and children's health, in which maternal mortality remains as a core indicator in emerging frameworks for accountability – the latest narrative in the politics of progress. The primary basis for this chapter is a structured review of published articles on maternal mortality in developing countries. The focus was on overviews and review articles on measurement options and on tracking progress.

The Development of the 'Measurement Mantra'

The history of measuring maternal mortality, in large part, reflects the evolution of two broader strategic priorities: maternal health (safe motherhood) and health information systems. Although the evolution of these two priorities differs in detail, with the latter going back further – to the 1970s and *Health for All* – for the purposes of exploring maternal mortality, their pathways can be grouped together into three main periods: mid-1980s to 2000, 2000–2010 and 2010 to the present day. Interestingly, these broadly coincide with the three phases in the recent history of international efforts to improve maternal health, wellbeing and survival first proposed by Fathalla (1999) over a decade ago: awareness, acknowledgement and enquiry, and commitment.

Informing progress and judging progress are inextricably linked, and this is reflected in the published literature. Using the crude metric of the volume of journal papers, Plate 2 shows the trends in articles found through a search using terms 'measuring maternal mortality in developing countries' for the period 1970 to 2010, which yielded a total of 749 articles. This indicates a marked upturn in the number of papers from the mid-1980s, as well as the presence of two subsequent phases: of slight expansion followed by a marked increase at the turn of the new millennium. Plate 2 also shows the number of papers from selected journals with the greatest contribution to the total. The graph reveals an interesting shift from those with a demographic and measurement mandate, such as the *International Journal of Epidemiology*, to those with a more clinical focus, such as the *International Journal of Gynaecology and Obstetrics*, and on to a sharp recent increase in papers published in the general medical journal the *Lancet* – reflecting its own broader commitment to global health. These trends in publications can in turn be linked to Fathalla's three broad phases, as now to be discussed.

Awareness: mid-1980s to 2000

The launch of the Safe Motherhood Initiative in Nairobi in February 1987 is widely regarded as the primary catalyst for propelling the burden of maternal mortality in developing countries on to the global health agenda (Starrs, 2006; Maclean, 2010). Prior to this, there was recognition at the national level of the need for care as seen in the provision of maternal and child health services across the vast majority of low income countries, albeit care widely varying in content and accessibility (Margolis *et al.*, 1997). Recognition of the comparative neglect of the maternal component in these services was highlighted in the mid-1980s in the seminal work by Rosenfield and Maine (1985) titled 'Where is the M in MCH?'. A further stimulus for the 1987 launch of the Safe Motherhood Initiative was the bringing together of country experience at a WHO Inter-Regional meeting. This event witnessed reports from a series of studies from nine countries on estimates of maternal mortality higher than expected given the levels of maternity service provision (WHO, 1986). What was also striking from this meeting was the balanced focus on the magnitude of maternal mortality, as reflected in numbers and ratios or rates, along with concern for the human tragedy of every single death, as captured in the famous story of 'Why did Mrs X die?' (Fathalla, 1987). The 1987 Call to Action made by the WHO Director-General in Nairobi set out an ambitious agenda for action, with explicit reference to tracking maternal mortality as the main parameter for judging progress (Mahler, 1987). This political call presented an immediate technical challenge given the limited range of options available for reliably showing levels and trends in the maternal mortality ratio (maternal deaths per 100,000 live births) in most low income countries – and so the politics of progress was born.

In the late 1980s, routine vital registration with reasonable coverage and reliable cause of death ascertainment was lacking for the vast majority of developing and for many transitional countries (Campbell and Graham, 1990). The alternative sources of population-based estimates were large scale household surveys or RAMOS, both of which needed significant technical and financial resources. Facility-based data on maternal deaths was recognized as unrepresentative of levels in the general population, but provided the basis for many papers published at this time, such as Walker and colleagues' work in Jamaica (Walker et al., 1990). Largely in response to the Call to Action and the heightened need for realistic options for providing estimates, new methods began to emerge, such as snowballing (Boerma and Mati, 1989), which uses key informant networks, and the sisterhood method, which identifies maternal

deaths among the sisters of adult respondents in population surveys (Graham et al., 1989). Crucially, this last development coincided with the launch of the first round of Demographic and Health Surveys, an international programme of household surveys focused initially on maternal, child and reproductive health services (ICF MACRO, 2011). This provided an opportunity to apply and adapt the sisterhood method, so enabling national estimates of the level of maternal mortality to be produced for the first time in many low income countries (Rutenberg and Sullivan, 1991).

From the outset, the Safe Motherhood Initiative acknowledged the importance of recognizing maternal health as not just a medical issue or just a matter of survival or death. This started to receive greater prominence when the broader context of reproductive health was highlighted in 1994 through the first International Conference on Population and Development (UNGA, 1994). This revised conceptualization of the 'burden' brought to light important gender and socio-economic inequities in health outcomes and access to care and made a clear link with rights to health and reproductive rights (Freedman, 2001). Recognition of the need to monitor a broader range of factors relevant to maternal health broadly coincided with an increasing emphasis on process indicators, in large part championed through the work of Maine and colleagues as part of the original Prevention of Maternal Mortality Network (subsequently to become the Averting Maternal Deaths and Disability initiative) (Maine, 1997; Paxton et al., 2005). These indicators not only encompassed measures of coverage of care for all pregnant women, such as the proportion of deliveries with skilled attendants, but also helped to increase attention to life-threatening complications and the essential need for EmOC (Wardlaw and Maine, 1999). For some of these process indicators, normative targets were set, as for the number of comprehensive EmOC facilities per 500,000 population, whilst others became elevated to international development targets, such as 80% of deliveries with skilled attendants by 2005 (UNGA, 1999; WHO, 2005). This shift in reliance on process indicators reflects once again the dual drivers of programmatic need – namely to inform and judge action, versus the realities of outcome measurement in low income countries. Indeed, one rationale given for developing what came to be known as the 'UN process indicators' (see Hounton *et al.*, Chapter 15 this volume) was the suggestion that maternal mortality was not a realistic outcome to monitor in the absence of complete and reliable vital registration (Maine, 1999). Nevertheless, reductions in the maternal mortality ratio continued to be proposed as a target, both in the World Summit for Children in 1990 (UNICEF, 1990) and as an international development target in 1999 (UNGA, 1999). The political and technical dilemma resulting from maternal mortality being proposed as a primary metric of progress was felt most acutely in the very countries where the burden was felt likely to be largest (AbouZhar and Wardlaw, 2001). Here there was an urgent need to achieve and maintain high-level political commitment to action by using the power of rates and ratios, yet the very reliability of such estimates cast doubt on the importance of the problem. The concept of a measurement trap was posed to describe this tension for maternal mortality and for other outcome indicators (Graham and Campbell, 1992), whereby weak measurement was both a cause and an effect of low prioritization of the burden itself. This interrelationship is essentially what is captured more recently in the commonly used phrase 'what you count is what you do' (WHO, 2005).

Within 10 years of the launch of the Safe Motherhood Initiative, the 'globalization' of maternal mortality was well underway as an international priority, if not as a universal national priority. As with other areas of global health, this progression also increased the political requirement for internationally comparative statistics (Byass, 2010). It was in this context that the first modelled estimates of maternal mortality were released by WHO and UNICEF in 1996, referring to levels in 1990 (WHO and UNICEF, 1996). This represented a significant development in the politics of progress, providing, for the very first time, estimates of a variety of maternal mortality measures (number of maternal

deaths, maternal mortality ratio and the lifetime risk of maternal death) for virtually all countries in the world. This modelling involved two distinct steps: assessment of the reliability and adjustment (typically upwards) of existing estimates, and use of a regression-based model to impute missing data and to create figures for countries without any empirical estimates. As the first experience of UN-generated global, regional and national estimates of maternal mortality, there were positive as well as negative reactions from countries – developing and developed (AbouZahr and Wardlaw, 2001). This prompted not only further refinements to the modelling methods, as discussed further below, but also the instigation of processes for engagement with country stakeholders. A further significant stimulus from these initial modelled estimates of maternal mortality was the encouragement to countries to strengthen the availability of their own empirical data from routine systems and surveys. This is reflected in the increased use in the Demographic and Health Surveys of the sisterhood method to estimate the maternal mortality ratio, as seen in Fig. 3.1, reaching a peak in the mid-1990s and then stabilizing at about 50–60% of surveys including the module of questions. Other approaches to investigating maternal deaths continued to be developed in parallel with methods for estimating levels, providing insights into avoidable factors and the broader socio-economic circumstances of deaths that are most relevant to action-oriented initiatives. These included, for example, confidential enquiry systems (Lewis, 2004), criterion-based audit (Graham and Bullough, 2004) and maternal death reviews (Bullough and Graham, 2004). Guidelines were produced by the WHO bringing together these and other in-depth approaches in a volume aptly called *Beyond the Numbers* (WHO, 2004).

By the end of the 1990s, the maternal mortality ratio remained the main international metric for describing the 'burden' of women's reproductive ill health. World maps provided a dramatic reminder of the concentration of the highest risks in sub-Saharan Africa and parts of South Asia, and of the geographical coincidence with other indices

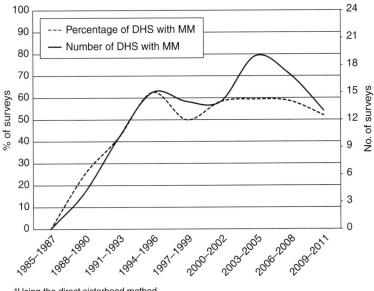

*Using the direct sisterhood method
DHS, Demographic and Health Surveys; MM, maternal mortality

Fig. 3.1. Percentage and number of Demographic and Health Surveys measuring maternal mortality* (1985–2011).

of development, such as women's education, poverty and child mortality (AbouZahr and Wardlaw, 2001). Maternal mortality estimates thus became seen as proxies for development and, in particular, as markers of the functioning of the wider health system (Goodburn and Campbell, 2001). The demand for data showing international and national trends in the maternal mortality ratio arose from an increasingly diverse set of stakeholders – those directly concerned with maternal survival and those dealing with a broader agenda of health and development. The new estimates for the maternal mortality ratio released by WHO, UNICEF and UNFPA at the turn of the new millennium referred to 1995 (AbouZahr *et al.*, 2001). However, as the modelling methods had changed since the earlier figures, statistically reliable trends could not be drawn between 1990 and 1995, and the wide boundaries of uncertainty around the central estimates meant that regional and national comparisons were problematic too. This state of heightened demand and political pressure to use the maternal mortality ratio to help judge progress from a broader development perspective as well as in terms of health

outcomes characterizes the end of the 20th century. It also provides an indication that Fathalla's (1999) awareness phase in 'building safe motherhood' had run its course.

Acknowledgement and enquiry: 2000–2010

The Millennium Declaration announced on 1 January 2000 included maternal mortality as the focus of one of just eight high-level targets (UNGA, 2000). MDG 5 was articulated as 'Improving maternal health' and the initial sole target set as a 75% reduction in maternal mortality ratio between 1990 and 2015. Subsequently a second target was set, referred to as MDG 5b – universal access to comprehensive reproductive health services (see McCaw-Binns and Hussein, Chapter 2 this volume). In recognition of the lack of maternal mortality ratio estimates for many low income countries, a proxy indicator was also agreed for MDG 5 – the proportion of births with skilled attendants, although the definition of 'skilled attendant' was not made explicit. The basis for setting the 75% reduction goal for the maternal mortality ratio is not documented. One suggestion is that it reflects an extension to the earlier maternal mortality ratio target from the Child Survival Summit of a 50% reduction between 1990 and 2000 (C. AbouZahr, Geneva, 2011, personal communication), which itself was simply based on the size of the decline seen historically in the global North and more recently in transitional countries, such as Malaysia, Sri Lanka and Thailand (Cross *et al.*, 2010). Compared with the targets for the other seven MDGs, and especially those for health, a three-quarters reduction was highly aspirational – some would argue unrealistically so (Shiffman and Smith, 2007) – for what could be achieved over the remaining 15 years up to 2015. This was regarded as particularly challenging for those countries where the level of maternal mortality ratio was highest and where only minimal progress was likely to have occurred since 1990. Indeed, for some countries in sub-Saharan Africa, the emergence of HIV/AIDS was already being considered before the turn of the new millennium as a likely driver of increases in the maternal mortality ratio (Graham and Newell, 1999; Bicego *et al.*, 2002).

The difficulty of tracking progress without a reliable baseline for the maternal mortality ratio in 1990 and without reliable vital registration was also acknowledged by some authors from the outset, with comments like 'A millennium development goal which cannot be monitored cannot be met nor missed' (Johannson and Stewart, 2002). The measurement challenges of MDG 5 became part of wider and renewed calls for strengthening information systems. A variety of new initiatives were launched in the early 21st century specifically in response to this call, such as the Health Metrics Network (HMN) (Boerma and Stansfield, 2007), along with others with a focus on tools for measuring maternal mortality and other maternal outcomes in order to evaluate major intervention strategies, such as the Initiative for Maternal Mortality Programme Assessment (Immpact) (http://www.immpact-international.org). Indeed, much of the rationale for Immpact was laid out in a paper published in the *Lancet* in 2002 entitled 'Now or never: the case for

measuring maternal mortality' (Graham, 2002). Lessons were also beginning to emerge from decennial censuses conducted in selected low income countries. These showed the potential of a census platform to overcome the usual concern with sample surveys of inadequate size to produce stable estimates of the maternal mortality ratio, but also emphasized the complex analytical adjustments needed (Stanton *et al.*, 2001). Alternative approaches to investigating maternal mortality at the national level at this time essentially remained the Demographic and Health Surveys and, in a few countries, confidential enquiries or RAMOS, for example in Egypt and Turkey (Campbell *et al.*, 2005; Graham *et al.*, 2008a). The latter have significant resource requirements and, unless conducted where there is already complete capture of all deaths to women of reproductive age, cannot produce population estimates of the maternal mortality ratio (Yazbak, 2007). The importance of the Demographic and Health Surveys in providing national-level maternal mortality ratio estimates cannot be overstated during this first half of the decade, as seen in Fig. 3.1. However, the retrospective nature of the maternal mortality ratio estimate from the direct sisterhood method, being time-located 0–6 years before the survey, remained poorly understood outside narrow technical circles, as did the wide uncertainty boundaries and the implications for monitoring trends (Graham *et al.*, 2008a; AbouZahr, 2011).

By mid-decade, the trends data available on national maternal mortality ratios were those produced by the UN Interagency group comprising WHO, UNICEF and UNFPA (AbouZahr and Wardlaw, 2004). Released in 2004, estimates were presented for 1990, 1995 and 2000, all based on the same overall adjustment and modelling strategy. For specific countries, however, the strategy could vary for the different years owing to the changing availability of data, which placed them in different adjustment groups. Analyses comparing the latest maternal mortality ratio estimates with national figures on the proportion of deliveries with skilled attendants showed somewhat enigmatic patterns, with a weak statistical relationship when restricted to low and middle income countries (WHO,

2005). This mismatch had been highlighted using earlier data series for maternal mortality ratio and skilled attendants (Graham *et al.*, 2001; Shah and Say, 2007) and raised at the tenth anniversary of the Safe Motherhood Initiative conference in Sri Lanka in 1997, as part of a broader questioning of simplistic assumptions about declining mortality being caused by an increase in skilled attendants at birth (Weil and Fernandez, 1999). In the mid-2000s, these questions returned as part of a wider demand to revisit 'what works' in reducing maternal mortality. This demand was both politically and technically driven, and highlighted the inevitable tensions in 'knowing what works' from different perspectives – policy makers, scientists, donors and advocates (Miller *et al.*, 2003; Campbell and Graham, 2006; Graham and Hussein, 2007). A variety of international and high profile events and activities can be seen as responses in part to this demand and were aimed at different stakeholders. For example, at the end of 2005 the first Countdown to 2015 conference was held, with an initial focus on child survival, which was then expanded in 2006 to include indicators of maternal outcomes and services (Countdown Coverage Writing Group, 2008). The new Partnership for Maternal, Newborn and Child Health was launched in New York in September 2005 and its first Partners' Forum held in Tanzania in February 2007 (Starrs, 2006). In September 2006, a special series was published in the *Lancet* which attempted to summarize the current state of knowledge. The series revealed the lack of high-grade scientific evidence on interventions evaluated in terms of impact on maternal mortality (Ronsmans and Graham, 2006). This set of activities together marks the beginning of a period in which the politics of progress – or rather poor progress – became a driver of what Fathalla (1999) calls 'enquiry': asking hard questions on *why* avoidable maternal deaths still occur in spite of political awareness and acknowledgement.

In the last 3 years of the decade, strategic advocacy helped to drive enquiry around commitment and resources to improve the health and survival of women as a human right. The 2007 Women Deliver conference was one of a series of international events that provided a powerful forum for advocacy and for pressing for firm commitments at the highest political level (Starrs and Sankore, 2010). Coinciding with the first Ministers' Forum, this conference also saw the release of the next series of maternal mortality ratio estimates from the UN Interagency group (now comprising WHO, UNICEF, UNFPA and the World Bank) for 2005 and recalculated figures back to 1990 (WHO, 2007). The persistence of a global total of half a million maternal deaths per year – or one every minute – was communicated as a shared global responsibility for poor progress. The use of country 'success stories' of reductions in maternal mortality provided more positive messaging around 'knowing what works' and 'what needs to be done'. In parallel, the constituency of actors focused on the continuum of maternal, newborn and child health were interacting with major political platforms such as the G8 (group of eight most industrialized nations) and International Parliamentary Union, and pushing enquiry – asking hard questions – about levels of donor and government funding (Bustreo and Johnsson, 2008; Greco *et al.*, 2008). The Global Campaign for Health MDGs championed by the Norwegian Government added further momentum in 2007 (Murray *et al.*, 2007), and the Consensus Statement for PMNCH in 2009 provided an additional focus of unified energy at an international level (PMNCH, 2009). The increased attention this brought to innovative financing strategies, such as performance-based funding (Witter *et al.*, 2009), provided a different framework for judging progress, primarily based on coverage indicators with underlying assumptions on benefits to health outcomes like maternal and newborn mortality.

By the end of the decade, evidence of 'what works' – how progress can be achieved – had been generated from two distinct streams with appeal to different stakeholders: from ecological level analyses of country case studies of 'success' and from intervention research studies. Although the former often used maternal mortality as a marker of 'success', at a scientific level, rigorous enquiry – hard questioning – was often not applied to the reliability of the data. Conversely, the research studies, while able to provide stronger assurance of data quality and attribution, were often not powered to show 'progress' in terms of maternal mortality reduction (Hussein *et al.*, 2011). This state of measurement paradox presents a significant challenge to the current phase of building safe motherhood – what Fathalla (1999) called 'commitment'. The marshalling and monitoring of commitments, difficult as this is, places a stronger demand on being able to differentiate between 'robust evidence of *no progress*' versus '*no robust evidence* of progress' in reducing maternal mortality (Graham *et al.*, 2008b). The key question is whether this demand will be tackled or lost within the revitalized global health landscape in the run-up to 2015.

Commitment: 2010 to present day

Since 2010, there has undoubtedly been an unprecedented level of political support and activity to accelerate progress towards achieving MDGs 4 and 5 (Starrs and Sankore, 2010). This reflects a shift in the international and national landscape for both maternal and newborn health, characterized by stronger harmonization and alignment among major global actors, national governments, civil society organizations and other constituencies (Shiffman, 2010). Many events, organizations and indeed committed individuals have helped to catalyse and sustain this renewed energy (see Hussein *et al.*, Chapter 1 this volume). At the international level, events include the Pacific Health Summit on Maternal and Newborn Health, the 2010 Women Deliver and Countdown to 2015 conferences, the G8 Summit, the Global Maternal Heath conference, the PMNCH Partners' Forum and the Delhi Declaration in November 2010. Major ongoing regional initiatives have also sought positive synergies, such as the African Union's harmonization of the Maputo Plan of Action for MDGs 4 and 5 with the Abuja Call for Accelerated Action for MDG 6, reflecting wider efforts to link the health-related MDGs along the continuum of care (African Union, 2010).

Arguably the most significant development in is the launch of the United Nations Secretary General's Global Strategy for Women's and Children's Health (UNSG, 2010). Building on the Consensus Statement for MNCH referred to earlier, this new strategy was announced in September 2010 and reflects the joint efforts of many players to raise the political profile of women's and children's health at the highest level among Heads of State. Whilst called 'new', in fact it builds and relies upon existing initiatives but also seeks fresh commitments from an expanded constituency to 'accelerate progress, deliver results and ensure accountability'. The full range of mechanisms linked to the Global Strategy for supporting the poorest countries in their national plans to improve women's and children's health is still being defined, supported by the WHO-led Commission on Information and Accountability (WHO, 2011a) These mechanisms highlight, among other issues, the need to strengthen monitoring and accountability systems in order not only to generate reliable and powerful evidence but also to ensure its effective *use* in informing remedial actions at national and international levels.

2011 has also seen significant developments in the politics of progress around maternal mortality. These new developments are of two main types: in reported trends in the maternal mortality ratio and in the methods of estimation. Although the new findings on trends have featured prominently in the various events and activities described above, scrutiny of the new estimation methods has occurred somewhat separately and confined to a more technical constituency. This separation of the results from the methods is in some ways not surprising, but it does pose risks and challenges for the future in terms of judging progress, particularly at a country level. The history and circumstances of developments since mid-2010 around trends and methods have been described and analysed in a number of recent publications, such as Byass (2010) and AbouZahr (2011). Here, the focus is more on exploring the implications for the emerging frameworks for results and accountability linked with the Global Strategy given that the maternal mortality ratio is one of the 11 proposed core indicators (http://www.everywomaneverychild.org).

Since May 2010 and for the first time in the history of global maternal mortality statistics, two sets of estimates of the maternal mortality ratio at world, regional and country levels have become available (see Stanton and McCaw-Binns, Chapter 4 this volume). Prior to this, such figures were generated by the UN Interagency group, which, as described earlier, had evolved its adjustment and modelling strategies since 1995 along with country consultation processes. While the release of each new set of estimates by the UN has been met with a range of reactions, from full endorsement to outright rejection (AbouZahr, 2011), for the purposes of international monitoring of levels and trends these have been the figures most widely used. As for many other global health statistics, the production of these maternal mortality ratio estimates involves considerable time and technical resources and thus was presumed to fall beyond the capacity of any single institution and instead requires the political buy-in of multiple agencies with strong country presence and outreach. The emergence of the Seattle-based Institute of Health Metrics and Evaluation (IHME) changed this presumption. In late April 2010, the *Lancet* published a new set of maternal mortality ratio estimates for 1980 to 2008 at global, regional and country levels produced by a team at the IHME (Hogan *et al.*, 2010). These were significant in terms of using not only methods of estimation which differed from those used by the UN Interagency group, particularly around handling uncertainty and the HIV/AIDS envelope of deaths, but also the conclusions on levels and trends in maternal mortality. Released just prior to the 2010 Women Deliver conference, the lower global total number of maternal deaths and the downward trends in some regions and low income countries were warmly welcomed positive news. As a scientific journal was the venue used for first sharing these important findings, interested parties at country and global level only became aware of the figures on the day of online publication. Detailed

technical scrutiny of the methods and estimates before release fell to a journal peer-review process, and opportunities to comment subsequently were provided through the Letters column of the *Lancet* (see, for example, Graham *et al.*, 2010; McCaw-Binns and Lewis-Bell, 2010; Qomariyah and Anggondowati, 2010) and at various meetings, including the Women Deliver conference.

A few months later, the revised estimates from the UN Interagency group were made available, just prior to the United Nations General Assembly and the launch of the Global Strategy on Women's and Children's Health (WHO *et al.*, 2010). These new UN figures were developed from a further improvement in the adjustment and modelling strategy and covered a similar span of time to the IHME figures. The excitement around the new Global Strategy diverted immediate attention away from detailed comparison of the IHME and UN estimates at country levels, particularly given that the 2008 world and regional numbers of maternal deaths and the maternal mortality ratios were very similar, as discussed by AbouZahr (2011). Further commentary on the existence of two sets of maternal mortality figures and on the significant differences between them for some low income countries, as illustrated for one country – Nigeria in Fig. 3.2 – was primarily confined to scientific journals (Ross and Blanc, 2011) and to technical conferences. Behind these immediate issues lie fundamental questions about the future of global health statistics – the producers, the users and the independent brokers responsible for quality assurance both of estimation processes and of results (Boerma *et al.*, 2010; Byass, 2010; Graham and Adjei, 2010; Murray and Lopez, 2010; Sankoh, 2010). The politics of progress is entering new and challenging times as the dual nature of accountability is realized – accountability for women's and children's health, wellbeing and survival *and* for the robust measurement of these important outcomes. There are also uncertainties in the run-up to the 2015 MDG deadline. Will the long standing tensions between national and international needs for maternal mortality estimates finally be relieved or be further aggravated? Will the

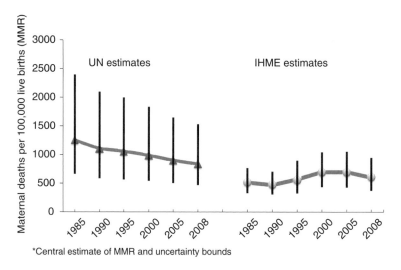

*Central estimate of MMR and uncertainty bounds

Fig. 3.2. Comparison of maternal mortality trends* for Nigeria, 1985–2008.

availability of different sources of country level figures – created through international estimation processes or nationally owned data capture – create confusion or confidence in reported progress?

Conclusion

Maternal mortality today has a political prominence in global health, which continues to exceed the technical capacity and resources available to provide robust estimates in most low-income countries. Inclusion of the maternal mortality ratio among the 11 core indicators provisionally recommended by the Commission on Information and Accountability represents the most recent example of this. However, unlike other global health priorities like HIV/AIDS, which have tended to develop dedicated sources of data for maternal mortality, major progress in measurement is largely dependent on investment in the broader information system and particularly vital registration. Although there has undoubtedly been significant advance over the last 25 years in the availability of methods and tools for capturing maternal deaths and for adjusting or modeling estimates, for most of the 11 low income countries projected to account for two-thirds of the global total

(WHO *et al.*, 2010), there are still no reliable empirical data since the routine information systems remain very weak. Whilst some may argue that ever more sophisticated models can continue to fill this gap, to use projections to hold country governments and donors to account – for no or poor progress – is not sound technically or politically.

The current unprecedented levels of political commitment to women's and children's health built incrementally over the last quarter-century and reinvigorated by the Global Strategy provide an opportunity to strengthen the information systems *within* countries to monitor births and deaths, health and wellbeing (WHO, 2011a) and to use the findings to inform progress – not just monitor it. Indeed, the provisional recommendations from the Commission on Information and Accountability place much emphasis on vital registration and, if implemented, could make a significant difference in the immediate term to data availability. The demand from stakeholders in-country – from civil society to governments – is not in question, and there is much optimism that commitment will be sustained and not replaced by apathy. But there remain knotty issues of harmonizing existing efforts to achieve lasting improvements and to avoid overburdening weak systems. There are also tensions remaining around different methods and models from different technical groups, which should not be ignored but rather marshalled to deliver the best measurement science. Models and modelling will continue to play a useful part, particularly at a global and world region level. This should not, however, be at the expense of investment or attention to strengthening country-owned information systems and capacity.

Given the continuing high demand for measuring maternal mortality, there is much room for innovation. The introduction of standards for monitoring, modelling and reporting, as used in other measurement-related fields (Braunholtz *et al.*, 2010), may help to assure the quality of products and practice. Techniques for assessing the boundaries of uncertainty around the central estimates of maternal mortality require further development, and more effective communication is needed with stakeholders about the implications of uncertainty for judging progress. The potential for developing alternative indicators should continue to be explored, such as combined measures of maternal mortality and near miss or of maternal and perinatal outcomes. Innovations in data capture using appropriate technologies, such as mobile phones (WHO, 2011b), must be nurtured but also evaluated, particularly in terms of their potential to facilitate local-level counting of *all* deaths and for the real-time monitoring most appropriate for accountability purposes. Identification of deaths must be linked to effective enquiry processes to illuminate the circumstances and the avoidable factors to inform future actions. The essential dynamic of 'monitor, review and act' highlighted in the interim recommendations of the Commission on Information and Accountability does not just apply at the level of aggregate statistics. Enquiry systems within countries and at local levels should enable individual adverse events among women, babies or children to inform action. Monitoring the maternal mortality ratio at a population level is thus a necessity but not a sufficient basis alone for judging progress. Measures of outcomes and processes are also needed to inform action on, for example, reducing the disproportionate burden of maternal deaths in the poorest families, along with clearer recognition of who is holding whom to account. The new and emerging frameworks for commitment and accountability will raise important issues about civil societies' role in defining and judging progress. This will present new challenges not only for measurement but also for communicating findings to diverse stakeholders. Delivering sound and effective messages on maternal mortality will remain an art and a science, given the politics of progress.

Acknowledgments

The author is funded by the University of Aberdeen and the UK Department for International Development. The views expressed in the paper are those of the author alone. WJG was a member of the former working group on Results and Accountability of the Commission on Information and Accountability.

The author would like to thank Ann Fitzmaurice for assistance in preparing the graphs and Lisa Davidson for support with the literature search. Acknowledgement is also given to Carla AbouZahr, Peter Byass, Julia Hussein and Ann Starrs for insightful comments on an earlier draft.

The paper was partly based on a seminar presentation 'War and Peace: the story of maternal mortality estimation' invited by the Maternal Health Task Force and given in New York in January 2011 (available for viewing at: http://maternalhealthtaskforce.org/discover/library/doc_view/1238-wendy-graham-war-and-peace-the-story-of-maternal-mortality-estimation?tmpl=component&format=raw).

References

AbouZahr, A. (2011) New estimates of maternal mortality and how to interpret them: choice or confusion? *Reproductive Health Matters* 19(37), 117–128.

AbouZahr, A. and Wardlaw, T. (2001) Maternal mortality at the end of the decade: what signs of progress? *Bulletin of the World Health Organization* 79, 561–573.

AbouZahr, A. and Wardlaw, T. (2004) *Maternal Mortality in 2000: estimates developed by WHO, UNICEF and UNFPA.* WHO, Geneva.

AbouZahr, C., Wardlaw, T. and Hill, K. (2001) *Maternal Mortality in 1995: estimates developed by WHO, UNICEF and UNFPA* (WHO/RHR/02.9). WHO, Geneva.

African Union (2010) Campaign on Accelerated Reduction of Maternal Mortality in Africa (CARMMA). Department of Social Affairs, African Union Commission. Available at: http://www.unfpa.org/africa/newdocs/maputo_eng.pdf (accessed 9 July 2011).

Bicego, G., Boerma, J.T. and Ronsmans, C. (2002) The effect of AIDS on maternal mortality in Zimbabwe and Malawi. *AIDS* 16, 1078–1081.

Boerma, J.T. and Mati, J.K.G. (1989) Identifying maternal mortality through networking: results from Coastal Kenya. *Studies in Family Planning* 20(5), 245–253.

Boerma, J.T. and Stansfield, S.K. (2007) Health statistics now: are we making the right investments? *Lancet* 369, 779–786.

Boerma, T., Mathers, C. and AbouZahr, C. (2010) WHO and Global Health Monitoring: The Way Forward. *PLoS Med* 7, e373. doi:10.1371/journal.pmed.1000373.

Braunholtz, D.A., Graham, W.J. and Hussein, J. (2010) Community based interventions to reduce maternal mortality. *Lancet* 375, 457

Bullough, C.H.W. and Graham, W.J. (2004) Clinical audit: learning from systematic case reviews assessed against explicit criteria. In: *Beyond the Numbers: Reviewing Maternal Deaths and Complications to Make Pregnancy Safer.* WHO, Geneva, pp. 125–140.

Bustreo, F. and Johnsson, A.B. (2008) Parliamentarians: leading the change for maternal, newborn and child survival. *Lancet* 371, 1221–1223.

Byass, P. (2010) The Imperfect World of Global Health Estimates. *PLoS* Med 7(11), e1001006.

Campbell, O.M.R. and Graham, W.J. (1990) *Measuring Maternal Mortality and Morbidity: levels and trends.* Maternal and Child Epidemiology Unit, London School of Hygiene and Tropical Medicine, London.

Campbell, O.M.R. and Graham, W.J. (2006) Strategies for reducing maternal mortality: getting on with what works. *Lancet* 368(9543), 1284–1299.

Campbell, O.M.R., Gipson, R., Issa, A.H. *et al.* (2005) National maternal mortality ratio in Egypt halved between 1992–93 and 2000. *Bulletin of the World Health Organization* 83, 462–471.

Countdown Coverage Writing Group (2008) Countdown to 2015 for maternal, newborn and child survival: the 2008 report on tracking coverage of interventions. *Lancet* 371, 1247–1258.

Cross, S., Bell, J.S. and Graham, W.J. (2010) What you count is what you target: the implications of maternal death classification for tracking progress towards maternal mortality in developing countries. *Bulletin of the World Health Organization* 88, 147–153.

Drife, J.O. (2011) No news is good news: Confidential Enquiries into Maternal Deaths. *British Medical Journal* 342, d3390. doi: 10.1136/bmj.d3390.

Fathalla, M. (1987) Why did Mrs X die? *People* 14, 8–9.

Fathalla, M. (1999) Interview with Speyer R 'Reducing maternal mortality rate': Obgyn.net conference coverage. ACOG, Philadelphia, Pennsylvania. Available at: http://www.obgyn.net/women/women.asp?page=/avtranscripts/speyer_fathalla (accessed 4 July 2011).

Freedman, L.P. (2001) Using human rights in maternal mortality programs: from analysis to strategy. *International Journal of Gynaecology and Obstetrics* 75, 51–60.

Goodburn, E. and Campbell, O.M.R. (2001) Reducing maternal mortality in the developing world: sector-wide approaches may be the key. *British Medical Journal* 322, 917. doi: 10.1136/bmj.322.7291.917.

Graham, W.J. (2002) Now or never: the case for measuring maternal mortality. *Lancet* 359(9307), 701–704.

Graham, W.J. and Adjei, S. (2010) A call for responsible estimation of global health. *PLoS Med* 7(11), e1001003. doi:10.1371/journal.pmed.1001003.

Graham, W.J. and Bullough, C.H.W. (2004) Facility-based maternal death reviews: learning from deaths occurring in health facilities. In: *Beyond the Numbers: Reviewing Maternal Deaths and Complications to Make Pregnancy Safer.* WHO, Geneva, pp. 57–76.

Graham, W.J. and Campbell, OM.R. (1992) The measurement trap. *Social Science and Medicine* 35, 967–976.

Graham, W.J. and Hussein, J. (2007) Ethics in public health research: minding the gaps: a reassessment of the challenges to safe motherhood. *American Journal of Public Health* 97(6), 978–983.

Graham, W.J. and Newell, M.L. (1999) Seizing the opportunity: collaborative initiatives to reduce HIV and maternal mortality. *Lancet* 353, 836–839.

Graham, W.J., Brass, W. and Snow, R.W. (1989) Estimating maternal mortality: the sisterhood method. *Studies in Family Planning* 20, 125–135.

Graham, W.J., Bell, J.S. and Bullough, C.H.W. (2001) Can skilled attendance at delivery reduce maternal mortality in developing countries? In: DeBrouwere V. and Van Lerberghe, W. (eds) *Safe Motherhood Strategies: a review of the evidence. Studies in Health Services Organization & Policy* 17, 97–130.

Graham, W.J., Ahmed, S., Stanton, C., Abou-Zahr, C.L. and Campbell, O.M.R. (2008a) Measuring maternal mortality: an overview of opportunities and options for developing countries. *BMC Medicine* 6, 12. doi:10.1186/1741-7015-6-12.

Graham, W.J., Foster, L.B., Davidson, L., Hauke, E. and Campbell, O.M.R. (2008b) Measuring progress in reducing maternal mortality. *Best Practice and Research Clinical Obstetrics and Gynaecology* 22(3), 425–445.

Graham, W.J., Braunholtz, D.A. and Campbell, O.M.R. (2010) New modelled estimates of maternal mortality. *Lancet* 375(9730) 1963.

Greco, G., Powell-Jackson, T., Borghi, J. and Mills, A. (2008) Countdown to 2015: assessment of donor assistance to maternal, newborn, and child health between 2003 and 2006. *Lancet* 371, 1268–1275.

Hogan, M.C., Foreman, K.J., Naghavi, M. *et al.* (2010) Maternal mortality for 181 countries, 1980–2008: a systematic analysis of progress towards Millennium Development Goal 5. *Lancet* 375(9726), 1609–1623.

Högberg, U. and Wall, S. (1986) Secular trends in maternal mortality in Sweden from 1750 to 1980. *Bulletin of the World Health Organization* 64, 79–84.

Hussein, J., Bell, J., Dar Lang, M., Mesko, N., Amery, J. and Graham, W.J. (2011) An Appraisal of the Maternal Mortality Decline in Nepal. *PLoS ONE* 6(5), e19898. doi:10.1371/journal.pone.0019898.

ICF MACRO (2011) MEASURE Demographic and Health Surveys: Quality information to plan, monitor, and improve population, health, and nutrition. Celebrating 25 years. Available at: http://www.measuredhs.com/aboutdhs/document/about_dhs_booklet.pdf (accessed 9 July 2011).

Johansson, C. and Stewart, D. (2002) *The millennium Development Goals: commitments and prospects. Human Development Report Office Working Papers and Notes: Working Paper No 1.* UNDP, New York.

Lewis, G. (2004) Confidential enquiries into maternal deaths. In: *Beyond the Numbers: Reviewing Maternal Deaths and Complications to Make Pregnancy Safer.* WHO, Geneva, pp. 77–101.

Loudon, I. (1992) *Death in Childbirth. An international study of maternal care and maternal mortality 1800–1950.* Clarendon Press, Oxford.

Macfarlane, A. (2001) Enquiries into Maternal Deaths during the 20th century. In: Royal College of Obstetricians and Gynaecologists. *Why Mothers Die 1997–1999. The Confidential Enquiries into Maternal Death in the United Kingdom.* RCOG Press, London, pp. 346–357.

Maclean, G.D. (2010) An historical overview of the first two decades of striving towards Safe Motherhood. *Sexual & Reproductive Healthcare* 1, 7–14.

Mahler, H. (1987) The Safe Motherhood Initiative: a call to action. *Lancet* 668–670.

Maine, D. (1997) The strategic model for the PMM Network. *International Journal of Gynecology and Obstetrics* 59(Suppl. 2), S23–S25.

Maine, D. (1999) What's so special about maternal mortality. *Reproductive Health Matters* 175–182.

Margolis, L.H., Cole, G.P. and Kotch, J.B. (1997) Historical foundations of maternal and child health. In: Kotch, J.B. (ed.) *Maternal and Child Health: Programs and Policy in Public Health.* Aspen Publishers, Maryland.

McCaw-Binns, A. and Lewis-Bell, K. (2010) New modelled estimates of maternal mortality. *Lancet* 375, 1967–1968.

Miller, S., Sloan, N.L., Winikoff, B., Langer, A. and Fikree, F.F. (2003) Where is the 'E' in MCH? The need for an evidence-based approach in safe motherhood. *Journal of Midwifery and Women's Health* 48, 10–8.

Murray, C. and Lopez, A. (2010) Production and analysis of health indicators: the role of academia. *PLoS Med* 7, e1004. doi:10.1371/journal.pmed.1001004.

Murray, C.J.L., Frenk, J. and Evans, T. (2007) The Global Campaign for the Health MDGs: challenges, opportunities, and the imperative of shared learning. *Lancet* http://www.thelancet.com/journals/lancet/issue/vol370no9592/PIIS0140-6736(07)X6040-9 370, 1018–1020. doi:10.1016/S0140-6736(07)61458.

Partnership for Maternal, Newborn and Child Health (PMNCH) (2009) Consensus for MNCH. Available at: http://who.int/pmnch/events/2009/20090922_consensus.pdf (accessed 9 July 2011).

Paxton, A., Maine, D., Freedman, L., Fry, D. and Lobis, S. (2005) The evidence for emergency obstetric care. *International Journal of Gynaecology and Obstetrics* 88, 181–193.

Qomariyah, S.N. and Anggondowati, T. (2010) New modelled estimates of maternal mortality. *Lancet* 375, 1964–1965.

Ronsmans, C. and Graham, W.J. (2006) Maternal mortality: who, when, where and why. *Lancet* 368(9542), 1189–1200.

Rosenfield, A. and Maine, D. (1985) Maternal mortality – a neglected tragedy. Where is the M in MCH? *Lancet* 2, 83–85.

Ross, J.A. and Blanc, A.K. (2011) Why aren't there more maternal deaths? A decomposition analysis. *Maternal and Child Health Journal* doi: 10.1007/s10995-011-0777-x.

Rutenberg, N. and Sullivan, J.M. (1991) *Direct and Indirect Estimates of Maternal Mortality from the Sisterhood Method*. IRD/Macro International Inc., Washington, DC.

Sankoh, O. (2010) Global health estimates: stronger collaboration needed with low and middle income countries. *PLoS Med* 7, e1005. doi:10.1371/journal.pmed.1001005.

Setel, P., Macfarlane, S., Szreter, S. *et al.* (2007) A scandal of invisibility: making everyone count by counting everyone. *Lancet* 370(9598), 1569–77. doi: 10.1016/S0140-6736(07) 61307-5.

Shah, I. and Say, L. (2007) Maternal mortality and maternity care from 1990 to 2005: uneven but important gains. *Reproductive Health Matters* 15(30), 17–27.

Shiffman, J. (2010) Issue attention in global health: the case of newborn survival. *Lancet* 375, 2045–2049.

Shiffman, J. and Smith, S. (2007) Generation of political priority for global health initiatives: a framework and case study of maternal mortality. *Lancet* 370, 1370–1379.

Stanton, C., Hobcraft, J., Hill, K. *et al.* (2001) Every death counts: measurement of maternal mortality via a census. *Bulletin of the World Health Organization* 79, 657–664.

Starrs, A.M. (2006) Safe Motherhood Initiative: 20 years and counting. *Lancet* 368(9542), 1130–1132.

Starrs, A.M. and Sankore, R. (2010) Momentum, mandate and money: achieving health MDGs. *Lancet* 375, 1946–1948.

UN (2000) *UN Millennium Declaration*. United Nations, New York.

UN General Assembly (UNGA) (1994) *Programme of Action of the International Conference on Population and Development*. Doc A/CONF. 171.13. United Nations, Cairo.

UN General Assembly (UNGA) (1999) *Report of the Ad Hoc Committee of the Whole of the Twenty-first Special Session of the General Assembly*. (General Assembly document, No. A/S-21/5/Add.1) United Nations, New York.

UN General Assembly (UNGA) (2000) United Nations Millennium Declaration A/RES/55/2. United Nations, Geneva. Available at: http://www.un.org/millennium/declaration/ares552e.pdf (accessed 4 November 2011)

UNICEF (1990) World Declaration on the Survival, Protection and Development of Children. Available at: http://www.unicef.org/wsc/declare.htm (accessed 9 July 2011).

UN Secretary-General (UNSG) (2010) *Global Strategy for Women's and Children's Health*. United Nations, New York.

Walker, G.J.A., McCaw-Binns, A., Ashley, D.E.C. and Bernard, G.W. (1990) Identifying maternal deaths in developing countries: experience in Jamaica. *International Journal of Epidemiology* 19(3), 599–605.

Wardlaw, T. and Maine, D. (1999) Process indicators for maternal mortality programmes. *Reproductive Health Matters* 24–30.

Weil, O. and Fernandez, H. (1999) Is safe motherhood an orphan initiative? *Lancet* 354, 940–943.

WHO (1986) *Prevention of Maternal Mortality: report of the WHO inter-regional meeting, November 1985*. WHO/FHE/86.1. WHO, Geneva.

WHO (2004) *Beyond the Numbers: Reviewing Maternal Deaths and Complications to Make Pregnancy Safer*. WHO, Geneva.

WHO (2005) World Health Report 2005: make every mother and child count. WHO, Geneva. Available at: http://www.who.int/whr/2005/en/index.html (accessed 1 Feb. 2007).

WHO (2007) *Maternal Mortality in 2005: Estimates developed by WHO, UNICEF, UNFPA and the World Bank*. WHO, Geneva.

WHO (2011a) Accountability Commission for Health of Women and Children. Available at: http://www.who.int/topics/millennium_development_goals/accountability_commission/en/ (accessed 9 July 2011).

WHO (2011b) *mHealth: new horizons for health through mobile technologies: second global survey on eHealth*. WHO, Geneva.

WHO and UNICEF (1996) *Revised 1990 Estimates of Maternal Mortality: a new approach by WHO and UNICEF*. WHO, Geneva.

WHO, UNICEF, UNFPA and World Bank (2010) *Trends in maternal mortality: 1990 to 2008*. WHO, Geneva.

Witter, S., Adjei, S., Armar-Klemesu, M. and Graham, W.J. (2009) Providing free maternal health care: ten lessons from an evaluation of the national delivery exemption policy in Ghana. *Global Health Action* 2.

World Bank and International Monetary Fund (2011) *Global Monitoring Report 2011: Improving the Odds of Achieving the MDGs*. World Bank, Washington, DC.

Yazbak, A.S. (2007) Comment: challenges in measuring maternal mortality. *Lancet* 370, 1291–1292.

4 The Epidemiology of Maternal Mortality

Cynthia Stanton[1] and Affette McCaw-Binns[2]

[1]*Johns Hopkins Bloomberg School of Public Health, Baltimore, USA;*
[2]*University of the West Indies, Kingston, Jamaica*

Summary

- Three different definitions of maternal death should be distinguished: maternal deaths, pregnancy-related deaths and late maternal deaths.
- Four indicators are used to describe different aspects of the level of maternal mortality: maternal mortality ratio, maternal mortality rate, maternal proportion of female deaths and the lifetime risk of maternal death.
- Constraints related to the quality and completeness of vital registration systems and under-reporting of maternal deaths have resulted in the need to develop various data collection methods to estimate maternal mortality.
- The UN estimated that 358,000 maternal deaths occurred worldwide in 2008. The maternal mortality ratio was 260 maternal deaths per 100,000 live births. The rate of decline in the maternal mortality ratio varies from annual reductions of 1.3% to 2.3% between 1990 and 2008.
- The leading direct causes of maternal death are haemorrhage, hypertensive diseases of pregnancy, pregnancy-related sepsis, obstructed labour and unsafe abortion. Indirect causes of death are due to complications of medical conditions that can occur during pregnancy. The greatest risk of maternal death occurs near the time of delivery, with decreasing risk throughout the first week after delivery.

Introduction

This chapter provides an overview of the epidemiology of maternal mortality with a focus on low income countries, as more than 98% of maternal deaths occur there. The chapter describes the magnitude, geographical distribution, medical causes and timing of these deaths.

Definitions, Indicators and Measurement Issues

Definitions of maternal and pregnancy-related death

The International Classification of Diseases, Revision 10 (ICD10), specifies three different definitions for deaths occurring to pregnant or recently delivered women. According to the ICD10, the definition of a *maternal death* is:

> the death of a woman while pregnant or within 42 days of termination of pregnancy, irrespective of the duration and the site of the pregnancy, from any cause related to or aggravated by the pregnancy or its management but not from accidental causes. (WHO, 1994)

Thus, two criteria must be met when defining a maternal death. There must be a temporal relationship between the death and pregnancy (the death occurs at any point during pregnancy or within 42-days of the termination of pregnancy, regardless of the duration of pregnancy), and there must be a causal relationship between the pregnant state and death (death from accidents during pregnancy or the 42-day postpartum period do not constitute a maternal death).

A *pregnancy-related death* is defined as:

> the death of a woman while pregnant or within 42 days of termination of pregnancy, irrespective of the duration and the site of the pregnancy. (WHO, 1994)

This means that pregnancy-related deaths do include, for example, deaths to pregnant or recently delivered women from violence, suicide and accidents, all causes which would not meet the causal criterion required to categorize a death as maternal. However, data based on this definition are very often and erroneously referred to as maternal deaths even in journal articles and scientific reports, though this definition ignores information on cause of death. It should also be noted that the most frequently used data collection methods in low income countries tend to measure pregnancy-related, rather than maternal, deaths due to the difficulty in arriving at a clinical diagnosis of the cause of death in these settings.

The ICD10 also provides a definition for *late maternal deaths*, which it defines as:

> a death from direct or indirect obstetric causes more than 42 days but less than 1 year after termination of pregnancy. (WHO, 1994)

This extended reference period is particularly appropriate in low mortality settings where,

thanks to accessible high quality health care, women with direct or indirect obstetric complications may survive beyond the 42-day reference period for a maternal death.

Indicators of maternal and pregnancy related death

Four different indicators are used to describe different aspects of the level of maternal mortality. Measures of maternal mortality should refer to a clearly specified time period and ideally reflect each of the following factors:

- The risk of maternal death per birth;
- The risk of maternal death per woman of reproductive age;
- The proportion of all adult female deaths due to maternal causes;
- The cumulated risk of maternal death across the reproductive lifespan.

The indicators are described below. Pregnancy-related deaths can be substituted for maternal deaths in all of these indicators.

The most commonly used indicator is the maternal mortality ratio (MMRatio), which refers to the number of maternal deaths per live birth, multiplied by a conventional factor of 100,000:

$$MMRatio = \frac{\text{Number of maternal deaths}}{\text{Number of live births}} \times 100,000$$

(4.1)

The MMRatio was designed to express obstetric risk. In fact, the MMRatio may overestimate obstetric risk by excluding from the denominator pregnancies that do not terminate in a live birth (for example, spontaneous and induced pregnancy terminations, and fetal deaths, but which may be responsible for a maternal death). In theory, it would be preferable to refine the denominator to include all pregnancies. In practice, it is rare that suitable data on pregnancies not resulting in a live birth are available.

The MMRatio is frequently, though erroneously, referred to as the maternal mortality rate (MMRate). The MMRate is an indicator of the risk of maternal death among women of reproductive age (generally defined as 15–49 years, though often restricted to 15–44 years of age). It is simply a cause-specific death rate. The MMRate is usually expressed per 1000 women:

$$MMRate = \frac{\text{Number of maternal deaths}}{\text{Number of women aged } 15-44 \text{ or } 49 \text{ years}} \times 1000$$

(4.2)

While the MMRate provides an indication of the risk of maternal death in the adult female population, it conceals the effect of differing levels of fertility in cross country comparisons. The relationship between the MMRate and the MMRatio is as follows:

$$MMRatio = \frac{MMRate}{\text{General Fertility Rate}} \times 100$$

(4.3)

The General Fertility Rate is the ratio of live births to women aged 15–49 (or 44) years.

A third indicator that expresses the salience of maternal deaths relative to other causes of death among women of reproductive age is the proportion of maternal female deaths (PMFD) among women of reproductive age:

$$PMFD = \frac{\text{Number of maternal deaths}}{\text{Number of deaths among women aged } 15-49 \text{ years}}$$

(4.4)

A fourth indicator of maternal mortality, primarily used for advocacy purposes, is the lifetime risk of maternal death (LTR). The LTR reflects the chances of a woman dying from maternal causes over the course of her 35-year reproductive lifespan. This indicator takes into account the probability of a death due to maternal causes each time a woman becomes pregnant. A common way of calculating an *approximation* of the LTR is included below. This calculation, however, does not take into account the

risks of death from other competing causes over the reproductive lifespan. The technically correct approach is described by Wilmoth (2009).

$$LTR = 35 \times MMRate$$

(4.5)

For advocacy purposes, the reciprocal of the LTR is often used (1/LTR). For example, an LTR of 17% could be described as one woman in six dying of maternal causes at some point during her reproductive lifespan.

Among the four indicators, the maternal mortality ratio has received the most attention from policy makers, programme managers and the donor community. But, even with highly precise data, a variety of indicators are needed to understand the level of maternal mortality. The interplay between changes in maternal mortality and fertility may produce unexpected results, which may be misinterpreted if relying on one indicator. For example, a decrease in the MMRate may simply be reflecting a decline in fertility, particularly in settings where the risk of maternal death per birth has remained constant. Fewer births result in fewer maternal deaths, even if no new maternal health interventions are in place. Likewise, the PMFD may change substantially if there are changes in the overall distribution of causes of death (for example, due to AIDS mortality). Thus, trends in maternal mortality should be interpreted in light of the risk per woman and per birth and with consideration of changes in fertility and the distribution of deaths by cause.

Table 4.1 provides examples from several countries of these four indicators using pregnancy-related mortality data, and also provides neonatal and infant mortality rates, for comparative purposes. By comparing the pregnancy-related mortality ratio per 1000 live births (instead of 100,000 births) to the neonatal and infant mortality rates per 1000 births, one has a better sense of the burden of pregnancy-related mortality in the population than from focusing on the pregnancy-related mortality ratio alone. In all of these countries, infant deaths occur

Table 4.1. Pregnancy-related and early childhood mortality indicators from demographic and health surveys (Macro International, 2009).

Country	Reference period	Pregnancy-related mortality ratio per 1000 live births	Pregnancy-related mortality rate per 1000 women	Adult female deaths due to pregnancy-related causes (%)	Lifetime risk of pregnancy-related death	Neonatal mortality per 1000 live births	Infant mortality per 1000 live births
Benin	2001–2006	3.97	0.77	24	0.023	32	67
Dem. Republic of Congo	2000–2005	7.81	1.20	19	0.036	33	75
Zimbabwe	1996–2005	5.55	0.76	7	n/a	24	60
Indonesia	2002–2007	2.28	0.18	10	n/a	19	34
Cambodia	2000–2005	4.72	0.50	17	0.017	28	66
Peru	1995–2000	1.85	0.18	20	n/a	18	33

n/a, not available.

10 to 18 times more often than pregnancy-related deaths, even in very high maternal mortality settings. However, the proportion 'pregnancy-related' reminds one that pregnancy-related death is probably the leading or second leading cause of death among women of reproductive age in all of these countries except Indonesia and Zimbabwe. Each of these indicators provides a different perspective on pregnancy-related death that is lost when focusing on one indicator only.

Measurement issues related to maternal mortality

The maternal mortality ratio has been included on select lists of indicators to be monitored for multiple key global initiatives going back 20 years. The most recent such initiative and the drive behind the greatly increased demand for data on country-specific maternal mortality ratios is the 2001 United Nations Millennium Declaration. This declaration requires annual reporting on indicators associated with eight MDGs covering social development, health and the environment (UN, 2010) (see McCaw-Binns and Hussein, Chapter 2 this volume). The fifth MDG is a reduction in the maternal mortality ratio by three-quarters between 1990 and 2015. Hence, as signatories to the declaration, countries are under strong pressure to produce annual estimates of the maternal mortality ratio.

The quality of vital registration data is considered sufficient when systems register more than 90% of deaths, there is medical certification of death following ICD coding standards and there are less than 10% of deaths with ill-defined causes. Such criteria were fulfilled in only 23 of 115 countries reporting data to the World Health Organization in 2003. Death registration in African countries was less than 10% (Mathers *et al.*, 2005). Even high income countries with complete coverage of reporting on the number of deaths by age and on live births may have inadequate data on cause of death. Under-reporting of maternal deaths in these settings is often due to the absence of specific information on the death certificate indicating that the deceased was pregnant or recently delivered at the time of death. Consequently, very specific cause of death codes may be recorded indicating, for example, death from cardiac disease but without additional data specifying the timing of this death relative to pregnancy or delivery. These maternal deaths are not counted as maternal unless special efforts are in place to link adult female death certificates to infant birth and stillbirth certificates. Table 4.2 provides data from studies showing the under-registration of maternal deaths from vital registration systems in eight developed countries.

Table 4.2. Studies documenting under-reporting of maternal deaths in vital registration data (Hill *et al.*, 2007).

Country	Method	Year	ICD revision no.	No. of maternal deaths from vital registration	No. of maternal deaths from in-depth study	Ratio
Australia	Confidential enquiry	2000–2002	10	39	84	2.2
Austria	Confidential enquiry	1980–1998	9	119	191	1.6
Canada	Record linkage	1988–1992	9	72	105	1.5
Canada	Record linkage	1997–2000	9–10	42	64	1.5
Finland	Record linkage	1987–1994	9	31	29	0.9
Finland	Record linkage	1999–2000	10	3	6	2.0
France	Record linkage	1999–2000	9–10	53	58	1.1
The Netherlands	Confidential enquiry	1983–1992	9	133	180	1.4
United Kingdom	Confidential enquiry	2000–2002	10	148	261	1.8
USA – North Carolina	Record linkage	1999–2000	10	27	30	1.1
Total				667	1008	1.5

In response, a number of data collection methods have been developed or adapted over the years. Examples of these approaches are: sample registration systems, national population censuses, several methods relying on large retrospective household surveys using indirect and direct sisterhood methods, reproductive age mortality studies and verbal autopsies focusing on maternal death and prospective surveillance of deaths of reproductive age women using community-based informants. All of these methods, as well as their advantages, disadvantages and appropriate contexts, have been described in detail elsewhere (Graham *et al.*, 2008) (a comprehensive source of information on measuring maternal mortality can be found on the website: http://www.maternal-mortality-measurement. org). Regardless of the method used, identification of maternal or pregnancy-related deaths all require questions that identify: (i) deaths; (ii) the timing of the woman's death relative to a pregnancy or the postpartum period; and, if maternal deaths are being identified, (iii) the medical cause of the death. Data from studies suggest that between 2% and 56% of maternal deaths occur at home (Ronsmans and Graham, 2006). Thus, in many settings, eliciting information on medical cause of death must be based on questions addressed to a family member, preferably one who was present at the death, regarding signs and symptoms associated with various causes of maternal death. This method of investigation is known as a verbal autopsy. The sensitivity and specificity of verbal autopsy questions for maternal cause of death vary by setting, the questions, whether the death is due to direct or indirect causes and the algorithms used to classify maternal deaths (Chandramohan *et al.*, 1998). However, in any setting with weak death registration and in which a large proportion of maternal deaths occur at home, verbal autopsy is the only option available for identifying causes of maternal death.

Several of the methods listed above collect data on pregnancy-related and not maternal deaths, although results are often described in terms of maternal mortality. The largest sources of national empirical data on pregnancy-related or maternal mortality are the Demographic and Health Surveys and the Reproductive Health Surveys of the Center for Disease Control and Prevention, which have collected pregnancy-related mortality data in approximately 100 national surveys in over 50 countries (Hogan *et al.*, 2010). The Demographic and Health Surveys (available at: http://www.measuredhs.com) are nationally representative household surveys, which cover key issues such as family planning practices, fertility, child health, childhood vaccination, maternal health-care utilization, nutrition and mortality. In the majority of these surveys, such data are collected by asking reproductive-aged women about the survival of their sisters. For each adult sister who has died, respondents are asked if the death occurred during pregnancy, during childbirth or within 2 months of the end of pregnancy (Rutenberg and Sullivan, 1991). This is what is referred to as the direct sisterhood method.

Although the availability of maternal mortality data has increased over the past decade, as of 2007 there were still 61 low income countries, representing one-quarter of global births, with no empirical estimate of maternal mortality for the previous 10 years (WHO *et al.*, 2007). Even fewer low and middle income countries have multiple and comparable estimates of maternal mortality to provide indications of trends. This reality, in the context of strong demand for maternal mortality data, has led UN agencies to develop statistical models to predict maternal mortality ratios, particularly for countries lacking a recent national empirical maternal mortality ratio. Until 2010, these estimates remained in the domain of UN agencies, which produced global, regional and country-specific maternal mortality ratios for 1990, 1995, 2000 and 2005 (WHO and UNICEF, 1996; WHO, 2001; WHO *et al.*, 2004, 2007). However, as of 2010, two series of global, regional and country-specific maternal mortality ratio estimates became available. A group of UN agencies has published estimates

for 1990 to 2008 (Who *et al.*, 2010) and Hogan and colleagues at the Institute of Health Metrics and Evaluation at the University of Washington have published estimates for 1980 to 2008 (Hogan *et al.*, 2010).

The data compilation and statistical analyses supporting each of these series are based on the principles that, where data are lacking, one should make the best possible use of existing data; and that strong demand for data will improve the availability and the quality of data over time. Given the quality of the underlying data to support such estimates and the different methods of estimation used, it is not surprising that the estimates of the maternal mortality ratio, particularly at the country level, differ across these two series of estimates (Fig. 4.1). Some key differences between the two series of estimates include: the regression techniques used; the extent to which analysts relied on maternal mortality data from vital registration; and how indirect maternal deaths from HIV were handled.

The existence of the two series of estimates has led to a lively debate regarding the best way forward. The questions asked include the following. Is there a role for academia in the production of these estimates, given that previously UN agencies took on this responsibility? How can one increase the contribution of scientists from low income countries into these estimation exercises? Who are these estimates intended

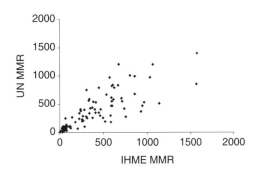

IHME, Institute of Health Metrics;
UN, United Nations; MMR, maternal mortality ratio

Fig. 4.1. Comparison of two sets of estimates for the maternal mortality ratio for 171 countries, 2008 (Graham and Adjei, 2010).

to serve – international agencies or country-level health programmers? And how can one ensure transparency of global estimates? Recommendations for the development of global estimates for health-related indicators have been outlined, emphasizing the importance of transparency of methods, accessibility of the dataset on which the series was developed and external peer review of methods and results (Shibuya *et al.*, 2005; Boerma *et al.*, 2010; Byass, 2010; Graham and Adjei, 2010; Murray and Lopez, 2010; Sankoh, 2010). Such recommendations are most welcome. However, there are no hard and fast rules for many other decisions. For example, the team of analysts must decide which existing maternal mortality ratio estimates are of sufficient quality to use as are, which countries require model-based estimates, which countries have existing estimates that could be used but require adjustment, how various types of adjustment should be calculated and on what basis, and when one has an insufficient number of 'good' observations to go forward in developing a global series of estimates. One variable of import is whether and how international organizations will support strategies to improve the ability to produce high quality, valid and reliable estimates in those countries with the capacity to do so.

Magnitude, Geographical Distribution and Trends in Maternal Mortality

As described above, global series of maternal mortality estimates have been produced by UN agencies and by Hogan *et al.* (Hogan *et al.*, 2010; WHO *et al.*, 2010). For 2008, at the global level, the number of maternal deaths and the maternal mortality ratio are fairly consistent across the two series, with UN estimates of 358,000 maternal deaths and 260 maternal deaths per 100,000 live births (uncertainty interval: 200–370) and the estimates by Hogan *et al.* (2010) of 342,900 maternal deaths and 251 maternal deaths per 100,000 live births (uncertainty interval: 221–289). However, there are important differences in the estimates of the maternal mortality ratio at the country level, particularly in high mortality settings (Fig. 4.1), and in the pace of the decline in the maternal mortality ratio since 1990 (Fig. 4.2).

The Hogan *et al.* (2010) estimates suggest a decline in the global maternal mortality ratio from 320 per 100,000 live births (uncertainty interval: 272–378) to 251 per 100,000 live births (uncertainty interval: 221–289), representing an annual 1.3% decline. The UN estimates show a decline in the global maternal mortality ratio from 400 in 1990 to 260 in 2008, representing an annual decline of 2.3%.

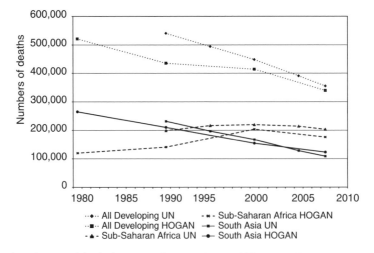

Fig. 4.2. Number of maternal deaths by area and source (Ross and Blanc, 2011).

Table 4.3 presents summarized maternal mortality data by world region from the 1990 and 2008 UN series. In both time periods, sub-Saharan Africa has the highest maternal mortality ratios in the world (870 and 640 maternal deaths per 100,000 live births in 1990 and 2008, respectively). South Asia has the second highest maternal mortality ratios (590 and 280 maternal deaths per 100,000 live births in 1990 and 2008, respectively). In 1990, sub-Saharan Africa and South Asia contributed approximately 36% and 43% of global maternal deaths, respectively. Over this approximate 20-year period, these data suggest an important shift in the distribution of maternal deaths with sub-Saharan Africa contributing 57% of global maternal deaths versus 30% by South Asia. The same general pattern is shown in the Hogan *et al.* (2010) estimates.

Ross and Blanc (2011) have decomposed maternal mortality ratios and rates to illustrate the contribution of the growth in the population of women of reproductive age,

changes in fertility and the risk of maternal death to the global number of maternal deaths. They show that the number of women aged 15–49 years in low income countries increased by 42% from 1990 to 2008. This increase in women of childbearing age was offset by a decline in fertility, which resulted in an unchanged annual number of births in 2008 relative to 1990, and a decline of 35% in the risk of maternal death per birth. The result is a 34% decline in the number of maternal deaths in low income countries.

The trends in these components vary substantially in sub-Saharan Africa as compared to South Asia. For example, in sub-Saharan Africa, the number of women of reproductive age rose by 66% between 1990 and 2008. Although fertility declined somewhat, the annual number of births associated with this fast growing number of women resulted in a 37% increase in the number of births. The increase was offset by only a moderate decline of 26% in the risk of maternal death. The result is an annual number of

Table 4.3. 1990 and 2008 UN estimates of the maternal mortality ratio and number of maternal deaths by regions (WHO *et al.*, 2010).

Region	1990		2008		Change in MMR between 1990 and 2008 (%)
	Maternal mortality ratio per 100,000 live births	No. of maternal deaths	Maternal mortality ratio per 100,000 live births	No. of maternal deaths	
World	400	546,000	260	358,000	−34
Developed countries	16	2,000	14	1,700	−13
CIE countries	68	3,200	40	1,500	−41
Developing countries	450	540,000	290	355,000	−34
Africa	780	208,000	590	207,000	−25
North Africa	230	8,600	92	3,400	−59
Sub-Saharan Africa	870	199,000	640	204,000	−26
Asia	390	315,000	190	139,000	−52
Eastern Asia	110	29,000	41	7,800	−63
South Asia	590	234,000	280	109,000	−53
South-east Asia	380	46,000	160	18,000	−57
Western Asia	140	6,100	68	3,300	−52
Latin America/ Caribbean	140	17,000	85	9,200	−41
Oceania	290	540	230	550	−22

maternal deaths from sub-Saharan Africa that barely changed from 1990 to 2008 (199,000 to 204,000) (Fig. 4.2). In contrast, in South Asia, the number of women of reproductive age also increased dramatically (52%), but was effectively counterbalanced by impressive declines in fertility, which resulted in the same annual number of births in 2008 as in 1990. The maternal mortality ratio decreased by more than half (54%), resulting in nearly a 50% decrease in the number of maternal deaths. Their analyses underscore the critical role that family planning programmes play in complementing maternal health interventions designed to reduce the risk of death in women who are already pregnant.

Causes and Timing of Maternal Death

Data from both high and low income countries show convincingly that the greatest risk of maternal death occurs near the time of delivery, with decreasing risk throughout the first week after delivery. The distribution of the timing of death does vary somewhat from country to country but this is primarily due to differences in level of abortion-related mortality earlier in pregnancy. Although the postpartum period is defined as 42 days following the termination of pregnancy, there is evidence that the risk of death is increased for 6 months postpartum (Ronsmans and Graham, 2006). Deaths beyond the postpartum period would only be accounted for when using the late maternal death definition.

Within the period from conception through to 42 days postpartum, the causes of maternal death are divided into two causal categories. Direct causes of death are those resulting specifically from pregnancy and childbirth. The leading direct causes of maternal death include: haemorrhage, hypertensive diseases of pregnancy (pre-eclampsia and eclampsia), pregnancy-related sepsis and obstructed labour. Unsafe abortion is often included as a cause of maternal death although deaths from unsafe abortion are predominantly from haemorrhage and/or sepsis. This is done for programmatic purposes since interventions to address unsafe abortion do

not differ greatly from the obstetric interventions required for the other four main direct causes of death. Indirect causes of death are due to complications of medical conditions, which may occur whether or not the mother is pregnant, and which are exacerbated by the pregnant state. Common indirect causes of maternal death include malaria, anaemia, hepatitis, HIV and cardiac and renal disease. Preparations for the 11th Revision of the International Classification of Diseases were underway at the time of the writing of this chapter and are to be published in 2015 (WHO, 2011). It is anticipated that substantial changes will be made to the classification of maternal deaths (Pattinson et al., 2009); thus readers are encouraged to seek the most up-to-date information.

The best information available on the distribution of causes of maternal death globally results from a systematic review of the literature by Khan et al. (2006), as even countries with empirical data on the maternal mortality ratio may well lack detailed data on medical causes of maternal death. Plate 3 summarizes data on cause of maternal death in four world regions.

The distribution of causes is fairly similar between Africa and Asia, which together contribute approximately 97% of global maternal deaths. Haemorrhage is the leading cause of maternal death, representing more than 30% of deaths in both regions. Haemorrhage subsumes bleeding during pregnancy (antepartum haemorrhage from ectopic pregnancy or induced or spontaneous abortion), during birth (intrapartum bleeding from placenta praevia or placenta abruption) and postpartum bleeding (due to uterine atony, retained placenta, genital tract lacerations or inverted uterus). Data in this review were insufficient to identify proportions from each, though it is generally accepted that the majority of cases of haemorrhage occur during the immediate postpartum period and are due to uterine atony (failure of the uterine muscles to contract adequately to stop bleeding after delivery). Other indirect causes (particularly malaria), hypertensive disease of pregnancy and sepsis are leading causes in Africa and Asia. Key differences in the distributions between

Africa and Asia are the greater proportion of maternal deaths attributed to anaemia in Asia and HIV in Africa. In Latin America and the Caribbean, hypertensive disease of pregnancy is the leading cause of maternal death (26%), followed by obstructed labour and unsafe abortion at 12% and 13%, respectively. In all three developing country regions, the direct causes of maternal deaths account for at least 60% of all maternal deaths. The distribution of causes of maternal death in the developed world differs markedly from developing country regions: the leading cause of maternal death being 'other direct causes', which includes deaths from anaesthesia and Caesarean section. Hypertensive disease of pregnancy and embolism are the second and third leading causes of maternal death in industrialized countries.

Conclusion

Our need for global maternal mortality estimates is a reality that cannot be circumvented. Given the paucity of empirical, population-based maternal mortality data, particularly in high mortality settings, maternal mortality could not be on the international agenda without some global quantification of the problem. At the same time, model-based estimates or adjusted national estimates may undermine ownership of maternal mortality data at the national level and lead to confusion and frustration at national and international levels. Until the necessary investment is made to produce high quality, reliable, population-based data on maternal mortality in lower and middle income countries, global estimates of the levels, causes and distribution of maternal mortality will continue to be required.

References

Boerma, J.T., Mathers, C. and Abou-Zahr, C. (2010) WHO and global health monitoring: the way forward. *PLoS Medicine* 7(11), e1000373.

Byass, P. (2010) The imperfect world of global health estimates. *PLoS Medicine* 7(11), e1001006.

Chandramohan, D., Rodrigues, L.C., Maude, G.H. and Hayes, R.J. (1998) The validity of verbal autopsies for assessing the causes of institutional maternal death. *Studies in Family Planning* 29(4), 414–422.

Graham, W.J. and Adjei, S. (2010) A call for responsible estimation of global health. *PLoS Medicine* 7(11), e1001003.

Graham, W.J., Ahmed, S., Stanton, C., AbouZahr, C. and Campbell, O. (2008) Measuring maternal mortality: an overview of opportunities and options for developing countries. *BMC Medicine* 6(12).

Hill, K., Thomas, K., AbouZahr, C., Walker, N., Say, L., Inoue, M. and Suzuki, E. (2007) Estimates of maternal mortality worldwide between 1990 and 2005: an assessment of available data. *Lancet* 370(9595), 1311–1319.

Hogan, M.C., Foreman, K.J., Naghavi, M., Ahn, S.Y., Wang, J., Makela, S.M., Lopez, A.D., Lozano, R. and Murray, C.J.L. (2010) Maternal mortality for 181 countries, 1980-2008: a systematic analysis of progress towards millennium development goal 5. *Lancet* 375(9726), 1609–1623.

Khan, K.S., Wojdyla, D., Say, L., Gulmezoglu, A.M. and Van Look, P.F. (2006) WHO analysis of causes of maternal death: a systematic review. *Lancet* 367(9516), 1066–1074.

Macro International (2009) MEASURE DHS STATcompiler. Available at: http://www.measuredhs.com (accessed 26 July 2011).

Mathers, C.D., Ma Fat, D., Inoue, M., Chalapati, R., Lopez, M., Chalapati, R. and Lopez, A. (2005) Counting the dead and what they died from: an assessment of the global status of cause of death data. *Bulletin of the World Health Organization* 83(3), 171–177.

Murray, C.J. and Lopez, A.D. (2010) Production and analysis of health indicators: the role of academia. *PLoS Medicine* 7(11), e1001004.

Pattinson, R., Say, L., Souza, J.P., van den Broek, N. and Rooney, C. on behalf of the Working Group on Maternal Mortality and Morbidity Classifications (2009) WHO maternal death and near-miss classifications (editorial). *Bulletin of the World Health Organization* 87, 734.

Ronsmans, C. and Graham, W.J. on behalf of The Lancet Maternal Survival Series steering group (2006) Maternal mortality: who, when, where, and why. *Lancet* 368(9542), 1189–1200.

Ross, J.A. and Blanc, A.K. (2012) Why aren't there more maternal deaths? A decomposition analysis. *Maternal and Child Health Journal* 16(2): 456–63.

Rutenberg, N. and Sullivan, J. (1991) Direct and indirect estimates of maternal mortality from the sisterhood method. In: *Proceedings of the Demographic and Health Surveys World Conference*. Macro International Inc., Maryland, 1669–1696.

Sankoh, O. (2010) Global health estimates: stronger collaboration needed with low- and middle-income Countries. *PLoS Medicine* 7(11), e1001005.

Shibuya, K., Scheele, S. and Boerma, T. (2005) Health Statistics: Time to Get Serious. *Bulletin of the World Health Organization* 83(10), 722.

UN (2010) *Millennium Development Goals*. Available at: http://www.un.org/millenniumgoals (accessed 26 July 2011).

WHO (1994) *International Classification of Diseases and Related Health Problems*; 10th Revision, Vol. 2, 2nd edn. WHO, Geneva, pp. 139–141.

WHO (2001) *Maternal Mortality in 1995: Estimates Developed by WHO, UNICEF, UNFPA*. WHO, Geneva.

WHO (2011) The International Classification of Diseases, 11th Revision. Available at: http://www.who.int/classifications/icd/revision/en (accessed 30 June 2011).

WHO and UNICEF (1996) *Revised 1990 Estimates of Maternal Mortality: A New Approach by WHO and UNICEF*. WHO, Geneva.

WHO, UNICEF and UNFPA (2004) *Maternal Mortality in 2000: Estimates Developed by WHO, UNICEF and UNFPA*. WHO, Geneva.

WHO, UNICEF, UNFPA and World Bank (2007) *Maternal Mortality in 2005; Estimates Developed by WHO, UNICEF, UNFPA and the World Bank*. WHO, Geneva.

WHO, UNICEF, UNFPA and World Bank (2010) *Trends in Maternal Mortality: 1990–2008, Estimates Developed by WHO, UNICEF, UNFPA and the World Bank*. WHO, Geneva.

Wilmoth, J. (2009) The lifetime risk of maternal mortality: concept and measurement. *Bulletin of the World Health Organization* 87(4), 256–262.

5 The Epidemiology of Stillbirths and Neonatal Deaths

Cynthia Stanton[1] and Joy E. Lawn[2]

[1]*Johns Hopkins Bloomberg School of Public Health, Baltimore, USA;*
[2]*Save the Children, Cape Town, South Africa*

Summary

- Six million babies die each year either as late fetal deaths in the last trimester or the first month of life (neonatal deaths); 98% occur in developing countries and 75% in sub-Saharan Africa and South Asia, which is also where 87% of global maternal deaths occur.
- Between 1995 and 2008, stillbirths and neonatal deaths have decreased by 14.5% and 28.0%, respectively, mostly in East Asia. Unlike child deaths, there are no international goals for reducing stillbirths, making these 2.6 million deaths practically invisible to the international community.
- The term 'perinatal' is used to refer to outcomes that occur before or soon after the time of birth, so includes the unborn fetus and the newborn. Due to multiple definitions for the perinatal period, the term is unsuitable for epidemiological use, but for programmatic purposes it is helpful to consider stillbirths and early neonatal deaths jointly because many of the interventions to improve these outcomes are similar or related.
- While data on the causes of newborn deaths are widely available (leading causes: preterm birth, birth asphyxia, sepsis, pneumonia) the causes of stillbirth are less well documented. There is not even international consensus on how to document and report the causes of these deaths. At minimum, the timing of these deaths should be routinely reported (antepartum or before labour and intrapartum or during labour).
- Improved identification and management of infections such as syphilis, pregnancy complications, intrapartum care, antepartum steroid administration where preterm birth is inevitable, judicious use of Caesarean section where indicated, training in neonatal resuscitation, Kangaroo care, and early identification and treatment of respiratory infections have all been proven effective in improving perinatal survival.
- Improving the data for all outcomes around the time of birth – maternal and neonatal mortality and morbidity – and using these data for action in programmes is a fundamental challenge for progress towards the MDGs and beyond.

Introduction

This chapter provides an overview of the epidemiology of stillbirths and neonatal deaths, which have traditionally been grouped as perinatal mortality. The focus is on low income countries, where 98% of these deaths occur. We discuss the definitional issue embedded in the term 'perinatal' and its components. We also present analyses to estimate the number and rates of stillbirths and the most recent data on neonatal deaths. A brief overview of evidence-based interventions known to effectively reduce fetal and newborn deaths in developing countries is presented.

In the year 2009, there were an estimated 2.6 million stillbirths (Cousens *et al.*, 2011) and 3.3 million neonatal deaths (Oestergaard *et al.*, 2011) globally. These deaths are closely linked to maternal mortality and morbidity. An understanding of their epidemiology in terms of geography, timing and underlying conditions is critical to reducing this burden and maximizing returns on investments in care at the time of birth.

Definitions, Indicators and Measurement

Definitions

The term 'perinatal mortality' refers in general to deaths that occur to the fetus (stillbirths) or to the newborn infant (early or late neonatal deaths); in other words, deaths that occur before or soon after the time of birth. However, there are a variety of time periods included in the term 'perinatal', depending on the definitions used and the potential for fetal survival outside the womb, which is also influenced by the availability of means for advanced resuscitation, for example in developed countries. Consequently, stillbirths may be defined as fetal deaths occurring at 18, 20, 22, 23, 24 or 28 weeks of gestation. The neonatal component may include only early neonatal deaths (1–7 days) or all neonatal deaths (1–28 days) (Lawn *et al.*, 2011) (Plate 4). Epidemiologists now prefer the use of the two specific terms, stillbirths and neonatal deaths, rather than 'perinatal' deaths, due to these multiple definitions for the perinatal period (Kramer *et al.*, 1999).

Stillbirth is a colloquial term which refers more specifically to early and late fetal deaths. According to the *International Classificaton of Diseases* ICD 10, a *fetal death* is:

> a death prior to the complete expulsion or extraction from its mother of a product of conception, irrespective of the duration of

pregnancy; the death is indicated by the fact that after such separation the fetus does not breathe or show any other evidence of life, such as beating of the heart, pulsation of the umbilical cord or definite movement of voluntary muscles.

Early fetal deaths are defined by the ICD 10 as 'death to a fetus weighing at least 500 grams or if birth weight is unavailable, after 22 completed weeks gestation, or a crown-heel length of 25 centimeters or more'. A *late fetal death* is defined using the following parameters: 1000 g or more birth weight; or 28 weeks or more gestation; or a crown–heel length of 35 cm or more (WHO, 1993) (Plate 4).

For the purposes of international comparison, WHO recommends that stillbirths be defined as a late fetal death; that is '1000 grams or more birth weight; or 28 weeks or more gestation' (WHO, 1993). However, it is recognized that other definitions may be used within countries. High income settings, with increased likelihood of neonatal viability thanks to sophisticated intensive care, may define a stillbirth as a fetal loss from as early as 20 weeks gestation. In countries where neonatal intensive care is lacking, the survival of a fetus of less than 28–30 weeks is unlikely (Lawn *et al.*, 2011). In addition, the quality of stillbirth and neonatal death data differs, with fewer nationally reliable data for stillbirths. Thus, by combining the two outcomes under the term 'perinatal', these differences and the specific steps required to improve data capture of both outcomes may be masked (Lawn *et al.*, 2010). Hence, for epidemiologic reporting, it is preferable to record and report stillbirths separately from early neonatal deaths (Kramer *et al.*, 1999). For programmatic purposes, it is helpful to consider stillbirths and early neonatal deaths jointly because many of the interventions to improve these outcomes are similar or related. For this same reason, perinatal death data should also be linked to data on maternal outcomes.

Antepartum (or macerated) versus *intrapartum* (or fresh) stillbirths are further distinctions with very important programmatic implications. An intrapartum stillbirth describes a fetal death that is thought to have occurred within approximately 12 h before delivery or roughly after the onset of labour. Antepartum stillbirths are those that died more than 12 h before delivery or before the onset of labour. The distinction is determined based on physical characteristics of the fetal body and whether the fetal heart or other signs of life were present during labour. For example, peeling skin, a darkened umbilical cord and skull softening are signs of maceration associated with the deterioration that accompanies an antepartum fetal death. Intrapartum stillbirths are generally considered to be an indicator of the quality of or access to obstetric care. Antepartum stillbirths are considered to be an indicator of the quality of care during pregnancy and of fetal growth (Lawn *et al.*, 2009a). Plate 4 illustrates the definitional cut points.

Indicators of stillbirth and neonatal death

The indicators of stillbirth and early neonatal death are relatively straightforward once the definitional issues are specified. A stillbirth rate is the number of stillbirths divided by the number of all births (the sum of stillbirths and live births), and is expressed per 1000 total births:

$$SBR = \frac{\text{Number of}\ \text{stillbirths}}{\text{Number of stillbirths}\ \text{and live births}} \times 1000$$

(5.1)

The early neonatal mortality rate is simply the number of deaths within the first 7 days of life among live-born infants divided by the number of live births, and is expressed per 1000 live births.

$$ENMR = \frac{\text{Number of early}\ \text{neonatal deaths}}{\text{Number of}\ \text{live births}} \times 1000$$

(5.2)

The intrapartum case fatality rate is a health facility-based indicator intended to measure

the quality of obstetric care from the perspective of the fetus and neonate, independent of the mortality risks associated with very small size at birth. It examines the number of intrapartum stillbirths with a birth weight of 2.5 kg or more, plus the number of very early neonatal deaths (defined as live born infants weighing at least 2.5 kg who die within the first 24 h of life), divided by the number of all births (all stillbirths, late fetal deaths and live births). The numerator is confined to large infants at low risk of dying but who succumb to complications of labour and delivery eminently amenable to obstetric intervention. This indicator can be used in an individual health facility or aggregated across a number of health facilities (Fauveau, 2007). At the time of writing this chapter, this indicator is being refined and in the future will probably include weight cut-offs for the fetus and live-born infant and time cut-offs for very early neonatal deaths (24 versus 48 h).

$$IPCFR = \frac{\begin{array}{c}\text{Number of}\\ \text{intrapartum stillbirths}\\ + \text{very early}\\ \text{neonatal deaths}\end{array}}{\begin{array}{c}\text{Number of}\\ \text{all births}\end{array}} \times 1000$$

(5.3)

Measurement issues related to stillbirth and neonatal mortality

Where available and useable, mortality data from vital registration in developing countries report on under-5 and infant (first year of life) deaths and neonatal deaths, but less frequently report on early neonatal deaths. Nationally representative stillbirth data are available from some middle income countries, but are limited in high mortality settings in sub-Saharan Africa and South Asia, where 98% of stillbirths occur. For example, a systematic review of the literature on stillbirth rates by Cousens *et al.* (2011) identified only one country in these two regions – Mauritius – with a national stillbirth rate based on vital registration with adequate coverage (Lawn *et al.*, 2011).

Consequently, the large majority of national estimates of stillbirth, neonatal and under-5 child mortality in low income countries comes from demographic and health surveys (see Stanton and McCaw-Binns, Chapter 4 this volume). Data pertaining to live births are an important focus of these surveys, so neonatal mortality rates are available from every survey going back to 1985. In contrast, pregnancy loss and gestational duration of each pregnancy (the data components required to identify still-births in the absence of birth weight) have been collected in a subset of only about 50 surveys (Macro International, 2009). In these household surveys, it is necessary to rely on pregnancy loss and gestational age data to define stillbirths, as approximately 40–45% of births in low income countries occur at home (Macro International, 2009) and the babies are therefore not weighed. Furthermore, even among health facility births, it is not uncommon for babies not to be weighed or for the weight not to be recorded (Lawn *et al.*, 2010), especially if stillborn and macerated at birth.

Other sources of stillbirth data include health facility data (which, in settings with high institutional birth rates, may be very useful for programme planning), demographic surveillance sites, special studies and from high and selected middle income countries' vital registration systems. Misclassification of stillbirths and early neonatal deaths is common in vital registration data, even in high income countries, due to the challenges of establishing vital status at birth, as well as a number of cultural and certification practices that lead to over- or under-reporting of these outcomes. Misclassification is even more common in survey and health facility-based data in low income countries due to the difficulty in determining signs of life at birth, particularly where the mother is the respondent and yet may not be shown the baby in cases of stillbirth or death shortly after birth. Live-born infants who die very soon after birth may be recorded as stillbirths. It is also likely that perinatal deaths go completely unreported, where the pregnancy, stillbirth, live birth or subsequent early death is never reported at all.

Although demographic and health surveys provide the majority of available nationally representative data on stillbirth and early neonatal death, there is a clear need for additional methodological research to improve survey-based data collection for both outcomes. Two simple data quality assessments illustrate this point (Box 5.1 and Box 5.2).

Magnitude, Trends and Geographical Distribution of Stillbirths and Neonatal Deaths

Global data on stillbirth in low income countries are sparse relative to infant and child mortality data and even to maternal mortality. As late as 2005, very few national or international estimates of perinatal mortality or its components existed for many developing countries. Two publications by WHO provided perinatal mortality estimates for 1983 and 1995 (WHO, 1996). In 1983, WHO estimated the perinatal mortality rate at 64 per 1000 births for developing countries and 17 per 1000 births for developed countries. For 1995, these estimates were 57 for developing countries and 11 per 1000 births for developed countries. The 1995 report also estimated developing country stillbirth and early neonatal mortality rates of 32 and 26 per 1000 births, respectively. In 1995, the global totals for stillbirths and early neonatal deaths were 4.3 and 3.4 million respectively, with 97% of such events occurring in developing countries. These early exercises to estimate perinatal mortality suggested that approximately two-thirds of neonatal deaths occurred during the early neonatal period in developing countries while four-fifths of neonatal deaths occurred during the early neonatal period in developed countries (WHO, 1996). As infant mortality rates decline, increasing proportions of infant deaths will occur in the neonatal period because neonatal deaths are less susceptible to public health interventions such as immunization compared to infant deaths in the post-neonatal period (1–11 months of age).

Box 5.1. Ratio of stillbirth to early neonatal mortality rate as a marker of quality of stillbirth data.

A WHO review of historical vital registration data between 1900 and 1950 from Europe, the USA, Hong Kong, Japan, Singapore, Mexico and Chile was undertaken to assess the relationship between third-trimester stillbirth and early neonatal death rates. This period was selected because the early neonatal mortality rates in these countries at the time were similar to those seen in high mortality countries today. These historical data produced a median ratio of the stillbirth to early neonatal death of 1.2 for early neonatal mortality rates of 20–24 per 1000 births (WHO, 2006). This ratio can be used to assess data quality of reporting of events around birth. Figure 5.1 shows the ratio of the stillbirth rate to the early neonatal mortality rate for 50 demographic and health surveys from 41 countries (Macro International, 2010).

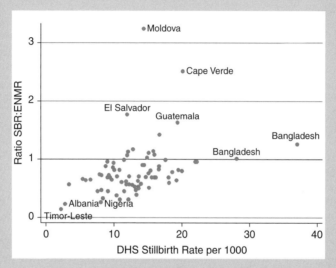

Fig. 5.1. Ratios of stillbirth to early neonatal mortality rate, by stillbirth rate for 50 countries. Demographic and Health Surveys (DHS) (Macro International, 2011).

The figure shows that the median ratio across demographic and health survey estimates is 0.76, with 20% of the sample below 0.50. Of these ratios, 96% are less than 1.2. In contrast, the observation from Moldova stands out as an extreme outlier with a ratio of 3.2. This comparison also assumes that the early neonatal death rates are valid, whereas the data in Fig. 5.2 (see below) suggest serious under-reporting of early neonatal deaths and even further under-reporting of stillbirths. Methodological research into the measurement of vital events at birth warrants increased attention, given that national and international programmes are likely to need to rely on survey-based mortality indicators for a number of years into the future.

Magnitude and trends in stillbirth rates

Although a literature review of stillbirth data was published in 2006 (Say *et al.*, 2006), up to that point no organization had reported regional or country-specific rates and numbers of stillbirths. Stillbirths were simply invisible. From the 1970s onward, tremendous attention was paid to interventions to reduce infant and child mortality, most of which occurred during the post-neonatal and childhood (1 through 4 years) periods. Consequently, there was great interest in monitoring change in infant and child mortality. Indeed, until the mid to late 1990s very little attention was paid to the distribution of infant deaths and the fact that approximately 35–40% of deaths of children under 5 occurred during the first 28 days of life and 30% occurred during the first week of life.

Box 5.2. Index of heaping for age at death as a marker of quality of neonatal mortality data.

In demographic and health surveys, women are asked the age of death for live-born children who died. Age at death is reported in days for deaths at less than 1 month, in months for deaths from 1 to 23 months and in years for deaths at age 2 or more. Heaping (the tendency to report common numeric responses) on day 7 would result in under counting of early neonatal deaths. The heaping index shown in Fig. 5.2 is the mean of responses for age at death at day 6 and day 8, divided by the number of responses for day 7.

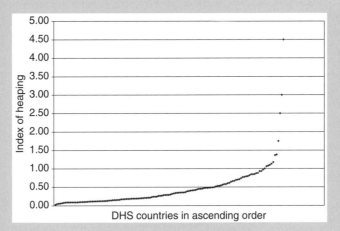

Fig. 5.2. Index of heaping for reporting age at death at day 7; 136 DHS surveys (Hill and Choi, 2006).

An index of one represents no heaping. Heaping on day 7 is severe in the reporting of age at death in many surveys. The mean and median heaping index is 0.30 and 0.47, respectively, for these 136 DHS surveys (Hill and Choi, 2006). This suggests that early neonatal mortality rates that are not adjusted for such heaping are likely to be seriously underestimated.

The general impression previously was that little could be done to avert stillbirths or save very ill babies (Shiffman, 2010; Froen *et al.*, 2011; Lawn *et al.*, 2011).

Similar to the situation with global maternal mortality estimates (see Stanton and McCaw-Binns, Chapter 4 this volume), in 2006, two sets of estimates of 2000 global, regional and country-specific stillbirth rates were published (Stanton *et al.*, 2006; WHO, 2006). These two global estimates, generated using different approaches, resulted in remarkably similar global totals: 3.2 and 3.3 million stillbirths annually, with stillbirth rates for developed and developing countries ranging from 5 to 6 and 25 to 26 per 1000 births, respectively. Like the 2008 maternal mortality estimates, there was substantial variation in the estimates for individual countries.

In 2011, a collaborative effort between WHO, academic institutions and the non-governmental agency Save the Children/Saving Newborn Lives resulted in a global series of estimates for 2009, with trend data from 1995 to 2009. The 2009 estimate of the global number of stillbirths was 2.64 million, with a global stillbirth rate of 18.9 per 1000 births (Cousens *et al.*, 2011). According to this analysis, whereas 87% of global maternal deaths are in sub-Saharan African and South Asian countries (WHO *et al.*, 2010), three-quarters of stillbirths originate from these countries. The trend analysis suggested a 14.5% decrease in the global stillbirth rate since 1995, with reductions in every world region. East Asia, predominated by China, nearly halved (48%) their stillbirth rate between 1995 and 2009. Oceania and sub-Saharan Africa showed the smallest reductions at 8 and 8.7%, respectively (Table 5.1). Ten

Table 5.1. Estimated stillbirth rates and numbers of stillbirths for 1995 and 2009 by region (Cousens et al., 2011).

World region	1995		2009		Change in the stillbirth rate from 1995 to 2009 (%)
	Stillbirth rate per 1000 births	Number of stillbirths	Stillbirth rate per 1000 births	Number of stillbirths	
World	22.1	3,031,300	18.9	2,642,000	−14.5
High income countries	3.9	45,800	3.1	36,400	−20.3
Eurasia (CIS in Europe)	10.9	22,800	9.0	19,700	−17.6
Eurasia (CIS in Asia)	10.5	17,900	8.8	13,800	−16.0
East Asia	18.5	414,300	9.7	188,500	−47.5
South Asia	30.2	1,248,400	26.7	1,080,300	−11.7
Southeast Asia	16.8	198,500	13.9	156,100	−17.1
West Asia	14.9	68,500	12.0	60,200	−19.2
Latin America and the Caribbean	12.1	141,900	8.7	97,100	−28.0
North Africa	17.7	61,800	13.6	51,300	−22.9
Sub-Saharan Africa	31.0	807,600	28.3	934,600	−8.7
Oceania	15.8	3,700	14.5	3,900	−8.0

highly populous countries account for two-thirds of global stillbirths. These are: India, Nigeria, Pakistan, China, Bangladesh, the Democratic Republic of the Congo, Ethiopia, Indonesia, Tanzania and Afghanistan (Table 5.2). The top five of these countries account for more than half of all stillbirths, maternal deaths and neonatal deaths. Increased attention to survival and health around the time of birth in these countries is clearly required to achieve global goals for these related outcomes (Lawn et al., 2011).

Cause of death in stillbirth

There are no global estimates of the distribution of causes of stillbirth. In contrast, information on neonatal causes of death has been estimated since 2005 by country, is published widely and is routinely updated by the Child Health Epidemiology Reference Group (CHERG) of the United Nations. National data profiles have been disseminated by Countdown to 2015 (Lawn et al., 2006; Black et al., 2010). Such data have focused attention

on the three leading causes of neonatal death (infections, intrapartum-related causes and preterm birth complications), which permits focused programmatic responses (Lawn et al., 2011).

Thirty-five different classification systems for cause of death in stillbirths have been identified in the literature (Reddy et al., 2009). Lack of comparability between these classification systems greatly limits their interpretation. The number of causes identified in these systems ranges from 6 to 37. Most of these systems reflect data from high income countries with fetal surveillance and sophisticated diagnostic testing, offering little to our understanding of the 98% of stillbirths that occur in developing countries. Data from a broader array of countries are available on time of fetal death, that is, antepartum and intrapartum stillbirths.

Recent estimates with wide uncertainty levels suggest that 30–56% of stillbirths in high mortality regions are intrapartum, occurring after the onset of labour (Lawn et al., 2011). Globally, the major cause of intrapartum stillbirth is fetal hypoxia. Other less

Table 5.2. Top ten countries accounting for the majority of the absolute numbers of stillbirths (66%), maternal deaths (62%) and neonatal deaths (67%) (Lawn et al., 2011).

Country	Rank for number of stillbirths	Rank for number of maternal deaths	Rank for number of neonatal deaths
India	1	1	1
Nigeria	2	2	2
Pakistan	3	7	3
China	4	12	4
Bangladesh	5	8	7
Democratic Republic of Congo	6	3	5
Ethiopia	7	5	6
Indonesia	8	9	8
Tanzania	9	6	10
Afghanistan	10	4	9

common causes include preterm labour, intrapartum infections and congenital abnormalities (Lawn et al., 2009a).

Common causes of antepartum stillbirth include maternal conditions such as infection (particularly, syphilis), hypertension, diabetes and antepartum haemorrhage. Congenital abnormalities are often assumed to be a major cause, but data suggest only 1–11% are attributed to this causal group, noting that diagnosis in low income settings may underestimate significant abnormalities such as congenital heart disease. Even in high income countries and in hospital-based studies, 30% or more of stillbirths, more so antepartum stillbirths, are often categorized as 'unexplained', limiting interpretation of the remaining distribution of causes. This is also very distressing for families who have experienced a loss for which the cause cannot be explained (Froen et al., 2011).

The Lancet stillbirth series team (Lawn et al., 2011) suggest that, in order to better understand why stillbirths occur, a classification system is needed that identifies causes of stillbirth with programmatic relevance and along with data on related maternal conditions, both of which can be identified via clinical observation or verbal autopsy. The development, acceptance and promotion of such a system will require consensus from a broad array of partners, such as UN agencies, programmes supporting large scale data collection, academics and non-government and advocacy organizations.

For illustrative purposes, stillbirth verbal autopsy (a means of collecting data on deaths through interviews, see Stanton and McCaw-Binns, Chapter 4 this volume) cause of death data from three data sources are provided in Table 5.3. These include a verbal autopsy module added to the demographic and health survey in Pakistan (2006–2007), verbal autopsy data reported by women who delivered in hospital in Chandigarh, India (2006–2008) and verbal autopsy data from women residing in a demographic surveillance site in Kintampo, Ghana (2003–2004). The results underscore the lack of comparability even between datasets using verbal autopsy and highlight the large proportion of deaths that are unexplained.

Magnitude, trends and causes of neonatal death

The increased recognition that the two-thirds reduction in child mortality of MDG 4 will not be achieved without substantial reductions in neonatal death has greatly increased attention on preventing newborn deaths (Lawn et al., 2005). There are two sets of national estimates of neonatal mortality rates, one by WHO and the Child Health Epidemiology Reference Group (Oestergaard et al., 2011) and one by the Institute for Health Metrics and Evaluation as part of an assessment of progress for under-5 deaths (Rajaratnam et al., 2010).

Rajaratum and colleagues (2010) estimate the number of global neonatal deaths at 3.1 million in 2010 and report annual declines in neonatal deaths at 2.1% between 1990 and 2010. Their data suggest an accelerating pace of decline in 13 of 21 world regions. In the WHO series, the global neonatal mortality rate fell from 33.2 in 1990 to 23.9 per 1000 live births with a global total of 3.3 million deaths in 2009. The average annual rate of reduction of the neonatal mortality rate is 1.7%

Table 5.3. Distribution of verbal autopsy cause of death data for stillbirths from three data sources, illustrating lack of comparability.

Pakistan; 2006–2007 Stillbirth cause of death (Bhutta *et al.*, 2008)		Chandigarh, India; 2006–2008 Stillbirth cause of death (Aggarwal *et al.*, 2011)		Kintampo, Ghana; 2003–2004 Stillbirth cause of death (Edmond *et al.*, 2008)	
Cause of death categories	Prevalence (%)	Cause of death categories	Prevalence (%)	Cause of death categories	Prevalence (%)
Antepartum stillbirths					
Congenital abnormalities	5	Congenital malformations	13.8	Congenital abnormalities	1.7
Antepartum maternal disorders	19	Underlying maternal condition	8.4	Maternal disease	14.0
		Pregnancy-induced hypertension	25.3		
		Antepartum haemorrhage	16.9	Maternal hemorrhage	4.1
		Obstetric complications	9.3		
		Multiple pregnancy	3.1		
Antepartum unexplained	33			Unexplained	57.4
				Other	22.8
Intrapartum stillbirths					
Intrapartum asphyxia	21	Asphyxia not explained by maternal condition	4.9		
		Other specific fetal problem	0.0	Congenital abnormalities	0.8
		Unexplained preterm stillbirth (<37weeks)	5.7	Obstetric complications	59.3
		Unexplained small size for gestational age	4.4	Maternal hemorrhage	4.8
Intrapartum unexplained	21	Unexplained stillbirth	8.0	Unexplained	31.5
Unclassified	1			Other	3.6

(Table 5.4), compared to 2.3% for maternal mortality rate reduction and 2.1% for under-5 mortality rate reduction (Oestergaard *et al.*, 2011). The data also show that the sub-Saharan African region is being left further and further behind in progress for reducing neonatal deaths, both because of slow progress in reducing risk (the average annual rate of reduction in sub-Saharan Africa is less than 1% per year) and because the birth rate remains very high. Increasing access to and use of contraception to prevent unwanted pregnancy remains underemphasized as a highly cost-effective approach to reducing maternal and neonatal deaths as well as stillbirths.

Both series of estimates highlight the fact that neonatal deaths constitute approximately

Table 5.4. Neonatal mortality trends 1990–2009 globally and by WHO region (Oestergaard *et al.*, 2011).

Region	Neonatal mortality rate per 1000 births	1990	1995	2000	2005	2009	Percentage change 1990–2009 (annual)
Global	Neonatal mortality rate	33.2	32.0	29.4	26.3	23.9	−28.0 (−1.7)
	Deaths in 1000s (% of global)	4574 (100)	4296 (100)	3913 (100)	3536 (100)	3265 (100)	−28.6
High-income	Neonatal mortality rate	6.0	4.9	4.2	3.9	3.6	−40.3 (−2.7)
	Deaths in 1000s (% of global)	79 (1.7)	63 (1.5)	52 (1.3)	48 (1.4)	45 (1.4)	−42.7
Africa[a]	Neonatal mortality rate	43.6	43.0	41.1	38.3	35.9	−17.6 (−1.0)
	Deaths in 1000s (% of global)	971 (21.2)	1047 (24.4)	1094 (27.9)	1119 (31.6)	1114 (34.1)	14.7
Americas[a]	Neonatal mortality rate	22.0	19.0	15.8	13.1	11.4	−48.3 (−3.4)
	Deaths in 1000s (% of global)	255 (5.6)	220 (5.1)	181 (4.6)	145 (4.1)	121 (3.7)	−52.7
Eastern Mediterranean[a]	Neonatal mortality rate	41.3	39.1	36.3	33.2	31.1	−24.6 (−1.5)
	Deaths in 1000s (% of global)	565 (12.4)	530 (12.3)	506 (12.9)	490 (13.9)	481 (14.7)	−14.9
Europe[a]	Neonatal mortality rate	21.0	20.1	17.0	13.2	10.7	−49.2 (−3.5)
	Deaths in 1000s (% of global)	148 (3.2)	118 (2.8)	90 (2.3)	72 (2.0)	60 (1.8)	−59.6
South-east Asia[a]	Neonatal mortality rate	46.9	43.6	39.2	34.2	30.7	−34.6 (−2.2)
	Deaths in 1000s (% of global)	1860 (40.7)	1738 (40.5)	1549 (39.6)	1326 (37.5)	1161 (35.6)	−37.6
Western Pacific[a]	Neonatal mortality rate	22.9	22.1	18.6	14.6	12.0	−47.5 (−3.3)
	Deaths in 1000s (% of global)	694 (15.2)	580 (13.5)	442 (11.3)	336 (9.5)	283 (8.7)	−59.3

[a]Includes only low and middle income countries

41% of under-5-year-old child deaths. Historical data suggest that as neonatal mortality falls the proportion of deaths occurring in the first week of life increases. Globally, it is estimated that approximately up to 50% of all neonatal deaths occur on the first day of life (Lawn et al., 2005). However, there are no recent estimates, using comparable methods, of early neonatal mortality rates or early neonatal causes of death. Based on these data, a conservative assumption that three-quarters of neonatal deaths occur in the first week of life would suggest that approximately 2.3 to 2.7 million early neonatal deaths occurred annually between 2008 and 2010.

Estimates of global, regional and country-specific neonatal cause of death data are available and widely disseminated (Lawn et al., 2011). The global distribution of neonatal causes of death for 2008 is shown in Fig. 5.3, with complications from preterm birth (29%), birth asphyxia (23%), sepsis (15%) and pneumonia (11%) as leading causes (Black et al., 2010).

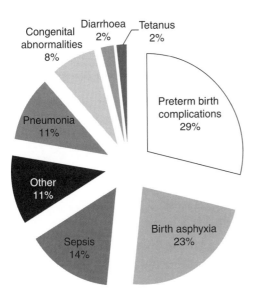

Fig. 5.3. Estimated distribution of the causes of death within the neonatal period for 192 countries in the year 2008 (Black et al., 2010).

Preventing fetal and neonatal deaths

Given the timing of onset of symptoms and death, complications from preterm birth and birth asphyxia predominate as causes of death during the early neonatal period with increased proportions from infections (pneumonia, tetanus, meningitis and diarrhoea) occurring in the late neonatal period. It has also been shown that the distribution of causes of neonatal death varies markedly by level of neonatal mortality. Proportions of neonatal deaths due to prematurity and congenital abnormalities increase as neonatal mortality decreases. Likewise, proportions of sepsis/pneumonia and tetanus decrease with decreasing neonatal mortality (Lawn et al., 2005).

Clinical obstetric interventions effective in saving mothers' lives are described in Langer et al., Chapter 8 this volume. Many of these – infection control, management of the hypertensive disorders of pregnancy, use of the partograph to prevent obstructed labour – will also prevent late fetal and early newborn deaths by reducing intrapartum complications that put the fetus and newborn at risk.

Some specific interventions can prevent fetal and early neonatal deaths. Where preterm birth is indicated either to save the mother's life or in the event of precipitate preterm delivery, antenatal corticosteroids have helped accelerate fetal lung maturity and reduce respiratory conditions, which contribute to many deaths in preterm infants (Peltoniemi et al, 2011). A review of the efficacy of neonatal resuscitation training to reduce term intrapartum-related deaths has been conducted. It suggests that in countries where most neonatal deaths occur such training would save newborn lives, although further evaluation is required for impact, cost and implementation strategies in various contexts (Lee et al., 2011).

Survival of very small babies in low income settings is improved by Kangaroo mother care. This technique consists of establishing skin-to-skin contact between a mother and her newborn to reduce hypothermia and enable frequent and exclusive or nearly exclusive breastfeeding, coupled with early discharge from hospital, as an alternative to conventional neonatal care for low birth weight infants. A review of Kangaroo care showed decreased mortality and severe infection but Kangaroo care was also associated with improving selected measures of infant growth, breastfeeding and mother–infant bonding (Conde-Agudelo *et al.*, 2011).

Conclusion

In total, almost 6 million babies died in 2009, either in the last trimester of pregnancy or in the first month of life. The losses are very real to the women and families affected, but have low visibility in programmes and policy – for example, there are no UN goals related to stillbirth reduction. The estimates for stillbirth and neonatal deaths have wide uncertainty ranges but have been improved in terms of inputs, methodology and transparency in the last few years. Further investment will allow improvements in the quantity and quality of data, especially on stillbirths, from low and middle income countries. This could be achieved through methodological assessment of the demographic and health survey modules and a commitment to include improved modules in all surveys. In order to prioritize interventions within maternal and neonatal programmes that would also address stillbirth, a proactive approach is required to develop a generic mapping of classifications.

In the meantime, there are more than enough data to show that this huge loss of life around birth is closely linked to the same conditions that affect maternal mortality and morbidity, and including these outcomes together makes a much stronger case for national and international investment (Lawn *et al.*, 2009b). The grief and stigma of the loss of a baby disproportionately affect women, even decades after the loss (Froen *et al.*, 2011). Improving the data for all outcomes around the time of birth and using these data for action in programmes are a fundamental challenge for progress towards the MDGs and beyond.

References

Aggarwal, A.K., Jain, V. and Kumar, R. (2011) Validity of verbal autopsy for ascertaining the causes of stillbirth. *Bulletin of the World Health Organization* 89, 31–40.

Bhutta, Z., Cross, A., Rizvi, A. and Raza, F. (2008) *Pakistan Demographic and Health Survey, 2006–07.* National Institute of Population Studies, Islamabad and Macro International, Calverton, Maryland.

Black, R.E., Cousens, S., Johnson, H.L., Lawn, J.E., Rudan, I., Bassani, D.G., Jha, P., Campbell, H., Walker, C.F., Cibulskis, R., Eisele, T., Liu, L. and Mathers, C. (2010) Global, regional, and national causes of child mortality in 2008: a systematic analysis. *Lancet* 375, 1969–1987.

Conde-Agudelo, A., Belizán, J.M. and Diaz-Rossello, J. (2011) Kangaroo mother care to reduce morbidity and mortality in low birthweight infants. *Cochrane Database of Systematic Reviews* 16(3), CD002771.

Cousens, S., Blencowe, H., Stanton, C., Chou, D., Ahmed, S., Steinhardt, L., Creanga, A.A., Tuncalp, O., Balsara, Z.P., Gupta, S., Say, L. and Lawn, J.E. (2011) National, regional, and worldwide estimates of stillbirth rates in 2009 with trends since 1995: a systematic analysis. *Lancet* 377, 1319–1330.

Edmond, K.M., Quigley, M.A., Zandoh, C., Danso, S., Hurt, C., Owusu Agyei, S. and Kirkwood, B.R. (2008) Aetiology of stillbirths neonatal deaths in rural Ghana: implications for health programming in developing countries. *Paediatric and Perinatal Epidemiology* 22, 430–437.

Fauveau, V. (2007) New indicator of quality of emergency obstetric and newborn care. *Lancet* 370, 1310.

Froen, J.F., Cacciatore, J., Mcclure, E.M., Kuti, O., Jokhio, A.H., Islam, M. and Shiffman, J. (2011) Stillbirths: why they matter. *Lancet* 377, 1353–1366.

Hill, K. and Choi, Y. (2006) Neonatal mortality in the developing world. *Demographic Research* 14(18), 429–452.

Kramer, M.S., Platt, R., Yang, H., Mcnamara, H. and Usher, R.H. (1999) Are all growth-restricted newborns created equal(ly)? *Pediatrics* 103, 599–602.

Lawn, J.E., Cousens, S. and Zupan, J. (2005) 4 million neonatal deaths: When? Where? Why? *Lancet* 365, 891–900.

Lawn, J.E., Wilczynska-Ketende, K. and Cousens, S.N. (2006) Estimating the causes of 4 million neonatal deaths in the year 2000. *Internation Journal of Epidemiology* 35, 706–718.

Lawn, J.E., Yakoob, M.Y., Haws, R.A., Soomro, T., Darmstadt, G.L. and Bhutta, Z.A. (2009a) 3.2 million stillbirths: epidemiology and overview of the evidence review. *BMC Pregnancy Childbirth* 9(Suppl. 1), S7.

Lawn, J.E., Kinney, M., Lee, A.C., Chopra, M., Donnay, F., Paul, V.K., Bhutta, Z.A., Bateman, M. and Darmstadt, G.L. (2009b) Reducing intrapartum-related deaths and disability: can the health system deliver? *International Journal of Gynaecology and Obstetrics* 107(Suppl. 1), S123–S140, S140–S142.

Lawn, J., Gravett M.G., Nunes, T.M., Rubens, C. and Stanton, C. (2010) Global report on preterm birth and stillbirth (1 of 7): definitions, description of the burden and opportunities to improve data. *BMC Pregnancy and Childbirth* 10(Suppl. 1), S1.

Lawn, J.E., Blencowe, H., Pattinson, R., Cousens, S., Kumar, R., Ibiebele, I., Gardosi, J., Day, L.T. and Stanton, C. (2011) Stillbirths: Where? When? Why? How to make the data count. *Lancet* 377, 1448–1463.

Lee, A.C., Cousens, S., Wall, S.N., Niermeyer, S., Darmstadt, G.L., Carlo, W.A., Keenan, W.J., Bhutta, Z.A., Gill, C. and Lawn, J.E. (2011) Neonatal resuscitation and immediate newborn assessment and stimulation for the prevention of neonatal deaths: a systematic review, meta-analysis and Delphi estimation of mortality effect. *BMC Public Health* 11(Suppl. 3), S12.

Macro International (2009) *DHS StatCompiler*. Calverton, Maryland.

Macro International (2010) *Demographic and Health Surveys*. Calverton, Maryland.

Macro International (2011) *DHS StatCompiler*. Calverton, Maryland. Accessed: 14 July 2011.

Oestergaard, M.I., Yoshida, S., Mahanani, W., Gore, F., Cousens, S., Lawn, J.E. and Mathers, C.D. on behalf of the United Nations Inter-Agency Group on Child Mortality Estimation and the Child Health Epidemiology Reference Group (2011) Systematic analysis of neonatal mortality levels for 193 countries in 2009 with trends since 1990; progress, projections and priorities. *PLoS Med*, 8(8): e1001080. doi:10.1371/journal.pmed.1001080.

Peltoniemi, O.M., Kari, M.A. and Hallman. M. (2011) Repeated antenatal corticosteroid treatment: a systematic review and meta-analysis. *Acta Obstetricia et Gynecologica Scandinavica* 90(7), 719–727.

Rajaratnam, J., Marcus, J., Flaxman, A., Wang, H., Levin-Rector, A., Dwyer, L., Costa, M., Lopez, A. and Murray, C. (2010) Neonatal, postneonatal, childhood and under-5 mortality for 187 countries, 1970–2010: a systematic analysis of progress towards Millennium Development Goal 4. *Lancet* 375(9730), 1988–2008.

Reddy, U.M., Goldenberg, R., Silver, R., Smith, G.C., Pauli, R.M., Wapner, R.J., Gardosi, J., Pinar, H., Grafe, M., Kupferminc, M., Hulthen Varli, I., Erwich, J.J., Fretts, R.C. and Willinger, M. (2009) Stillbirth classification – developing an international consensus for research: executive summary of a National Institute of Child Health and Human Development workshop. *Obstetrics and Gynecology* 114, 901–914.

Say, L., Donner, A., Gulmezoglu, A.M., Taljaard, M. and Piaggio, G. (2006) The prevalence of stillbirths: a systematic review. *Reproductive Health* 3, 1.

Shiffman, J. (2010) Issue attention in global health: the case of newborn survival. *Lancet* 375, 2045–2049.

Stanton, C., Lawn., J.E., Rahman, H., Wilczynska-Ketende, K. and Hill, K. (2006) Stillbirth rates: delivering estimates in 190 countries. *Lancet* 367, 1487–1494.

WHO (1993) *International Classification of Diseases and Related Health Problems*, 10th Revision, Vol. 2. WHO, Geneva.

WHO (1996) *Perinatal mortality; A listing of available information*. WHO, Geneva.

WHO (2006) *Perinatal and Neonatal Mortality for the Year 2000: Country, regional and global estimates*. WHO, Geneva.

WHO, UNICEF, UNFPA and World Bank (2010) Trends in maternal mortality: 1990–2008. In: World Health Organization (eds). WHO, Geneva.

6 Health Systems

Dileep V. Mavalankar and Parvathy Sankara Raman
Indian Institute of Public Health, Gandhinagar, India

Summary

- A functioning health system is crucial for maternal health programmes to achieve their goals of improving maternal and perinatal health.
- The six essential building blocks of a health system are service delivery, health workforce, information, equipment and supplies, financing and leadership and governance.
- Health systems are complex and interconnected social and political organizations. Although some of their core elements are tangible (infrastructure, equipment, supplies, vehicles and people), many are intangible or conceptual in nature, such as health sector reforms and governance.
- Maternity services are the means through which the health system provides care for mothers and their babies. Maternity services are usually organized in at least three levels – primary, secondary and tertiary.
- Acute problems exist in the recruitment, retention, deployment and distribution of people working in the health system. The problems are not restricted to doctors, nurses and midwives, but extend to paramedical and ancillary staff (such as laboratory technicians, radiographers) and professional managers.
- Health sector reforms are changes in policy and institutional arrangements of the health system and are required for a health system to be responsive to a range of external factors and ultimately to provide equitable and efficient health services.
- Some major reforms pertinent to maternity care in India are discussed in this chapter, including examples of public–private partnerships, financing health care and aid harmonization.

Introduction

The way health systems are designed, managed and financed affects people's lives and livelihoods. The difference between a well-performing health system and one that is failing can be measured in death, disability, impoverishment, humiliation and despair.

Gro Harlem Brundtland (WHO, 2000).

Why is the health system important for maternal health programmes to achieve their goals of improving maternal and perinatal health? The Alma-Ata declaration originally focused on primary level health services, but this focus shifted to vertical health programming for immunization, child survival activities and then maternal health interventions (Alma-Ata, 1978; Walsh and Warren, 1979;

Cueto, 2004). In spite of this internationally driven targeting of specific problem areas, the progress in maternal and perinatal mortality reduction has been slow (WHO and UNICEF, 2010). Many health systems in developing countries had deep rooted management, accountability and governance problems in addition to the financial constraints faced (Sachs, 2001). The vertical programming efforts did not strengthen the health system on which these programmes were dependent. A health system can be described as the 'cement' that binds together the health services and various technical interventions which contribute to improving maternal and perinatal health. If the health system is weak, the interventions cannot work together to achieve the desired goals (Achura, 2010). A variety of health system constraints can prevent rapid and complete scale up of maternal health interventions, including lack of human resources, unacceptable quality of care and poor infrastructure (Koblinsky et al., 2006). For example, a weak supply and maintenance system will result in unavailability of life-saving drugs (see Langer et al., Chapter 8 this volume) and surgical interventions for pregnant women. A poorly functioning health system cannot recruit, deploy and monitor the midwives necessary to make childbirth safe (Potter and Brough, 2004) and cannot maintain adequate referral systems (see Munjanja et al., Chapter 11 this volume) or address issues of demand for health care (see Mumtaz and Levay, Chapter 12 this volume).

This chapter takes the perspective of the health system as a basic foundation upon which the achievement of maternal and perinatal health depends. The functions of health systems and crucial concepts necessary to support and improve health system function are discussed with special attention to issues important for maternal health programmes.

Defining the Health System

A health system is comprised of 'all organizations, institutions and resources devoted to producing actions whose primary intent is to improve health. Most national health systems include public, private, traditional and informal sectors' (WHO, 2000).

Health systems should be effective, responsive and fair. They should be effective in contributing to better health for all and be responsive to people's expectations, safeguarding dignity, confidentiality and autonomy; and sensitive enough to cater to the specific needs and vulnerabilities of all population groups. A health system should be fair in how individuals contribute to funding the system (see Witter and Ensor, Chapter 7 this volume), so that everyone has access to the services available and is protected against potentially impoverishing levels of spending due to ill health (WHO, 2000).

The six essential functions or building blocks of a health system have been defined as service delivery, health workforce, information, inventory, financing and leadership and governance (WHO, 2007). For the system to work effectively and efficiently, there should be connections between and integration of all the six building blocks. The role of each building block is as follows:

1. *Service delivery*: a health system should provide effective and efficient services for all, wherever or whenever they are needed.
2. *Health workforce*: health workers provide services, and an effective system requires sufficient numbers of competent, responsive and productive people who are appropriately distributed across the levels of the health system.
3. *Information systems*: the information system analyses the requirements of health services, controls for the provision of the services and assesses their impact with respect to coverage, quality, accessibility and equity of services.
4. *Inventory*: the inventory ensures an uninterrupted supply of medical products, vaccines and equipment needed to provide services.
5. *Financing*: adequate and timely availability of financial resources is required to enable the smooth functioning of the health system.

6. *Leadership and governance*: at the heart of the health system are the processes and procedures which ensure that strategic policy frameworks, systems design, regulation and accountability work efficiently to deliver health care at all levels of the health system.

Organization of Maternity Services

Maternity services are the means through which the health system provides care for mothers and their babies. The availability, accessibility, acceptability and quality of these services directly impact on their health and all other components of the health system and in preparing for and performing care-related activities.

Health service delivery systems in countries are generally organized from the village level to the national level and maternity care is no exception. Table 6.1 gives a brief overview of the health service delivery system pertaining to maternal and perinatal health in a selection of South Asian countries. There are broad similarities across most countries in terms of primary, secondary and tertiary levels (see Phoya *et al.*, Chapter 10 this volume).

The health system in India is controlled by the Ministry of Health and Family Welfare at state and national level. The health system is organized from the sub-centre level to the tertiary care level. Each state in India has several medical college hospitals, which form the apex of the health-care delivery system. Below this lie the district hospitals, sub-district hospitals, primary health-care centres and sub-centres (Box 6.1). Outside the public health structure, there are many levels of private health services. They are large in number and are distributed in major urban areas and surrounding developed districts (De Costa *et al.*, 2009). At the village level there are traditional birth attendants and village healers, which are part of informal healing traditions.

On paper, health systems appear simple but in reality they are complex and interconnected social and political organizations. Smooth functioning of all components and levels of health care, including public and private health-care systems, is needed. The various elements of health-care systems may be tangible or intangible. The tangible elements are those that can be physically seen – infrastructure, medical equipment, supplies and vehicles – discussed elsewhere (see Phoya *et al.*, Chapter 10 this volume). The term

Table 6.1. Maternity service delivery in India, Bangladesh, Pakistan and Sri Lanka.

Health service delivery systems	India (Vora *et al.*, 2009)	Sri Lanka (Pathmanathan *et al.*, 2003)	Bangladesh (Mridha *et al.*, 2009)	Pakistan (Ministry of Health, undated)
Apex level	Medical college hospitals	Teaching hospitals	Post-graduate medical institutes Medical college hospitals	Medical college hospitals
Tertiary care level	District hospitals	Specialist maternity hospitals District hospitals	District hospitals	District headquarters hospitals
Secondary care level	First referral units Community health centres	Provincial or general hospitals Base hospitals Peripheral hospitals	Maternal and child welfare centres Sub-district health complexes	Headquarters hospitals
Primary care level	Primary health centres	Cottage hospitals, rural hospitals	Sub-centres Health and family welfare centres	Rural health centres
	Sub-centres	Maternity homes		Basic health units

Box 6.1. Overview of the maternity service delivery system in India.

The sub-centre is the most peripheral level of government service; it provides maternal and child health services for a group of villages. This level is generally staffed by an auxiliary nurse midwife or a female health worker, who provides services such as immunization, vaccination, conducting delivery and counselling for family planning.

The primary health centre provides both preventive and curative services and is generally staffed by a medical officer supported by nurses or health assistants. This level can provide basic EmOC and some neonatal care.

The next level of care is the sub-district hospital, which is the first referral unit. This level of facility provides specialist care including life-saving surgery and Caesarean sections. First referral units are generally staffed by specialists (including obstetricians) and supported by medical doctors and nurses.

The third level is the district hospital, which provides a range of speciality services and will have round the clock teams of specialists and other medical doctors. These hospitals handle most of the referred patients from the other facilities.

'human resources' refers to the all important health workers who provide health services, as well as support staff, administrators and managers who work within the health system. Intangible elements such as service delivery, reforms and governance are conceptual in nature but are nevertheless crucial in influencing the performance of the health system.

Human Resources for Health

The health system is dependent upon its health workforce. A severe health workforce crisis exists. WHO estimates that 57 countries, most of them in Africa and Asia, are experiencing acute problems in recruitment, retention, deployment and distribution of health personnel. At least 2,360,000 health service providers and 1,890,000 management support workers, i.e. a total of 4,250,000 health workers, are needed to fill the existing gaps (WHO, 2010). The international norm suggested to achieve a minimum of 80% coverage of skilled care attendance at birth is a minimum of 2.28 health workers (doctors, nurses and midwives) per 1000 population (African Working Group, 2006). A recent international report on midwives indicated that many low and middle income countries have insufficient numbers of midwives to meet a benchmark of six midwives to attend every 1000 births annually, with 111,880

midwives needed by 2015 to close the gap (UNFPA, 2011).

Table 6.2 provides an international comparison of the human resource situation for the years 2002–2009 (WHO, 2010). From the table it is evident that the health workforce scarcity is worse in lower income countries, but even in developed countries such as the USA shortages exist.

Some countries with the highest maternal mortality ratios such as Afghanistan are not the worst off in terms of health workforce while other countries like Bhutan have lower levels of maternal mortality despite the acute lack of human resources for health. This suggests that other system weaknesses and factors are important determinants of maternal health outcomes.

Across all countries, the median level of doctors per 10,000 population is 11 and for nurses and midwives 27. India lies below this median for both types of health workers. Indeed, the demise of the professional midwife in India has been highlighted (Sankara Raman *et al.*, 2010). Sri Lanka provides an example of a country that is highly successful in reducing its maternal mortality, yet has a doctor density ratio the same as India but a higher nurse-midwife ratio. Countries such as Brazil, Egypt and the Philippines have densities of health professionals above the median. Norway has one of the highest nurse/midwife densities in the world and Cuba the highest doctor to population density (WHO, 2010).

Table 6.2. Density of doctors and nurses/midwives per 10,000 population, international comparison, selected countries: 2002–2009, ranked by density of physicians to population (WHO, 2010).

	Physicians		Nurses and midwives	
	Number	Density (per 10,000 population)	Number	Density (per 10,000 population)
Selected countries				
Niger	288	<0.5	2115	1
Bhutan	52	<0.5	545	2
Chad	345	<0.5	2,499	3
Guinea	940	1	401	<0.5
Afghanistan	5,970	2	14,930	5
India	643,520	6	1,372,059	13
Sri Lanka	10,479	6	33,431	17
The Philippines	90,370	12	480,910	61
China	1,862,630	14	1,259,240	10
Brazil	320,013	17	549,423	29
Egypt	179,900	24	248,010	34
USA	793,648	27	2,927,000	98
Denmark	17,226	32	53,133	98
France	227,683	37	494,895	81
Norway	18,143	39	76,173	163
Cuba	72,416	64	97,800	86
Countries by income				
Low income	332,034	4	899,015	10
Lower middle income	3,464,085	10	4,917,127	14
Upper middle income	2,126,466	24	3,566,218	40
High income	2,825,205	28	8,166,399	81

The lack of doctors, nurses and midwives does not show the full extent of the problem. Paramedical personnel, laboratory technicians, radiographers and operation theatre assistants also have a key role to play in providing maternity care but their training and recruitment are poorly supported. Many of the key services which should be provided in these areas are done by unqualified and untrained support staff or not done at all – for example, only 25% of maternity units surveyed in Gujarat (a state in India with progressive indicators for health and development) could offer blood culture services for detection of infection (Mehta *et al.*, 2011). Many private hospitals are known not to employ fully qualified nurses but train women 'on the job' to provide nursing and midwifery services. Certain high level skills such as providing anaesthesia and intensive care for the newborn are in particularly short supply yet are needed for providing safe and effective care for emergencies during child-

birth (Mavalankar and Sriram, 2009). The available specialists are especially reluctant to go to rural and remote areas. To overcome this problem, countries with diverse settings such as the USA, Nepal and Tanzania have used nurses and other technicians to provide anaesthesia by 'task shifting' (see below).

Inability to recruit and retain health personnel in low resource and rural settings has contributed to the human resource crisis. One concern is the movement of skilled workers across international boundaries. Despite higher health professional densities in developed countries (Table 6.2), the health workforce gap is a global one, which has led to migration of skilled workers from developing countries to developed countries – referred to as a 'brain drain'. Multiple factors contribute to this leaching of skilled workers from developing countries and include low remuneration, low recognition and high workloads in their countries of origin (Green, 2008). Another problem leading to uneven distribution of skills is the unwillingness of health workers to practise and live in rural areas. A number of strategies have been tried out in an attempt to incentivize health workers or compensate for the difficulties of living in remote and rural locations (Box 6.2).

Task shifting

Given the shortage of highly skilled professionals, there have been various efforts to train nurses, midwives, paramedical staff and medical officers to take up higher levels of clinical work normally done by specialists. This is called task shifting or task sharing (Mavalankar, 2002; Bergstrom, 2005; AMDD, 2010). With proper training and supportive supervision the health workers can perform highly skilled, life-saving maternity functions such as performing Caesarean sections and administering anaesthesia. Task shifting ensures that health staff based in rural areas have the requisite skills to save the lives of mothers and children. Even though this practice is improving access to services in rural and remote areas there are many challenges: legal authorizations and administrative orders for task shifting are not clear or well circulated; specialist professionals (obstetricians and anaesthesiologists)

and their associations object to task shifting; people may hesitate to accept services from newly trained personnel; and the posting and transfers of the trained people may not be aligned to service delivery (Berer, 2009).

Many of these factors hinder the provision of emergency obstetric care (EmOC) and newborn care services. Nevertheless, task shifting has been practised for over 20 years in parts of Africa. In selected cases, the outcome of the procedures done by medical technicians is no different from those done by obstetricians (Pereira, 2010). There has also been experience built up for task shifting in family planning programmes. India, Bangladesh, Bhutan and Nepal have recently initiated task-shifting initiatives to increase the provision of life-saving EmOC skills (Iyengar and Iyengar, 2009; Mavalankar and Sriram, 2009; Nick Simons Institute, undated) resulting in an increase in the number of surgeries performed (Cherian *et al.*, 2010).

Task shifting requires ongoing supportive supervision for the newly trained personnel (Mavalankar and Sriram, 2009). The danger arises when they are placed in rural areas with little supervision and experience, which can result in mishandling of cases and substandard care. A loss of confidence and demotivation can occur along with loss of trust among the community they serve.

Box 6.2. Strategies for the retention of the health workforce in rural areas.

- Tamil Nadu, India: the Government of Tamil Nadu retained doctors in remote locations by making it mandatory to complete service postings in rural primary health centres before applying for postgraduate training. Of the training slots for postgraduate courses, 50% are reserved for doctors who have completed their postings in rural areas (Padmanaban *et al.*, 2009).
- Indonesia: to attract more qualified health workers to rural areas, the Indonesian government provides incentives such as doubling the salary, subsidizing tuition fees, free clothing, room and board and learning materials (Pereira, 2010).
- South Africa and Zambia: special allowance packages are provided for staff working in rural health facilities, such as increases in salary by up to 30%, renovation of accommodation facilities, contribution to the school fees, housing loans and vehicle loans (Cumbi *et al.*, 2007).
- Pakistan: a female postgraduate rotation scheme placed recently qualified female medical graduates on rotations in rural hospitals. The doctors take on responsibilities (such as performing Caesarean sections) beyond those usually undertaken by fresh graduates. They receive special supervision to conduct these duties and recognition of their activities for specialist training. The female doctors receive a stipend in addition to their normal salary, are provided with furnished accommodation and given transportation for training activities (Hussein *et al.*, 2010).

Health systems managers

Most discussion on human resources has focused on health workers who directly provide health services, yet an efficient health system needs professional managers. Traditionally, senior doctors and nurses were promoted to take up management positions, while generally trained civil servants and elected politicians were placed in bureaucratic positions within health departments and ministries. There is limited literature available on management capacity in health in developing countries. In India, there are few managers in the health system for maternal and reproductive and child health – with its 1 billion population and 25 million births, there are only three technical managers for maternal health and no state-level maternal health managers. Those who manage maternal health programmes may not be trained in management sciences and are generally promoted as managers because of their seniority (Vora *et al.*, 2009). Only a handful of centres provide training for public health managers. This affects the planning, implementation and quality of services (De Costa *et al.*, 2009; Ramani and Mavalankar, 2009). With expansion of programmes and provision of development aid targeted to maternal and perinatal health, wastage of resources and non-achievement of goals may result if insufficient attention is given to improving management capacity (USAID, 2009).

Health Sector Reforms

The WHO defines health sector reforms as 'sustained processes of fundamental change in the policy and institutional arrangements in the health sector' (WHO/SEARO, 2011). The reasons for reforms are multiple. They may take place in response to donor requirements, cost considerations and demographic transitions, but usually have the ultimate goal of ensuring health systems are responsive to the needs of the population in an equitable and efficient manner.

After publication of the World Development Report of 1993 (World Bank, 1993),

many countries instituted health reforms in various ways. The key direction of the health reforms was to develop newer financing mechanisms and pooling of donor funding (sector-wide approach), encouragement for public–private partnerships and contracting of health services, restructuring of health departments with creation of semi-autonomous bodies and improvement of human resource management. These reforms change the structure and functioning of the health system, which have direct impact on maternal and perinatal health (Sachs, 2008).

Public–private partnerships

The services provided by public health institutions are weakening due to various reasons, which include the scarcity of human resources and lack of proper infrastructure but could be improved through broadening the healthcare system base by including private and non-government groups (Sachs, 2001). The private sector plays an important role in maternal health-care services. In Africa faith-based organizations have traditionally provided such essential health services while in India and many other Asian countries the private health sector has evolved rapidly in the last few decades. In Latin America social security organizations provide a substantial part of health care. Public–private partnerships are emerging as a new way to provide services for the community with more governments contracting the private sector to provide services for the people. Ideally, private sector facilities should also be considered within the health system but many public health planners do not explicitly include them (Loevinsohn and Harding, 2005).

Public–private partnerships assume an important role in the social sectors as resources for health increase. People's expectations of the private health sector are increasing and their use of services is shifting from public to private facilities as quality of care is perceived to be better in the private sector (Peters *et al.*, 2002). In countries such as Egypt, India, Indonesia and Nigeria, more births occur in private than in public facilities (Private health care in developing countries, 2008). There are many examples of the two sectors working synergistically in India. Blood bank services and emergency transport services are run in collaboration with the Red Cross (Indian Red Cross Society, undated). An extensive referral and communications network is operating as a private–public partnership (see Munjanja *et al.*, Chapter 11 this volume). Since 2005, the state government of Gujarat has involved the private sector in providing delivery services for the poor through a social health programme called the 'Chiranjeevi scheme' (Box 6.3)

These kinds of partnerships can help support health systems in developing countries. Contracting out health services has numerous attractive features, including (Baru, 1998):

- Ensuring a greater focus on the achievement of measurable results, especially if contracts define objectively verifiable outputs and outcomes.
- Overcoming constraints that prevent governments from effectively using the resources made available to them (often referred to as absorptive capacity issues).
- Using the private sector's greater flexibility and generally better morale to improve services.
- Increasing managerial autonomy and decentralizing decision making to managers on the ground.

- Using competition to increase effectiveness and efficiency.
- Allowing governments to focus on other roles that they are uniquely placed to undertake, such as planning, standard setting, financing and regulation.

Financing mechanisms

Financing mechanisms such as the Chiranjeevi programme in Gujarat, India (Box 6.3) have improved access to maternity services for the poor in some areas. Incentives or conditional cash transfers provide resources for the poor and help them to overcome the financial barriers to health. In the Janani Suraksha Scheme in India, the government provides Rs1500 (US$30) for pregnant women for nutritional supplements and to deliver in health facilities in some states. This has led to a sharp rise in institutional births in many parts of India where home births were originally a well-entrenched tradition. A sharp increase in health facility deliveries has been observed nationally, from 38.7% in 2005 to 73% in 2009 (IIPS, 2007; UNICEF, 2009). The increase is thought to be due to incentives paid under the scheme, with indication of associated decreases in neonatal and perinatal mortality (Lim *et al.*, 2010).

Box 6.3. The Chiranjeevi scheme, Gujarat state, India.

The scheme was launched in 2005 on a pilot basis in five districts with poor indicators of maternity care in Gujarat. The major objectives were to promote deliveries in health facilities and skilled care assistance during childbirth for needy and poor women in the state. As part of this scheme, the state government made an agreement with private obstetricians in Gujarat to provide delivery care services for poor women when needed.

The state government paid the specialists an advance of US$625 on signing the contract. As part of the package, Rs1795 (US$45) is paid for a single delivery (any type) conducted by the private obstetrician. Payment is received after completion of 100 deliveries. In return, the obstetricians are expected to provide free delivery services (normal or complicated) for poor women and give Rs200 (US$5) for transportation costs and Rs50 (US$1) as an honorarium for the woman's companion. The pregnant woman has to go for only one antenatal visit to the specialist before her delivery.

The scheme was scaled up for the whole state in 2007 (Singh *et al.*, 2009). Between January 2006 and March 2010, 467,969 poor women have delivered in private hospitals under the scheme – with 28,252 Caesarean sections or 6% of the total deliveries – this rate indicating that overuse of surgical interventions is not occurring. Over 700 private obstetricians have been enrolled in the scheme, which won the Asian Innovation award (http://www.wsj-asia.com/aia) in 2006.

Examples from other countries in the world indicate that removing financial barriers through various mechanisms such as conditional cash transfers, vouchers and social insurance can work effectively to protect the poor (ADB, 2009; see Witter and Ensor, Chapter 7 this volume).

Sector-wide approaches

In the 1990s, it became apparent that isolated projects funded by external donors were leading to fragmentation of the health system and resulting in islands of excellence. Individual projects were placing too many demands – for planning, implementation and monitoring – on the already overstretched health systems of developing countries. Policy and structural reforms to meet such demands were not being developed. To overcome these problems, a number of donors decided to redirect their aid support through a pooled funding mechanism with the 'Sector Wide Approach', or 'SWAp'. The approach describes a means for how governments and donors can work together. A prominent part of the SWAp is the pooling of funding from various donors, with priorities to be achieved through the funding discussed jointly between government and donor representatives. The SWAp was recognition of the need to harmonize aid from different donors to attain the MDGs. It was a strategy discussed internationally in various forums, and

the principles of aid harmonization were finalized in 2005 in Paris. This prestigious international meeting had participation from various developed and developing countries and civil society organizations and also delegates from various international donor agencies and resulted in the Paris Declaration (OECD, 2005). The declaration unanimously charted out guidelines and norms for the donors and development partners in how to move forward (Fig. 6.1).

In India, several donors joined the pooled funding mechanism to support the national Reproductive and Child Health programme, while others maintained separate funding arrangements, making it difficult to assess the impact of pooled funding in maternal health. In large countries like India, the bulk of funding for health comes from national government, so the impact of external funding is limited in terms of quantity, but could have substantial qualitative or priority setting impact. What has been observed is that key indicators of maternal health can get lost amongst other competing priorities such as child health, family planning and disease control. It seems that in the SWAp the sharp focus on specific programmes such as developing first referral units or improving skilled care at childbirth can get diluted.

At a global level, it is not clear whether the reforms have resulted in improved efficiencies and effectiveness overall. A recent evaluation report of the effects of the Paris

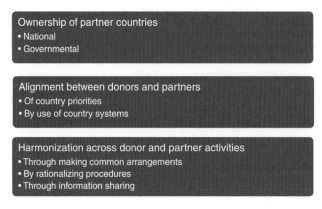

Fig. 6.1. Model for aid harmonization (WHO, 2006).

Declaration showed disappointing gains in the reduced burden of managing aid overall, although the management and use of aid seem to be improving slightly while the standards of partnership are being built up (Wood *et al.*, 2011).

Governance, Accountability and Corruption

In the development sector, the ability of governments to manage public services is a constant point of debate. There are various problems common across different departments and sectors within government. Public health systems tend to be hierarchical, bureaucratic, slow and inhumane in their interaction with their clients as well as their employees. Other key problems such as favoritism, nepotism, lack of accountability and monitoring systems hire and fire policies also affect government function. Managers complain of political interference in operational decisions and lack of clear policies, which hinder rational programming. For example, in India and South Asia (with notable exceptions like Sri Lanka) policies for recruitment, posting and transfer of health staff remain unclear or ambiguous. This leads to lack of accountability, arbitrary postings and transfers and, on occasion, corruption. One of the common manifestations of lack of accountability of peripheral health workers is absenteeism of health workers. The problems described affect maternity services directly with dysfunctional services and peripheral workers who do not stay at their place of posting (McPake and Koblinksy, 2009).

Other common forms of corruption are manifested in charging patients for free services through the government health system, the use of government infrastructure for private patients and corruption in procurement, appointment of staff and award of other contracts. There have been efforts in India to expose corruption with publication of data showing comparisons of corruption between states. The health sector is thought to be one of the most corrupt and unaccountable – with, for example, nearly 50% of the pharmacies without a qualified pharmacist out of which only 14 were prosecuted (Sudharshan, 2008).

Absenteeism in the health workforce is another major problem of governance, affecting especially health workers in rural areas. In some South Asian countries, 30% of health workers were found to be absent on any given day (World Bank, 2004). In Bangladesh, it was reported that health workers were available according to government records but were not available to provide services for the people in rural areas (Chaudhury and Hammer, 2003). In many countries, efforts are made to recruit people with rural backgrounds or with a specific reason to remain in rural areas as they are more likely to remain in post (Raha *et al.*, 2010; Sundararaman and Gupta, undated).

Removing corruption and bad governance takes top level commitment and systematic long term efforts alongside sector reforms. Given the sensitivity of the issue, major progress can only be made by open acknowledgement of the problem and specific focus on the problems. Within the health system one of the essential tools for improving governance and accountability lies in the development of a functional health management information system (see Hounton *et al.*, Chapter 15 this volume).

Conclusion

The provision of maternity care and maternal and perinatal mortality prevention needs effective functioning of all levels of the health service from the village level to the tertiary level, with a connecting referral system and supporting supply systems, human resources, information systems and good governance (Freedman *et al.*, 2005). Health systems are central in the achievement of maternal and perinatal health outcomes. If the various building blocks of the health system are weak and out of tune with each other, the investments made in maternal health programmes may not lead to desired improvements in health. Country-level policy makers, programme implementers and international partner agencies must carefully evaluate their programmes to see how they can make them supportive of the health systems, rather than allowing the programmes to weaken the system. Building up health systems is a long term endeavour involving visionary leadership and political will that should remain a crucial priority of health investments. A patchwork of small-scale projects and vertical schemes cannot be maintained by resource-constrained health systems and can detract from the need to invest in the system. Larger developing countries such as India may take longer and require considerable resources to evolve a credible and comprehensive health-care system that delivers quality health services. Bipartisan political consensus will contribute to development of plans that are robust enough to survive change of political leadership. MDGs 4 and 5 cannot be achieved if health systems remain weak and fragmented.

References

Achura, B.M. (2010) Strong health system key to achieving MDGs. Available at: http://www.endpoverty2015. org/en/maternal-health/news/strong-health-system-key-achieving-mdgs/24/aug/09 (accessed 8 October 2010).

African Working Group (2006) *Joint Learning Initiative on Human Resources for Health and Development. The health workforce in Africa: challenges and prospects*. WHO, Geneva.

Alma-Ata (1978) Declaration of Alma-Ata International Conference on Primary Health Care, Alma-Ata, USSR, 6–12 September 1978. Available at: http://www.who.int/hpr/NPH/docs/declaration_almaata.pdf (accessed 4 November 2011).

Asian Development Bank (ADB) (2009) Regional Forum on Social Assistance and Conditional Cash Transfer. Available at: http://www.adb.org/Documents/Speeches/2009/ms2009053.asp (accessed 15 September 2010).

Averting Maternal Deaths and Disability (AMDD) (2010) Task-sharing: Non-physician clinicians step in for doctors with equal success. Available at: http://www.amddprogram.org/d/content/task-sharing (accessed 15 September 2010).

Baru, R.V. (1998) Privatization in Medical care: an Overview. In: *Private Health Care in India: Social Characteristics and Trends*. Sage Publications, New Delhi.

Berer, M. (2009) Editrorial: Task-shifting: exposing the cracks in public health systems. *Reproductive Health Matters* 17(33), 4–8.

Bergstrom, S. (2005) Who will do the caesareans when there is no doctor? Finding creative solutions to the human resource crisis. *An International Journal of Obstetrics and Gynaecology: BJOG* 112, 1168–1169.

Chaudhury, N. and Hammer, J.S. (2003) *Ghost Doctors Absenteeism in Bangladeshi Health Facilities. Policy research working paper No. 3065*. The World Bank Development Research Group Public Services, Washington, DC.

Cherian, M., Choo, S., Wilson, I., Noel, L., Sheikh, M., Dayrit, M. and Groth, S. (2010) Building and retaining the neglected anaesthesia health workforce: is it crucial for health systems strengthening through primary health care? *Bulletin of the World Health Organization* 88, 637–639.

Cueto, M. (2004) The origins of primary health care and selective primary health care. *American Journal of Public Health* 11, 1874–1876.

Cumbi, A., Pereira, C., Malalane, R., Vaz, F., McCord, C., Bacci, A. and Bergström, S. (2007) Major surgery delegation to mid-level health practitioners in Mozambique: health professionals perceptions. *Human Resources for Health* 5, 27.

De Costa, A., Al-Muniriac, A., Diwan, V.K. and Eriksson, B. (2009) Where are healthcare providers? Exploring relationships between context and human resources for health in Madhya Pradesh province, India. *Health Policy* 93, 41–47.

Freedman, L.P., Waldman, R.J., de Pinho, H., Wirth, M.E., Chowdhury, A.M.R. and Rosenfield, A. (2005) Transforming health systems for women and children. *Lancet* 365, 997–1000.

Green, A. (2008) Health systems: a 2010 vision. In: Ramani, K.V., Mavalankar, D.V. and Govil, D. (eds) *Strategic Issues and Challenges in Health Management*. Sage Publishers, New Delhi, pp. 7–24.

Hussein, J., Newlands, D., D'Ambruoso, L., Thaver, I., Talukder, R. and Besana, G. (2010) Identifying practices and ideas to improve the implementation of maternal mortality reduction programmes: findings from five South Asian countries. *BJOG* 117(3), 304–317.

Indian Red Cross Society (undated) Programmes and Activities. Available at: http://www.indianredcross.org/program.htm (accessed 20 November 2010).

International Institute of Population Sciences (IIPS) (2007) *National Family Health Survey 3, 2005–2006*. International Institute of Population Sciences, Mumbai, 208 pp.

Iyengar, K. and Iyengar, S.D. (2009) Emergency obstetric care and referral: experience of two midwife-led health centres in rural Rajasthan, India. *Reproductive Health Matters* 17, 9–21.

Koblinsky, M., Matthews, Z., Hussein, J., Mavalankar, D., Mridha, M.K. and Anwar, I. (2006) Going to scale with professional skilled care. *Lancet* 368(9544), 1377–1386.

Lim, S.S., Dandona, L., Hoisington, J.A. and James, S.L. (2010) India's Janani Suraksha Yojana, a conditional cash transfer programme to increase births in health facilities: an impact evaluation. *Lancet* 375, 2009–2023.

Loevinsohn, B. and Harding, A. (2005) Buying results? Contracting for health service delivery in developing countries. *Lancet* 366, 676–681.

Mavalankar, D.V. (2002) Policy and management constraints on access to and use of life-saving emergency obstetric care in India. *Journal of the American Medical Women's Association* 57, 165–168.

Mavalankar, D. and Sriram, V. (2009) Provision of anaesthesia services for emergency obstetric care through task shifting in South Asia. *Reproductive Health Matters* 17, 21–31.

McPake, B. and Koblinsky, M. (2009) Improving maternal survival in South Asia – what can we learn from case studies? *Journal of Health, Population and Nutrition* 27(2), 93–107.

Mehta, R., Mavalankar, D.V., Ramani, K.V., Sharma, S. and Hussein, J. (2011) Infection control in delivery care units, Gujarat state, India: A needs assessment. *BMC Pregnancy and Childbirth* 11, 37.

Ministry of Health, Government of Pakistan (undated) *National Programme for Family Planning and Primary Health Care: Promoting Health by bridging the gap between the health services and communities by providing quality integrated health service to the doorsteps of our communities*. Government of Pakistan, Pakistan.

Mridha, M.K., Anwar, I. and Koblinsky, M. (2009) Public sector maternal health programmes and services for rural Bangladesh. *Journal of Health Population and Nutrition* 27, 124–138.

Nick Simons Institute (undated) Anesthesia Assistants. Available at: http://www.nsi.edu.np/aa.php (accessed 20 November 2010).

OECD (2005) Paris declaration on aid effectiveness: Ownership, Harmonisation, Alignment, Results and Mutual Accountability. Available at: http://www.oecd.org/dataoecd/11/41/34428351.pdf (accessed 20 August 2011).

Padmanaban, P., Raman, P. and Mavalankar, D.V. (2009) Innovations and challenges in reducing maternal mortality in Tamil Nadu. India. *Journal of Health Population and Nutrition* 29, 202–219.

Pathmanathan, I., Liljestrand, J., Martins, J.M., Rajapaksa, L.C., Lissner, C., de Silva, A., Selvaraju, S. and Singh, P.J. (2003) Sri Lanka. In: *Investing in Maternal Health: Learning from Malaysia and Sri Lanka*. Health Population and Nutrition Series, World Bank, Washington, DC.

Pereira, C. (2010) Task shifting of major surgery to midlevel providers of health care in Mozambique and Tanzania – a solution to the crisis in human resources to enhance maternal and neonatal survival. Doctoral Thesis, Karolinska Institute, Stockholm, Sweden.

Peters, D.H., Yazbeck, A.S., Sharma, R.R., Ramana, G.N.V., Pritchett, L.H. and Wagstaff, A. (2002) Problems of the public and private sectors. In: *Better Health Systems for India's Poor – Findings, Analysis, and Options*. Health, Nutrition and Population Series, Human Development Network, World Bank, Washington, DC.

Potter, C. and Brough, R. (2004) Systematic capacity building: a hierarchy of needs. *Health Policy and Planning* 189, 336–345.

Private health care in developing countries (2008) Maternal and child health services: Dying to give birth. Available at: http://ps4h.org/maternal_and_child.html (accessed 12 June 2010).

Raha, S., Bossert, T. and Vujicic, M. (2010) *Political Economy of Health Workforce Policy. The Chhattisgarh Experience with a Three-year Course for Rural Health Care Practitioners*. World Bank, Washington, DC.

Ramani, K.V. and Mavalankar, D.V. (2009) Management capacity assessment for national health programs – a study of RCH program in India. *Journal of Health Organization and Management* 23(1), 133–142.

Sachs, J.D. (2001) Macroeconomics and Health: Investing in Health for Economic Development. Report of the Commission on Macroeconomics and Health. Available at: http://whoindia.org/LinkFiles/Commision_on_Macroeconomic_and_Health_CMH_Final_Report.pdf (accessed 9 October 2010).

Sachs, J.D. (2008) Scaling up health in low income settings. In: Ramani, K.V., Mavalankar, K.V. and Govil, D. (eds) *Strategic Issues and Challenges in Health Management*. Sage Publishers, New Delhi, pp. 1–6.

Sankara Raman, P., Sharma, B., Mavalankar, D.V. and Upadhyaya, M. (2010) *Operationalization of First Referral Units in Gujarat: Midwifery and Maternal Health in India: Situation Analysis & Lessons from the field. Monograph 1.* Centre for Management of Health Systems, New Delhi.

Sankara Raman, P., Mavalankar, D.V. and Vora, K. (2011) Midwives of India: missing in action. *Midwifery* 27(5), 700–706.

Singh, A., Mavalankar, D.V., Bhat, R., Desai, A., Patel, S.R., Singh, P.V. and Singh, N. (2009) Providing skilled birth attendants and emergency obstetric care to the poor through partnership with private sector obstetricians in Gujarat, India. *Bulletin of the World Health Organisation* 87(12), 885–964.

Sudharshan, H. (2008) Health systems: A 2010 vision. In: Ramani, K.V., Mavalankar, K.V. and Govil, D. (eds) *Strategic Issues and Challenges in Health Management.* Sage Publishers, New Delhi.

Sundararaman, T. and Gupta, G. (undated) Human Resources for Health: The crisis, the NRHM response and the policy options. National Health Systems Resource Centre, New Delhi. Available at: http://nhsrcindia. org/pdf_files/resources_thematic/Human_Resources_for_Health/NHSRC_Contribution/174.pdf (accessed October 2011).

UNFPA (2011) *State of the World's Midwifery: Delivering Health, Saving Lives.* UNFPA, New York.

UNICEF (2009) Coverage Evaluation Survey: national fact sheet. Available at: http://www.unicef.org/india/ National_Fact_Sheet_CES_2009.pdf (accessed 17 November 2010).

USAID (2009) Overview: USAID support to Health System strengthening. Available at: http://www.usaid.gov/ our_work/global_health/hs/index.html (accessed 9 October 2010).

Vora, K.S., Mavalankar, D.V., Ramani, K.V., Upadhyaya, M., Sharma, S., Iyengar, S., Gupta, V. and Iyengar, K. (2009) Maternal health situation in India: a case study. *Journal of Health, Population and Nutrition* 27(2), 184–201.

Walsh, J.A. and Warren, K.S. (1979) Selective primary health care: an interim strategy for disease control in developing countries. *New England Journal of Medicine* 301, 967–974.

WHO (2000) World Health Report 2000: Health Systems Improving Performance. Available at: http://www. who.int/whr/2000/en/whr00_dgmessage_en.pdf (accessed 17 June 2010).

WHO (2006) A guide to WHO's role in sector-wide approaches to health development. Available at: http:// www.who.int/countryfocus/resources/guide_to_who_role_in_swap_en.pdf (accessed 21 June 2010).

WHO (2007) Everybody's business: Strengthening Health Systems to Improve Health outcomes. WHO framework for Action, Geneva, Switzerland. Available at: http://www.who.int/healthsystems/strategy/everybodys_business.pdf (accessed 18 June 2010).

WHO (2010) World Health Statistics. Available at: http://www.who.int/whosis/whostat/2010/en/index.html (accessed 20 August 2011).

WHO and UNICEF (2010) *Countdown to 2015 Decade Report (2000–2015): Maternal, Newborn and Child Survival.* WHO, Geneva.

WHO/SEARO (2011) Health sector reforms. Available at: http://www.searo.who.int/en/Section980/ Section1162/Section1167/Section1171_4813.htm (accessed 20 August 2011).

Wood, B., Betts, J., Etta, F., Gayfer, J., Kabell, D., Ngwira, N., Sagasti, F. and Samaranayake, M. (2011) *The Evaluation of the Paris Declaration, Final Report.* Danish Institute for International Studies, Copenhagen.

World Bank (1993) *World Development Report 1993.* World Bank, Washington, DC.

World Bank (2004) *World Development Report 2004: Making Services Work for Poor People.* World Bank, Washington, DC.

7 Financing Maternity Care

Sophie Witter[1] and Tim Ensor[2]
[1]*University of Aberdeen, Scotland, UK;*
[2]*University of Leeds, Leeds*

Summary

- The cost of accessing maternity care in low and middle income countries falls heavily on users, contributing to the low uptake of key services such as deliveries in health facilities and limited access to emergency obstetric care. This is a particular challenge for poor households.
- Different strategies have been piloted in recent years to reduce out of pocket payments of various kinds for maternity services. These include demand-side mechanisms such as user fee removal or reduction, community subsidies, social health insurance and provision of vouchers. Paying providers for performance, use of contracts and budget reforms are among the supply-side measures intended to increase access to services.
- These strategies have resulted in a degree of success in some contexts, depending on localized factors such as implementation capacity, external support and local ownership of the policy.
- Countries which have performed most strongly in improving access to maternity services have combined a range of strategies addressing provider incentives as well as consumer costs.
- Using pooled funds (such as taxation) to finance emergency obstetric care should be a priority, given the unpredictability, urgency and potentially catastrophic nature of these costs.
- Addressing core health systems issues such as the capacity to deliver reliable funds and drugs to facilities and reliable and adequate salaries to staff are critical to the quality, cost and sustainability of maternity services.

Introduction

Maternity care is integral to the health system and is therefore directly affected by the way in which funds are raised, pooled and allocated within the wider health system. It is well established that health systems are under-resourced at present, especially in countries with a high burden of maternal mortality. One study found that for 75 low and middle income countries to achieve 75% coverage of essential obstetric care requires an increase in spending of US$6.2 billion per year until 2015, whilst 95% coverage would need additional spending of US$9.5 billion (Johns *et al.*, 2007). In per capita terms, this represents between $0.73 and $1.03, an apparently modest sum but funding that needs to compete with other important claims on the health budget, such as spending on malaria, tuberculosis and HIV/AIDS.

The burden of financing health care can fall heavily on users of the health service who make direct out-of-pocket payments. A recent mapping exercise of 49 countries with high mortality found that 46% of all funding for health care (public and private) came from out-of-pocket payments, with 24% coming from governments' domestic resources, 21% from aid and only 9% from private risk-pooled systems such as insurance (Witter, 2010). Based on 2004 levels, donor funding would have to increase 11-fold to achieve the investment that the WHO estimates is needed by 2015 to meet the MDG goals 4 and 5 (Borghi et al., 2006; Powell-Jackson et al., 2006).

This chapter considers the implications of different ways of raising funds for maternity care and health systems generally, and then reviews recent experiences in addressing financial barriers from the demand and supply side. These experiments have been closely linked to maternal health programmes and indicators, largely because of the recognition that progress in expanding access to maternity care and reducing mortality and morbidity has been so slow and so uneven. We conclude with the lessons to date on the most promising avenues for financing appropriate and high-quality maternity services for all.

Common Mechanisms for Raising and Pooling Funds

There are two principal ways in which health care can be financed: direct and pooled mechanisms.

Direct payments

Direct payments are those where users pay for services at the time or just after treatment as user charges. Direct payments are often criticized because they impact on users at the time of illness when they are often least able to afford services. There is good evidence in rich and poor countries that direct payments act to deter or delay the use of services with a knock-on effect on health status. Evidence from large scale natural experiments in the USA demonstrated the negative impact of user fees on access to services, leading to delayed treatment and increased seriousness of the illness (Newhouse, 1993). Studies in

Asia and Africa have demonstrated the tendency of user fees to reduce utilization, especially amongst the poorest groups (Gertler and van der Gaag, 1990; Gilson, 1997; Witter, 2005). A recent simulation study across 20 African countries suggested that abolishing user fees could potentially eliminate 233,000 child deaths annually (James et al., 2005). Some of the two-directional linkages between poverty and ill health are illustrated in Fig. 7.1.

It is important to realize that the total payment for health care by a user may be determined by more than the official charge levied by a facility or health-care practitioner. In many countries unofficial payments are ubiquitous and can easily exceed formal charges for service. In addition, users incur other costs such as transport charges, loss of earnings and expenses of companions.

Pooled payments

In pooled payments, individuals are encouraged to put money aside on a regular basis in order to finance the costs of treatment in the event of illness. There are two main pooling mechanisms and prepayment: savings schemes and insurance systems.

Prepayment and savings schemes

Prepayment and savings schemes help an individual to pool resources over time.

Prepayment systems help individuals manage regular payments for health care. Individuals are able to buy a card providing an entitlement to a specific level of service (e.g. numbers of consultations, numbers of drug prescriptions) during a specified period, usually a year. The advantage is that payment can be made when an individual has resources, for instance, just after harvest time.

Medical savings schemes have gained popularity in a number of countries including South Africa, Singapore and the USA following their initial adoption in Singapore (Thomson and Mossialos, 2008). Savings schemes are more sophisticated than prepayment since they permit an individual to make regular contributions into a personal account

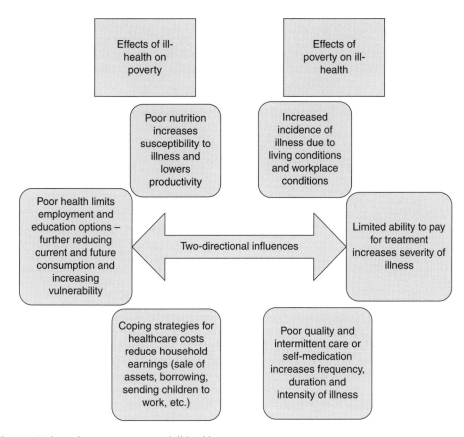

Fig. 7.1. Linkages between poverty and ill-health.

over a long period. This is then utilized in the event of illness. Individuals are spared having to pay a large bill at the time of treatment. Savings accounts are unsuitable for those unable to save and for paying for expensive treatment, for which an individual savings account will be insufficient. In general, both prepayment and saving schemes are most suitable for financing of low cost predictable services. Most countries introducing these systems use them to finance items such as consultations and outpatient medicines, but insurance systems are employed to finance more expensive services.

Insurance systems

Insurance systems provide much greater scope for pooling since they spread the financial risk across a group of individuals. As with savings schemes, individuals contribute

a regular sum. Rather than going into an individual account, the contribution is pooled with those of other members. Generally speaking, the bigger and more diverse the risk pool the better, since this improves the likelihood that ill health of members can be covered from the resources available.

The basis for computing the contribution for any one member varies according to the type of scheme. The simplest method is an average or community premium, where all members make the same contribution. This is commonly used in *community based health insurance* schemes, much used in low and middle income countries to provide insurance for a small local community. A problem is that those who consider themselves as unlikely to require services may choose not to join, which may result in only higher risk individuals joining, (adverse risk selection) which can quickly become financially unsustainable.

Private insurance commonly overcomes the problem of adverse risk selection by establishing higher contributions for those likely to use more services. Alternatively, they may disqualify more expensive or pre-existing conditions. The effect of this is that the less healthy, who often have less income, can be prevented from obtaining adequate cover. In this respect private insurance is likely to be a regressive form of funding, taking a proportionately greater proportion of income in contributions from the poor than from the rich. This contrasts with progressive funding, where a proportionately greater proportion of income is taken in contributions from the rich than from the poor. In proportional funding, the rich and poor pay the same proportion of income although the rich still pay more than the poor in absolute value.

General tax funding and social insurance provide a way of financing a pooled system of financing. Because both systems are usually compulsory for a defined group, it is possible to collect contributions that increase with individual income without the adverse selection that results from a voluntary scheme.

Social insurance is usually obtained through payroll (wage) contributions from those in formal employment. A proportional contribution ensures that individual premiums increase with income. Although maximum premiums are often capped, social insurance usually ensures that the rich pay more than the poor for similar cover.

General taxation also usually collects more from the rich than from the poor. The balance depends on the mix of taxation. Direct taxes are levied on income from employment, investments, profits and other sources and are generally progressive or proportional. Indirect sources are those taxes levied on goods and services. Since these are generally levied in proportion to

the price of the goods, they can be regressive since price represents a larger proportion of the income of the poor than of the rich. Many countries correct the deleterious impact of indirect taxes by focusing them on luxury goods, which are used mainly by the rich. There is evidence across a variety of Asian countries that taxation is likely to be a more progressive form of financing for health care than social insurance (Rannan-Eliya and Somananathan, 2006).

International development assistance contributes a substantial proportion of pooled public funding in many low income countries. A recent review, based on national health accounts data, found that donors contribute around one-third of total public spending on health care in low income countries (Farag *et al.*, 2009). Development assistance comes in many forms ranging from: budget support, where funds are allocated directly to the Ministry of Finance for across government purposes; health sector support, where funds are allocated to the Ministry of Health for across the sector programming; and direct support, where funds are allocated for specific projects or interventions. Donors may also bypass government entirely by spending on programmes that are run by non-governmental agencies. Where domestic resources are severely constrained, development assistance offers an important route for subsidizing services to poor and vulnerable communities.

Which system is best for maternal health services?

Maternity care covers a complex group of services ranging from low cost predictable services such as antenatal care or normal deliveries with a skilled birth attendant to high cost unpredictable services like intensive care (Table 7.1).

Table 7.1. Types of maternity care.

Cost	Predictable and/ or frequent	Unpredictable/ infrequent	Financing systems
Low	Antenatal care	Some types of supplementation	Prepayment or direct payment
Medium	Normal delivery with skilled birth attendant	Primary care for potential pre-eclampsia	Saving schemes for non-poor
High	Planned surgical delivery	Assisted/surgical delivery, postpartum complications, neonatal intensive care	Pooled insurance systems

Different financing systems are appropriate for each of these services. Direct user charges or a prepayment card could finance antenatal care. A safe normal delivery, which is a planned event for most households, might be financed through savings. The most potentially significant costs of delivery care are associated with complications during or immediately after delivery for the mother or child, which are mostly not predictable. These costs are only incurred for a minority of deliveries but are potentially catastrophic both in medical terms, if no medical care is forthcoming, and in financial terms. For complications, pooled insurance-based financing is the preferred funding option.

Whilst separate financing for different types of maternity care is possible, such mechanisms fail to take sufficient account of the overlap in demand for services. Antenatal care may help to pick up some conditions that, if undetected, could lead to more serious and expensive problems later in pregnancy. Antenatal care also affords an opportunity to encourage women to obtain delivery care from a skilled attendant. Similarly, delivery at a facility or with a skilled provider is likely to make it easier to access more sophisticated care if complications occur. A more sophisticated arrangement is to develop funding for all these services together by including safe normal delivery and antenatal care in an insurance package that also mitigates the potential costs of complications. In this way women can take steps to minimize the impact of later complications.

A funding package for maternity care may also need to include mitigation for large demand-side costs of services if it is to have a substantial impact on overall costs to the user. These costs include both the initial self-referral costs of getting to a birthing centre for safe delivery and onward referral for emergency obstetric care. The costs incurred may vary according to setting and context, as illustrated in Fig. 7.2.

Addressing Financial Barriers for Users

Financial barriers are not the only factor that prevents access to maternity services. In some contexts, they are not even the most

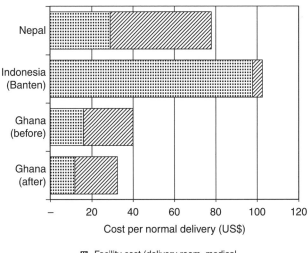

Fig. 7.2. Facility and non-facility costs of delivery care in Nepal, Indonesia and Ghana, before and after introduction of a fee exemption strategy.

important but they are major barriers in many contexts. Globally, skilled attendance at delivery shows the largest rich–poor gap, compared with other interventions (Gwatkin *et al.*, 2005), indicating that poverty and socio-economic status play an important role in determining access.

Reducing the cost (including access costs) and increasing the predictability of those costs can be an important part of addressing the complex and interrelated demand-side barriers (Fig. 7.3).

As well as reducing access to care, high costs and the absence of risk-sharing mecha-

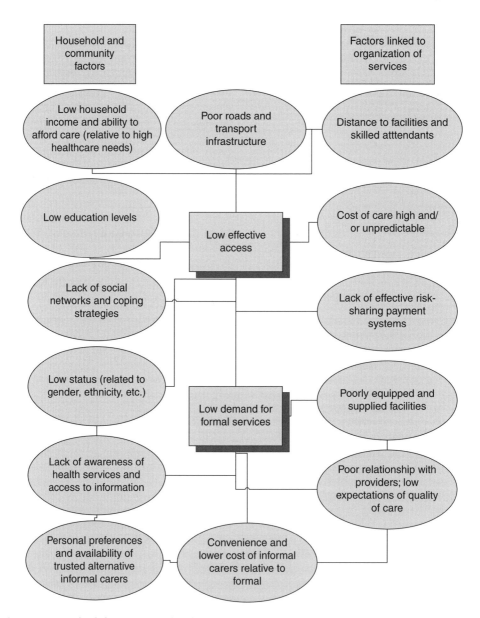

Fig. 7.3. Demand-side barriers to uptake of services.

nisms can force households into, or deeper into, poverty. The direct costs of maternity care range from 1 to 5% of total annual household expenditure, rising to between 5 and 34% if the woman suffers a maternal complication (WHO, 2006).

There are a variety of approaches, both direct and indirect, to reducing financial barriers to obstetric care. All have common objectives of improving coverage of skilled delivery care and reducing maternal mortality and inequalities of access.

The main characteristics of the direct approaches are summarized in Table 7.2. Although these are presented as independent options, they can be combined in schemes that will then have mixed characteristics.

In addition to direct approaches to reducing financial barriers, there are a variety of actions which, while not usually framed in those terms, do in reality bring down the real costs of accessing services for clients. These include, for example, bringing services closer to clients or improving the quality of care. These and wider organizational issues can play an important part in improving the supply of maternal healthcare services (Ensor and Ronoh, 2005; Gilson et al., 2007).

Supply-side approaches to reducing financial barriers for users

Fee exemption

An exemption is defined as an official reduction in direct payments for health care, which is targeted by group, area or service. The current literature distinguishes between waivers, which are granted to individuals, entitling them to free or reduced costs to access all services; and exemptions, which make certain services free or available at reduced cost for all individuals (Bitran and Giedion, 2003).

A mapping exercise on user fees found that 28 out of 50 countries included had introduced reforms to their user fee regimes in recent years (Witter, 2010). In many cases, the focus was on priority groups, particularly pregnant women and young children. West African countries feature prominently in this prioritization, but the approach extends to other parts of the world. Table 7.3 lists the 28 countries which introduced reforms (some have had more than one reform), of which half focus on delivery care (either exclusively or together with curative services for young children). Most of the fee exemption policies are national in scope, while the demand-side programmes such as vouchers are typically piloted at sub-national level.

Many fee exemption policies are now in the process of being evaluated. A review of evaluation evidence from Ghana and Senegal (Witter, 2009) concluded that funded service or group-based exemptions offered a promising way to mitigate inequities and inefficiencies in the health system. However, a number of constraints were noted which made this financing mode inherently unstable and likely to be transitional.

Wholesale removal of user fees

The desirability and realism of removing user fees for all basic health care have been examined in the literature. Conclusions emphasize the importance of tackling supply-side issues at the same time as removing fees so as to address bottlenecks in finance, appropriate staffing and drug supply (Bataringaya, 2003; Pearson, 2004; Witter, 2005). User fees commonly provide one of the few reliable and flexible sources of money at facility level so any change to user fees needs to address the failure of resources to reach facilities in a timely way.

The process of removing user fees also needs to include and 'buy in' key constituencies, including health staff, who often have most to fear due to the combination of reduced flexible income and increased workload (Walker and Gilson, 2004). Official fees should not be replaced by informal payments and alternative financing mechanisms replacing user fees need to be managed well (James et al., 2006).

Table 7.2. Summary of direct strategies to reduce financial barriers for users.

Strategy	Funding	Targeting	Which costs?	Purchasing	Payment systems
Supply side					
Fee exemption or reduction	Public finance or donors	Service based; possible geographical targeting and self-selection	Official fees for services and goods	Health facilities – public, private, private not for profit	Subsidies to inputs or retrospective payment per case to facilities
Waivers	Public finance or donors	Individual or household targeting	Official fees for services and goods	Health facilities – public, private, private not for profit	Payments per case or per capita to facilities
Reducing informal payments	User fees, with possible subsidy component	All services within specific facilities or facility types	Unofficial payments for services and goods	Health facilities – especially public	Internal to facility budget: substitution of official for unofficial payments
Demand side					
Conditional cash transfers	Public finance or donors	Individual or household targeting	Any cost component, potentially – fees, transport, food, opportunity costs	Health facilities – public, private, private not for profit	Payment per client, subject to specified attendance at facilities
Vouchers	Public finance or donors, with possible co-payments	Individual or household targeting usually, though could be geographical	Official fees for services and goods including non-facility costs such as transport	Health facilities – public, private, private not for profit	Payment per case to facilities in exchange for redeemed vouchers
Loans	Public finance, donors, community contributions	Individual and needs-based (sometimes based on credit-worthiness too)	May be restricted to certain costs or situations, or general	Generally administered by community-based organization	Loans to clients with or without fixed limits and interest
Prepayment/ community and social health insurance	Public finance or donors, with possible co-payments	Individual or household targeting usually, though could be geographical	Official fees for services and goods	Health facilities – public, private, private not for profit	Subsidy payment to insurance fund per target client

Waivers

Some of the challenges which waiver systems face are similar to those for exemptions: the need to raise awareness of the scheme; to fund it adequately; to monitor it effectively; and to avoid a conflict of interest for health workers. In addition, waivers raise difficulties of individual targeting, with its associated problems of information asymmetry, stigmatization and

Table 7.3. Recent reforms to user fee regimes in the selected countries (Witter, 2010).

Type of reforms to user fee regime	Countries	Number
Fee exemption for priority groups (delivery care, under-fives, in one case – Senegal – also for elderly)	Senegal, Ghana, Mali, Niger, Benin, Burkina Faso, Burundi, Kenya, Madagascar, North Sudan, Nepal, Sierra Leone	12
Making all basic health care free (either defined by health service level or by a package of care)	Nepal, Zambia, South Africa, Lesotho, Liberia	5
Addressing financial barriers via social health insurance and community health insurance	Tanzania, Kenya, Rwanda, Ghana	4
Insurance programmes targeted at/subsidized for the poor	Indonesia, China, Vietnam	3
All care in the public sector free	Uganda, South Sudan	2
Vouchers for demand-side costs of delivery care	Bangladesh, Cameroon	2
Area-based exemptions	Afghanistan	1
National programmes free (and demand-side incentives for priority areas such as delivery care)	India (and Nepal for delivery care)	1
Health equity funds	Cambodia	1

penalizing the near-poor. The design has to be more complex, including decisions about who grants waivers, what the eligibility criteria are and how they are assessed, how often they are re-assessed, whether they are granted at household or individual level, and what the penalties are for cheating (Bitran and Giedion, 2003). The increased accuracy of targeting has to be traded off against the additional costs (financial, social and political) of targeting.

There is a large body of literature that documents the failure of waiver policies, especially in Africa. Many waiver policies have been almost entirely non-functional, unfunded and granted at the whim of health staff. Coverage has often been low and leakage high (Gilson *et al.*, 1995; Garshong *et al.*, 2001; Bitran and Giedion, 2003; Witter, 2005). In Burkina Faso, extremely impoverished patients suffering a serious obstetric complication should, in theory, be exempt from paying. In practice, few informants were aware of the policy. Those who knew of the policy explained that it was almost impossible to access such schemes due to administrative hurdles. Health-care providers conveyed that it was not uncommon for poor patients to abscond from the hospital (Filippi *et al.*, 2007; Storeng *et al.*, 2008).

One of the most successful waiver schemes has been the health equity fund movement in Cambodia (Hardeman *et al.*, 2004). In order to avoid the conflict of interest for health staff of granting waivers and seeking to maximize revenue, the health equity funds are managed by staff of non-government organizations or other actors external to the health facilities. There is evidence that these have been effective, although they continue to rely heavily on external support and management. Administrative costs were also high – around 30–40% of the subsidies.

Reducing informal payments

Unofficial payments for nominally free government-financed obstetric care have been documented in countries such as Nepal (Borghi *et al.*, 2004), Tanzania (Mamdani and Bangser, 2004), Bangladesh (Nahar and Costello, 1998) and Mauritania (Renaudin, 2007). In ex-communist countries where public funding has collapsed, the growth of informal payments has been particularly severe. In Tajikistan, for example, increasing income inequalities combined with reduced spending and increases in informal payment for health care resulted in a reduction in facility deliveries from 90% in 1989 to 74% in 1998 (Falkingham, 2003). Unofficial payments are made for basic supplies, to provide an incentive to staff and to gain 'better' services.

The relationship between formal fees and informal fees has been debated: does the removal of formal fees lead to increased informal fees (e.g. to supplement health worker incomes) or does the end to formal charging remove an excuse for various additional payments to be levied? Or are they independent variables? Studies have found no pattern of relationship between the proportion of revenues raised from user fees and the reported levels of informal charging (Witter, 2010).

In a well-managed scheme, user fees replaced informal payments and were combined with quality improvements and effective exemptions. This lowered real costs to patients and increased utilization, as seen in a hospital in Cambodia (Akashi, 2004). Any measure to reduce informal payments has to tackle issues of funding, quality and regulation. To eliminate unofficial payments, the bulk of the revenue from official payments should be retained within the facility to finance supplies and salary top-ups. Without retention of fees, there is little motivation for staff to cease their payment collection practices. Fee retention is, however, not sufficient. There is evidence in Latin America that an increase in staff salaries without strong enforcement has little impact on unofficial activities (Di Tella and Savedoff, 2001).

Demand-side approaches to financial barriers

Conditional cash transfers and vouchers

These social transfers aim to reduce financial demand-side barriers while targeting resources to the poorest. This reflects the recognition that supply-side subsidies tend to be captured disproportionately by the better off groups in society. Demand-side measures also have the added potential benefit that they can stimulate competition and improve quality from suppliers. Transfers may be made conditional on the use of particular services. They can take the form of cash, in-kind benefits or 'near cash' benefits such as vouchers.

A review of experiences of social transfers found that their success relies on effective targeting of the poor and on providing subsidies of sufficient value to change behaviour (Chapman, 2006). The transfers were effective at increasing utilization of preventive services, but assumed a functioning health-care system and required substantial management capacity. An overview of conditional cash schemes relating to health in low and middle income countries (mostly drawn from Latin America) concluded that they have potential to increase service uptake, but that their impact on health outcomes is less sure, given quality and supply constraints (Lagarde et al., 2007).

A number of large-scale conditional cash transfer and voucher schemes focused on maternal health care have recently been rolled out in Asia, including in India, Nepal, Cambodia and Bangladesh. One of the largest is the Janani Suraksha Yojana (JSY) programme in India, which was launched in 2005 to increase deliveries in health facilities among the poor. A recent process evaluation concluded that there had been an increase in utilization of health services, but that the local decision to include home deliveries had led to a perversion of the original goals (Devadasan et al., 2008). An evaluation of a policy in Nepal, which combined fee exemption with conditional cash transfers and payments to health workers, concluded that the payments had affected behaviour (Powell-Jackson et al., 2008). Women exposed to the scheme were 24% more likely to use government health institutions, 5% less likely to deliver at home and 13% more likely to have a skilled attendant at delivery. However, there was no evidence that the scheme increased use of life-saving obstetric surgery (Caesarean sections).

An evaluation of a pilot voucher scheme for deliveries in Cambodia concluded that utilization was increased but that there were problems of targeting and uptake (Por et al., 2008). In its first year of operation 43% of the pregnant women (pre-identified at village level as poor) who were given vouchers used them to deliver in facilities. This relatively low uptake may be linked to other barriers of access (such as the non-availability of transport at night), concerns over staff attitudes and the difficulty of leaving home unattended. The authors of the study also estimate that 75–85% of poor pregnant women were excluded, probably because of poor preselection by village volunteers and chiefs and also because of the low frequency of visits to villages by voucher management agents.

An evaluation of the maternal healthcare voucher pilot in Bangladesh has concluded it significantly increased deliveries by skilled birth attendants at home, institutional deliveries and antenatal and postnatal services in intervention areas as compared to control health facilities (Schmidt et al., 2010). In addition, there was a significant reduction in out-of-pocket expenditures for antenatal, postnatal and delivery care in intervention areas compared to control areas (Hatt et al., 2010). On the other hand, operational and financial management issues were highlighted, including compliance with eligibility criteria for beneficiaries, delays in disbursement of cash incentives and gift box to voucher users, inadequate quality of care at facilities, limited involvement of private and non-government facilities and insufficient monitoring. Choice of provider has not been increased because in most areas there is only one facility providing services of adequate standard. The evaluation also suggests that the cost per extra delivery provided through the scheme is substantially above the usual average cost of a delivery. Much of the additional outlay is explained by the high costs of administering the system.

The social transfer approach presupposes a network of suppliers with the capacity to offer services of reasonable quality. There are also relatively high costs incurred to identify target groups, administer the disbursements and independently verify outputs. A recent systematic review found that the value of transfers as a proportion of the overall programme cost ranged from 4% in Mexico to 8% in Nicaragua, 16% in Colombia and 28% in Honduras (Lagarde et al., 2007). An evaluation of a cash transfer scheme in Ecuador found that child health improved, despite the unconditional nature of the transfers, raising questions over the importance of conditionalities (Paxson and Schady, 2007).

Loan schemes and revolving funds

One alternative to exemption schemes is loans. Loan schemes to assist with the costs associated with childbirth have been piloted in several countries, including Sierra Leone (Fofana et al., 1997) and Nepal (Neupane, 2004). One scheme in Nigeria offered loans for costs related to complications in pregnancy, repayable with an interest rate of 2% (Chiwuzie et al., 1997). It was administered by the local clans and four-fifths of the funds were raised by local communities. After 1 year of operation, repayment rates were 93%. Loans were used to pay for transport, fees, blood and drugs.

In general, loans enable repayment of costs incurred over a longer time frame with incremental repayments with or without interest. There have been some initial successes but implementation depends on strong community leadership and mobilization. Scaling up on a significant scale has not been reported. Access for the poorest is also a problem as such groups are not regarded as credit worthy.

Revolving drug funds have been implemented widely under the Bamako Initiative but not usually for maternity care. However, in Nebbi, Nigeria, a revolving fuel fund was established to pay for emergency obstetric referrals by commercial transport. It was found to improve the speed of access, though within the course of 2 years the funds were depleted due to defaulting (Shehu et al., 1997). This reflects a common challenge faced by revolving funds (Cross et al., 1986; Gamaleldin, 2000; Witter, 2007).

Community health insurance and prepayment schemes

Community health insurance and prepayment schemes are terms that are often used interchangeably. Their aim is to spread risks across members and over time, but many depend substantially on donor and government support for their financial sustainability. In Rwanda, for example, only 11% of costs were covered by members' premia (Schneider et al., 2001).

A review of community health insurance schemes found evidence that most reduce out-of-pocket payments by members, while increasing their utilization of health care (Jakab and Krishnan, 2001; Ekman, 2004; Franco *et al.*, 2006; Schneider and Hanson, 2006). Other studies have found more mixed results. In Ghana women who were beneficiaries were more likely to deliver in a hospital but in Mali and Senegal association between delivery with a modern provider and insurance coverage could not be demonstrated (Diop *et al.*, 2006). A review of three West African countries found that membership in a scheme was positively associated with the use of maternal health services, particularly in areas where utilization rates were very low, and more expensive care (Smith and Sulzbach, 2008).

The scale of community health insurance and its role in improving maternity care access is less documented in Asia. A scheme in China was started in the 1980s to help women set aside sufficient funds for childbirth. Services covered and payment levels varied across the scheme, but one study found a willingness to pay more for a wider range of services (Xu *et al.*, 2002).

Social health insurance

Social health insurance is distinguished from community health insurance by being a national scheme with mandatory contributions taken from the pay of the formally employed. It tends to focus on a broader package of health care, rather than being specifically focused on maternity care. However, by including protection against delivery costs it is a potentially useful tool to increase access to skilled care at delivery. A number of developing countries are currently introducing or developing social health insurance models.

A scheme directed at maternity care was introduced in Bolivia in 1996 (Dmytraczenko *et al.*, 1998). The overall percentage of births attended by skilled personnel rose from 42% in 1998 to 54% in 2002 (Nanda *et al.*, 2005). Although it was labelled an insurance scheme, it has more in common with a large-scale exemption scheme as the funding is largely public, rather than based on members' contributions. The equity gap has been closing but remains high, while increases in coverage have been slowing down in recent years. The

scheme is thought to have contributed to declines in maternal, infant and child mortality (PAHO/WHO, 2007). A similar scheme is being developed in Paraguay (World Bank, 2006). Other social health insurance programmes reporting improvements in maternity coverage are found in Chile (PAHO/WHO, 2007). Peru's integrated health insurance fund for pregnant women and children reported a 10% rise in skilled delivery care attendance between 2000 and 2004 but documented implementation problems included budget shortfalls, uneven implementation, lack of support for access costs, variations in staffing and poor referral systems.

Varying successes have been reported in reaching marginalized groups. Colombia's use of a refined individual targeting technique to provide subsidized health insurance for the disadvantaged raised insurance coverage in the poorest quintile of the population from well under 10% in the early 1990s to nearly 50% 4 years later (Gwatkin *et al.*, 2004). Indonesia has had a government-funded health insurance programme targeted at the poor ('Askeskin') since 2005, which includes maternal health benefits. Three-quarters of midwives in an evaluation study did not use the fee-exemption scheme (Makowiecka *et al.*, 2008). The incentives to providers may in part explain the differing performance of these schemes. At the referral level, however, the insurance was found to be more effective. Insurance for the poor covered 51% of women at Serang Hospital and 73% of the women at Pandeglang (Quayyum *et al.*, 2010). Without the insurance for the poor, many households would have been pushed into poverty: around 68% of the poorest users would have had to make catastrophic payments.

In Africa the country with the highest uptake of social health insurance is Ghana, which launched its National Health Insurance Scheme (NHIS) in 2005. Since then, membership has increased to 45% of the population, fuelled in large part by the inclusion of large exempted population groups. From July 2008, this included all pregnant women. While uptake of services is increasing for members, there are concerns about the financial sustainability of the scheme and other operational features, such as reimbursing providers on time.

A recent review article concluded that 'some trade-offs will be necessary between the existing wide benefits package of the NHIS and the laudable desire to reach universal coverage' (Witter and Garshong, 2009).

In general, evidence suggests that 'social health insurance schemes can achieve high coverage rates in middle-income settings with a large formal sector and when the institutional and administrative capacity exists to enforce the payment of premiums' (Borghi and Lissner, 2006).

Addressing Financial Barriers for Providers

Reforms that aim to reduce financial barriers for users have to ensure that provider income is maintained. In order to provide an effective service of adequate quality, it is critical that resources (especially wages, funds for drugs and other supplies and investments in equipment and facilities) reach the providers in adequate quantities and in a timely and predictable way. As maternity care is an integral part of the health system, it is very much affected by shortfalls and weaknesses in delivering these resources. These have knock-on effects on the demand side: if facilities are underfunded, there is a high probability of costs being passed on to users, in the form of increased user fees, increased informal payments and/or the requirement to purchase items such as drugs and supplies outside facilities. Costs to households vary by context but one study in Ghana found that in some cases facilities were charging more than the full cost of services to clients (Levin et al., 2003).

Using data from Ghana in 2002, a scenario from a district hospital is illustrated in Plate 5. All funding sources were low and irregular apart from administrative costs (low but regular) and user charges, which filled the gap and constituted the main financing source for the facility.

It is also recognized that motivating health workers is a key step in providing high quality maternity care. The World Health Report 2005 states that doctors in low income countries can often earn as much as six or seven times their salary in private practice (WHO, 2005). The 'coping strategies' adopted by health workers in under-funded situations is well documented (Van Leberghe et al., 2002) and can work against public policy objectives. In many African countries an absolute shortage of key health workers is also a major constraint for the health sector (Dovlo, 2003).

The three areas of current focus for improving provider motivation are:

1. Budget and public system finance reforms, which focus on improving the reliability and adequacy of resources at facility level, particularly for primary care.
2. Contracting out and in of services.
3. Paying for performance.

All three rely for their success on the overall adequacy of resources. All three are responses to core system weaknesses, which typically include: resource allocation systems which favour higher level facilities and urban areas; cumbersome financial systems, which limit the flexible use of resources; unpredictable flows from government and donors; and financial systems that do not reward performance. All of these inhibit good service planning and delivery.

Public finance reforms

Public finance reforms tackle the core problem driving all other reforms. If health systems could target and deliver resources efficiently according to needs and provider activities, there would be no need for parallel channels, which contracting out and paying for performance tend to establish. Contracting out offers additional potential to harness competitive forces (if alternative competent providers exist) and paying for performance can focus on aligning the incentives of providers with public policies. However, no reform mechanism can succeed (or be sustained without considerable external inputs) without a minimal degree of systemic capacity. Public finance reforms, allied with other managerial changes, are therefore a bed-rock for all initiatives to improve the supply of care.

One of the weaknesses of many public finance systems is the strict control of line budgets. This often prevents facilities spending without high-level approval. Although these controls are often in place because of genuine worries about weak governance, they severely constrain a facility's ability to provide effective services. Public finance reforms often focus on providing facilities with the ability to utilize budgets according to their own local plans through the provision of facility cash balances. Facility funds, for example, provide small cash budgets for health centres that allow them to undertake minor maintenance and replacement of broken consumables. These funds appear to have had a positive impact on service availability in Kenya (Opwora *et al.*, 2009).

A further change is to take a longer term perspective on programming budgets, vital when addressing medium- to long-term goals such as a reduction in maternal or child mortality. The Medium Term Budgeting or Expenditure Frameworks were introduced in low-income countries such as Uganda, Malawi and Cambodia. They enabled ministries to plan capital and recurrent budgets over an extended planning period, with annual budgets reflecting these longer term commitments (Fozzard and Foster, 2001). The approach encourages the setting and funding of longer term strategic priorities rather than lurching from annual budget to annual budget.

Contracting out and in

Contracting involves the specification of services to be provided and an agreed price, allowing creation of a clear agreement between purchaser and provider. The strategy usually relies on the existence of a strong non-government service network to channel resources more effectively and/or more equitably than public services. Competitive tendering permits an element of competition (contestability) to be introduced into the provision of services even when there is only one provider. One well known example is PROSALUD in Bolivia, which provides health services in six regions of the country, subsidized by payments in middle-class areas and subsidize funding (Newbrander *et al.*, 2001). In Brazil, the government subsidizes non government organization services, including reproductive health services in poorer areas of the country (Krasovec and Shaw, 2000). Similar schemes operate in Guatemala and a number of other Latin American countries (Rosen, 2000) and in

Cambodia (Gwatkin *et al.*, 2004). A systematic review of contracting out of health care in low and middle income countries found some evidence of increased utilization in underserved areas but it was not clear what strategies had contributed to that effect (Lagarde and Palmer, 2009).

Paying for performance

Pay for performance refers to the transfer of money or material goods conditional on taking a measurable action or achieving a predetermined performance target (Eichler, 2006). Paying for performance is also referred to as results-based financing, performance-based funding and output-based aid.

In high income countries paying for performance is used as a tool for improving quality (Christianson *et al.*, 2007) but it has wider objectives in developing country settings (Eldridge and Palmer, 2009), including:

- to increase the allocative efficiency of health services by encouraging the provision of high priority and cost effective services;
- to increase the technical efficiency by making better use of existing resources such as health staff;
- to improve equity of outcomes, for example, by encouraging expansion of services to hard-to-reach groups.

Paying for performance for providers is clearly premised on the assumption that for these three dimensions to shift a change in behaviour on the provider side is required. If, however, the barriers are more connected with demand-side factors (such as low affordability of services), then paying for performance for providers alone will not be effective.

In low and middle income countries paying for performance of providers can be offered directly to health workers, linked to facility budgets or used to set or supplement budgets in higher organizational units such as health districts or regions. It can also be used at national level, in particular by donor organizations negotiating aid for a national health sector. Clearly, incentives would be expected to operate differently at these different levels. For example, incentives to individuals are likely to be more directly motivating but may undermine cooperation, while organizational incentives might be expected to reinforce cooperation.

A systematic review of paying providers for performance in low and middle income settings (Witter *et al.*, 2012) concluded that the current evidence base is too weak to draw general conclusions, and that more robust and comprehensive studies are needed. However, a robust study from Rwanda found a positive impact on institutional deliveries, preventive care for young children and improved quality of prenatal care (Basinga *et al.*, 2010). The authors found no effect on the number of prenatal care visits or on immunization rates and concluded that the approach had the greatest effect on those services that had the highest payment rates and needed the lowest provider effort.

Conclusion

This overview suggests that most mechanisms for addressing financial barriers to accessing maternal health care in middle and low income countries have some potential for success, if implemented well and in a context-sensitive way. Countries that combine a range of strategies tend to perform strongly as evidenced in Rwanda and Nepal. Much of the research on financing equity underlines the importance of expanding the role of risk pooling mechanisms, preferably financed predominantly from general taxation (Rannan-Eliya and Somananathan, 2006).

A strategy for financing maternal health care aiming ultimately for universal coverage should include the following dimensions. These should be realistically costed and phased in according to local priority needs.

1. Focus on the main financing barrier for households

- Assess affordability of normal delivery costs and emergency obstetric care.
- Break down costs into facility and non-facility components as different strategies are implied for each.
- Address facility costs for normal deliveries by removal of fees or user fee exemptions.

- Where targeting is used, a hierarchy of strategies can be employed that begins by focusing on geographical characteristics that are strongly correlated to poverty, vulnerability and need.
- Address facility costs for emergency obstetric care via universal fee exemption policies.
- Fee exemption requires adequate, reliable and sustained funding of the additional recurrent costs of providing services by providers.
- For non-facility access costs, where these are significant, geographically targeted support in the form of transport or assistance with transport costs may be a high priority.
- Where distances are so large that safe care is simply not within reach even if finance is available, then a combination of moving supply closer to patients and subsidizing patient demand-side costs may be required.

2. Focus on the main supply barriers

- Develop a medium- and long-term plan to extend service infrastructure where significant geographical gaps are identified, planning for both capital costs and recurrent cost implications of such developments.
- Address 'core systems' weaknesses in allocating and channelling public resources to facilities and staff.
- Use clinical assessment tools to identify key quality of care bottlenecks and develop strategies with health professionals to address these.
- Provide the right financial and non-financial package of incentives for health workers to remain in post over time, particularly in underserved areas.
- Bring on board informal providers through incentives to refer women to facilities.
- Identify and address key barriers in service acceptability through participatory research and mobilization at community level.

A pragmatic but effective approach to extending coverage for maternity services is to focus on the main costs of care and target resources on the most vulnerable areas, while developing a health system environment that permits speedy access to emergency obstetric services for all.

References

Akashi, H. (2004) User fees at a public hospital in Cambodia: effects on hospital performance and provider attitudes. *Social Science and Medicine* 58(3), 553–564.

Basinga, P., Gertler, P., Binagwaho, A., Soucat, A., Sturdy, J. and Vermeersch, C. (2010) Paying primary health centres for performance in Rwanda. *Policy research working paper 5190.* World Bank, Washington, DC.

Bataringaya, J. (2003) The abolition of user fees – the Ugandan experience. Conference presentation: Available at: http://www.fic.nih.gov/dcpp/ppts/bataringya2.ppt; http://www.fic.nih.gov/dcpp/ppts/bataringya1.ppt.

Bitran, R. and Giedion, U. (2003) *Waivers and Exemptions for Health Services in Developing Countries.* World Bank, Washington, DC.

Borghi, J. and Lissner, C. (2006) *A Review of Options for Financing Maternal and Newborn Health Care in Less Developed Countries.* WHO, Geneva.

Borghi, J., Ensor, T., Neupane, B. and Tiwari, S. (2004) *Coping with the Burden of the Costs of Maternal Health.* DFID and Options Nepal Safer Motherhood Project, London.

Borghi, J., Ensor, T., Somanthan, A., Lissner, C. and Mills, A. (2006) Mobilising financial resources for maternal health. *Lancet* 368(9545), 1457–1465.

Chapman, K. (2006) *Using Social Transfers to Scale up Equitable Access to Education and Health Services: background paper.* DFID, London.

Chiwuzie, J., Okojie, O., Okolocha, C., Omorogbe, S., Oronsaye, A., Akpala, W., Ande, B., Onoguwe, B. and Oikeh, E. (1997) Emergency loan funds to improve access to obstetric care in Ekpoma, Nigeria. *International Journal of Gynaecology and Obstetrics* 59, S231–S236.

Christianson, J., Leatherman, S. and Sutherland, K. (2007) *Financial Incentives, Healthcare Providers and Quality Improvements: a review of the evidence.* The Health Foundation, London.

Cross, P., Huff, M., Quick, J. and Bates, J. (1986) Revolving drug funds: conducting business in the public sector. *Social Science and Medicine* 22(3), 335–343.

Devadasan, N., Elias, M., John, D., Grahacharya, S. and Ralte, L. (2008) A process evaluation of the Janani Suraksha Yojana in India. In: Richard, F., Witter, S. and De Brouwere, V. (eds) *Financing Obstetric Care.* ITM, Antwerp, pp. 257–274.

Diop, F., Sulzbach, S. and Chankova, S. (2006) *The Impact of Mutual Health Organisations on Social Inclusion, Access to Health Care and Household Income Protection: evidence from Ghana, Senegal and Mali. Working paper.* Abt Associates, Bethesda, Maryland.

Di Tella, R. and Savedoff, W.D. (2001) *Diagnosis Corruption: fraud in Latin America's public hospitals.* Latin American Research Network, Inter-American Development Bank, Washington, DC.

Dmytraczenko, T., Aitken, I., Carrasco, S., Capra Seonane, K., Holley, J., Abramson, W., Valle, A. and Effen, M. (1998) *Evaluation of the National Security Scheme for Mothers and Children in Bolivia.* Abt Associates for PHR, Bethesda, Maryland.

Dovlo, D. (2003) *The Brain Drain and Retention of Health Professionals in Africa.* ADEA Working Group on Higher Education, Accra.

Eichler, R. (2006) *Can Pay for Performance Increase Utilisation by the Poor and Improve the Quality of Health Services? Discussion paper.* Center for Global Development, Washington, DC.

Ekman, B. (2004) Community-based health insurance in low-income countries: a systematic review of the evidence. *Health Policy and Planning* 19, 249–270.

Eldridge, C. and Palmer, N. (2009) Performance-based payment: some reflections on the discourse, evidence and unanswered questions. *Health Policy and Planning* 24(3), 160–166.

Ensor, T. and Ronoh, J. (2005) Impact of organizational change on the delivery of reproductive services: a review of the literature. *International Journal of Health Planning and Management* 20(3), 209–225.

Falkingham, J. (2003) Inequality and changes in women's use of maternal health-care services in Tajikistan. *Studies in Family Planning* 34(1), 32–43.

Farag, M., Nandakumar, A.K., Wallack, S.S., Gaumer, G. and Hodgkin, D. (2009) Does funding from donors displace government spending for health In developing countries? *Health Affairs* 28(4), 1045–1055.

Filippi, V., Ganaba, R., Baggaley, R., Marshall, T., Storeng, K., Sombie, I., Ouattara, F., Ouedrago, T., Akoum, M. and Meda, N. (2007) Health of women after severe obstetric complications in Burkina Faso: a longitudinal study. *Lancet* 370, 1329–1337.

Fofana, P., Samai, O., Kebbie, A. and Sengeh, P. (1997) Promoting the use of obstetric services through community loan funds, Bo, Sierra Leone. *International Journal of Gynaecology and Obstetrics* 59, S225–S230.

Fozzard, A. and Foster, M. (2001) *Changing Approaches to Public Expenditure Management in Low-income Aid Dependent Countries*. United Nations University/World Institute for Development Economics Research, Helsinki.

Franco, L., Dmytraczenko, T., Simpara, C., Burgert, C. and Smith, K. (2006) *Evaluation of the Impact of Mutual Health Organisation and Information, Education and Communication on Utilisation of Maternal Health Care Services in Bla District, Mali. Working paper*. Abt Associates, Bethesda, Maryland.

Gamaleldin, K.M.A. (2000) Management of the revolving drug fund: experience of Khartoum State, Sudan. Dissertation for Masters, University of Bradford, School of Pharmacy, UK.

Garshong, B., Ansah, E., Dakpallah, G., Huijts, I. and Adjei, S. (2001) *'We are still paying': a study on factors affecting the implementation of the exemptions policy in Ghana*. Health Research Unit, Ministry of Health, Accra.

Gertler, P. and van der Gaag, J. (1990) *Modelling the Demand for Health Care: The Willingness to Pay for Medical Care*. World Bank, Washington, DC.

Gilson, L. (1997) The lessons of user fee experience in Africa. *Health Policy and Planning* 12(4), 273–285.

Gilson, L., Russell, S. and Buse, K. (1995) The political economy of user fees with targeting: developing equitable health financing policies. *Journal of International Development* 7(3), 369–401.

Gilson, L., Doherty, J., Loewenson, R. and Francis, V. (2007) *Challenging Inequity through Health Systems, Final report, Knowledge Network on Health Systems*. WHO Commission on the Social Determinants of Health, Geneva.

Gwatkin, D., Bhuiya, A. and Victora, C. (2004) Making health systems more equitable. *Lancet* 364, 1273–1280.

Gwatkin, D., Wagstaff, A. and Yazbeck, A. (2005) *Reaching the Poor with Health, Nutrition and Population Services: what works, what doesn't and why*. World Bank, Washington, DC.

Hardeman, W., Van Damme, W., Van Pelt, M., Por, I., Kimvan, H. and Meessen, B. (2004) Access to health care for all? User fees plus a Health Equity Fund in Sotnikum, Cambodia. *Health Policy and Planning* 19(1), 23–32.

Hatt, L., Nguyen, H., Sloan, N., Miner, S., Magvanjav, O., Sharma, A., Chowdhury, J., Islam, M. and Wang, H. (2010) *Economic Evaluation of Demand-side Financing Program for Maternal Health in Bangladesh*. Abt for GTZ, Bethesda, Maryland.

Jakab, M. and Krishnan, C. (2001) *Community Involvement in Health Care Financing: a survey of the literature on the impacts, strengths and weaknesses*. World Bank, Washington, DC.

James, C., Morris, S.S., Keith, R. and Thompson, A. (2005) Impact on child mortality of removing user fees: simulation model. *British Medical Journal* 331, 747–749

James, C., Hanson, K., McPake, B., Balabanova, D., Gwatkin, D., Hopwood, I., Kirunga, C., Knippenberg, R., Meessen, B., Morris, S., Preker, A., Souteyrand, Y., Tibouti, A., Villeneuve, P. and Xu, K. (2006) To retain or remove user Fees? Reflections on the current debate in low- and middle-income countries: review article. *Applied Health Economics and Health Policy* 5(3), 137–153.

Johns, B., Sigurbjornsdottir, K., Fogstad, H., Zupan, J., Mathai, M. and Tan-Torres Edejer, T. (2007) Estimated global resources needed to attain universal coverage of maternal and newborn health services. *Bulletin of the World Health Organization* 85(4), 256–263.

Krasovec, K. and Shaw, P. (2000) *Reproductive Health Care: linking outcomes to action, WBI working paper*. World Bank Institute, Washington, DC.

Lagarde, M. and Palmer, N. (2009) The impact of contracting out on health outcomes and use of health services in low and middle-income countries. *The Cochrane Database of Systematic Reviews* 7(4), CD008133.

Lagarde, M., Haines, A. and Palmer, N. (2007) Conditional cash transfers for improving uptake of health interventions in low- and middle-income countries: a systematic review. *Journal of the American Medical Association* 298, 1900–1910.

Levin, A., Dmytraczenko, T., McEuen, M., Ssengooba, F., Mangani, R. and Van Dyck, G. (2003) Costs of maternal health care services in three anglophone African countries. *International Journal of Health Planning and Management* 18(1), 3–22.

Makowiecka, K., Achadi, E., Izati, Y. and Ronsmans, C. (2008) Midwifery provision in two districts in Indonesia: how well are rural areas served? *Health Policy and Planning* 23(1), 67–75.

Mamdani, M. and Bangser, M. (2004) Poor people's experiences of health services in Tanzania: a literature review. *Reproductive Health Matters* 12(24), 138–153.

Nahar, S. and Costello, A. (1998) The hidden cost of 'free' maternity care in Dhaka, Bangladesh. *Health Policy and Planning* 13(4), 417–422.

Nanda, G., Switlick, K. and Lule, E. (2005) *Accelerating Progress Towards Achieving the MDG to Improve Maternal Health: a collection of promising approaches.* World Bank, Washington, DC.

Neupane, B. (2004) *Community-based Emergency Funds: an assessment of performance, management, utilisation and sustainability.* National Safer Motherhood Project, Kathmandu.

Newbrander, W., Cueller, C. and Timmons, B. (2001) *The PROSALUD Model for Expanding Access to Health Services.* Management Sciences for Health, Boston, Massachusetts.

Newhouse, J.P. (1993) *Free for all? Lessons from the RAND Health Insurance Experiment.* Harvard University Press, Cambridge and London.

Opwora, A., Kabare, M., Molyneux, S. and Goodman, C. (2009) *The Implementation and Effects of Direct Facility Funding in Kenya's Health Centres and Dispensaries.* Kenya Medical Research Institute funded by Consortium for Research on Equitable Health Systems, Nairobi.

PAHO/WHO (2007) *Social Protection in Health Schemes for Mothers, Newborn and Child Population. Lessons learned from the Latin American regions.* PAHO/WHO, Washington, DC.

Paxson, C. and Schady, N. (2007) *Does Money Matter? The effects of cash transfers on child health and development in rural Ecuador, Impact evaluation series No. 15.* World Bank, Washington, DC.

Pearson, M. (2004) *Issues Paper: The Case for Abolition of User Fees for Primary Health Services.* DFID Health Systems Resource Centre, London.

Por, I., Horeman, D., Narin, S. and Van Damme, W. (2008) Improving access to safe delivery for poor pregnant women: a case study of vouchers plus health equity funds in three health districts in Cambodia. In: Richard, F., Witter, S. and De Brouwere, V. (eds) *Reducing Financial Barriers to Obstetric Care.* ITG Press, Antwerp.

Powell-Jackson, T., Borghi, J., Mueller, D., Patouillard, E. and Mills, A. (2006) Countdown to 2015: tracking donor assistance to maternal, newborn and child health. *Lancet* 368, 1077–1087.

Powell-Jackson, T., Neupane, B., Tiwari, S., Morrison, J. and Costello, A. (2008) *Final Report of the Evaluation of the Safe Delivery Incentive Programme.* DFID, London.

Quayyum, Z., Nadjib, M., Ensor, T. and Sucahya, P.K. (2010) Expenditure on obstetric care and the protective effect of insurance on the poor: lessons from two Indonesian districts. *Health Policy and Planning* 25(3), 237–247.

Rannan-Eliya, R. and Somananathan, A. (2006) Equity in health and health care systems in Asia. In: Jones, A. (ed.) *The Elgar Companion to Health Economics.* Edward Elgar, Cheltenham, UK.

Renaudin, P. (2007) Ensuring financial access to emergency obstetric care: Three years of experience with Obstetric Risk Insurance in Nouakchott, Mauritania. *International Journal of Gynaecology and Obstetrics* 99(2), 183–190.

Rosen, J. (2000) *Contracting for Reproductive Health: a guide.* World Bank, Washington, DC.

Schmidt, J.O., Ensor, T., Hossain, A. and Khan, S. (2010) Vouchers as demand side financing instruments for health care: A review of the Bangladesh maternal voucher scheme. *Health Policy* 96(2), 98–107.

Schneider, P. and Hanson, K. (2006) Horizontal equity in utilisation of care and fairness of health financing: a comparison of micro-health insurance and user fees in Rwanda. *Health Economics* 15, 19–31.

Schneider, P., Diop, F., Maceira, D. and Butera, D. (2001) *Utilization, Cost and Financing of District Health Services in Rwanda.* Partnerships for Health Reform Project, Abt Asociates, Bethesda, Maryland.

Shehu, D., Ikeh, A. and Kuna, M. (1997) Mobilizing transport for obstetric emergencies in northwestern Nigeria. *International Journal of Gynaecology and Obstetrics* 59, S173–S180.

Smith, K. and Sulzbach, S. (2008) Community-based health insurance and access to maternal health services: evidence from three West African countries. *Social Science and Medicine* 66, 2460–2473.

Storeng, K., Baggaley, R., Ganaba, R., Ouattara, F., Akoum, M. and Filippi, V. (2008) Paying the price: The cost and consequences of emergency obstetric care in Burkina Faso. *Social Science and Medicine* 66(30), 545–557.

Thomson, S. and Mossialos, E. (2008) Medical savings accounts; can they improve health system performance in Europe? *Euro Observer* 10(4), 1–4.

Van Leberghe, W., Conceicao, C., Van Damme, W. and Ferrinho, P. (2002) When staff is underpaid: dealing with the individual coping strategies of health personnel. *Bulletin of the World Health Organization* 80(7), 581–584.

Walker, L. and Gilson, L. (2004) We are bitter but we are satisfied: nurses as street-level bureaucrats in South Africa. *Social Science and Medicine* 59, 1251–1261.

WHO (2005) *Make Every Mother and Child Count.* WHO, Geneva.

WHO (2006) *Moving Towards Universal Coverage Series.* WHO, Geneva.

Witter, S. (2005) *An Unnecessary Evil? User fees for health care in low income countries.* Save the Children (UK), London.

Witter, S. (2007) Achieving sustainability, quality and access – lessons from the world's largest revolving drug fund. *East Mediterranean Health Journal* 13(6), 1476–1485.

Witter, S. (2009) Service- and population-based exemptions: are these the way forward for equity and efficiency in health financing in low income countries? *Advances in Health Economics and Health Services Research* 21, 249–286.

Witter, S. (2010) *Mapping User Fees for Health Care in Low-income Countries – evidence from a recent survey.* Health Resource Centre, London.

Witter, S. and Garshong, B. (2009) Something old or something new? Social health insurance in Ghana. *BMC International Health and Human Rights* 9, 20.

Witter, S., Fretheim, A., Kessy, F. and Lindahl, A.K. (2012) Paying for performance to improve the delivery of health interventions in low and middle-income countries. *Cochrane Database of Systematic Reviews* 2; CD00789.

World Bank (2006) *Health Service Delivery in Paraguay: A review of quality of care and policies on human resources and user fees. Report No. 33416-PY.* World Bank, Washington, DC.

Xu, L., Liu, X., Sun, X., Fang, L. and Hindle, D. (2002) Maternal and infant health prepayment schemes in Shandong, China: a survey of demand and supply. *Australian Health Review* 25(3), 15–25.

8   Implementing Clinical Interventions within Maternal Health Programmes

Ana Langer,[1] Hannah Knight,[2] Annabel Charnock,[3]
Mary Nell Wegner[4] and José Villar[2]
[1]*Harvard School of Public Health, Boston, USA;* [2]*University of Oxford, England, UK;*
[3]*Department for International Development, London, UK;* [4]*New York, USA*

Summary
- Safe and effective interventions exist to prevent and treat the major causes of maternal mortality and morbidity which are: postpartum haemorrhage, sepsis, pre-eclampsia/eclampsia, obstructed labour and unsafe abortion.
- To successfully introduce and adopt evidence-based clinical interventions within maternal health programmes, integrated care modalities, a functioning health system, the policy environment and legal and cultural factors have to be considered. An enhanced knowledge base for implementation is also required.
- The evidence-based clinical interventions for prevention and treatment of obstetric complications are as follows:

	Prevention	Treatment
Postpartum haemorrhage	Active management of the third stage of labour Administration of oxytocin or misoprostol	Administration of postpartum oxytocin or misoprostol Uterine massage and compression Balloon tamponade Surgery
Sepsis	Infection control Prophylactic antibiotics for Caesarean section	Antibiotics
Pre-eclampsia/eclampsia	Antenatal care and routine blood pressure monitoring Calcium supplementation Low dose aspirin Magnesium sulphate Delivery	Timely identification of danger signs (at the family, community, and primary health-care facility levels) Magnesium sulphate Delivery
Obstructed labour	Use of the partograph	Instrumental vaginal delivery Caesarean section Symphysiotomy
Unsafe abortion	Contraception Access to safe and legal medical and surgical abortion	Treatment of haemorrhage and infection Surgical procedures

Introduction

The focus of this chapter is on clinical interventions proven to be safe and effective, but which are widely under-utilized in many parts of the world. The challenges associated with improving access to life-saving medical technologies are explored. Recommendations are made on the research and implementation priorities that emerge, with particular emphasis on delivering clinical interventions in the context of maternal health programmes and health systems in developing countries.

The chapter covers best practices proven to be safe and effective during pregnancy and in the immediate postpartum period. The inextricable links between mother and baby mean that most interventions in this chapter, although directed at the mother and primarily intended to save the mother's life, will also have benefits for perinatal health.

The vast majority of maternal and perinatal deaths can be averted with timely access to a set of key clinical life-saving interventions. These evidence-based practices require equipment, procedures and drugs that enable healthcare providers, with appropriate training, to manage a variety of obstetric complications. Of course, these interventions do not function in isolation from the wider health system and the communities in which they are provided. The challenges that the wider health context poses to the provision of maternal health care will also be considered in this chapter.

Clinical Interventions to Reduce Maternal Mortality

Safe, effective and affordable clinical best practices for reducing maternal deaths are available for the five leading causes of maternal mortality: postpartum haemorrhage, sepsis, hypertensive diseases of pregnancy (pre-eclampsia/eclampsia), obstructed labour and unsafe abortion. We also consider innovative technologies that are on the horizon and could potentially contribute to a better quality of maternal care in low resource settings. The recent review by Tsu and Coffey (2009) provides the foundation for this analysis.

Postpartum haemorrhage

An estimated 14 million cases of postpartum haemorrhage occur every year (WHO, 2006a). Despite considerable international attention in recent years, postpartum haemorrhage continues to remain the leading cause of maternal death in developing countries, accounting for over 25% of pregnancy-related mortality (WHO, 2005).

Due to the increased awareness surrounding the condition in the last 5 years, there has been considerable improvement in the uptake of key interventions to prevent postpartum haemorrhage. Progress in identifying effective treatment has been relatively slower.

Prevention through active management of the third stage of labour (AMTSL)

Predicting which women will develop postpartum haemorrhage is difficult. Risk factors include high parity and multiple pregnancies, but most women will have no identifiable risk factors. Once the condition occurs, it quickly becomes life threatening. Since most women in the developing world deliver a considerable distance from well-resourced hospitals, it is essential to make simple preventive measures, such as AMTSL, routine practice for all deliveries. A Cochrane review of five randomized controlled trials involving over 6000 women shows that AMTSL reduces the occurrence of postpartum haemorrhage by 38% and the need for blood transfusion by 34% (Prendiville *et al.*, 2000). AMTSL is inexpensive and does not require the supervision of a doctor, making it applicable to low resource settings with limited access to highly skilled providers.

AMSTL consists of three interventions designed to facilitate the delivery of the placenta:

1. ADMINISTRATION OF UTEROTONIC DRUGS IMMEDIATELY FOLLOWING DELIVERY Oxytocin is the drug of choice and a dose of 10 IU intramuscularly has been shown to reduce the risk of postpartum haemorrhage by 50% compared to no uterotonics (Cotter *et al.*, 2001). A prefilled disposable syringe device (Uniject™) that delivers a precise dose of oxytocin, greatly reducing the potential

for error and misuse has been developed (PATH, 2011). A recent study in Indonesia has shown that these devices are highly user friendly, even for minimally skilled midwives (Tsu *et al.*, 2009). Steps have been made towards making the Uniject™ device commercially available. The first regulatory approval for the device was granted in Argentina in spring 2009 and other countries are following suit. Pilot and programme evaluation studies are currently underway in Honduras, Guatemala, Argentina, South Africa and India.

Although oxytocin requires refrigeration, the drug can be used for up to 3 months if stored at room temperature. PATH has recently added a time-temperature indicator (a small sticker indicating how much heat the product has been exposed to) on to the Uniject™ device. This indicator adds flexibility to the transport and storage of oxytocin in Uniject™, minimizing wastage of active formulations as well as inadvertent use of a heat-spoiled product (PATH, 2011).

2. CONTROLLED CORD TRACTION TO REMOVE THE PLACENTA Controlled cord traction involves traction on the umbilical cord, combined with counter-pressure on the uterus to remove the placenta. The technique is currently the subject of a randomized controlled trial to test whether a simplified package of AMTSL without controlled cord traction might be possible (Gülmezoglu *et al.*, 2009).

3. UTERINE MASSAGE AFTER DELIVERY OF THE PLACENTA, AS APPROPRIATE Abdel-Aleem *et al.* (2006) recently reported an 80% reduction in the need for additional uterotonics in women who received routine AMTSL plus uterine massage, compared with those receiving routine

AMTSL without uterine massage. Further evidence is needed to confirm this benefit.

Treatment

When postpartum haemorrhage occurs, steps to identify the cause of bleeding and interventions to stop it must begin as quickly as possible. Treatment options may be medical, non-medical or surgical and are presented in Table 8.1 in the order in which they should be attempted.

Two recent randomized controlled trials evaluated whether oral misoprostol might be a suitable alternative to oxytocin for the treatment of postpartum haemorrhage (Blum *et al.*, 2010; Winikoff *et al.*, 2010). Both studies concluded that, in settings where oxytocin is not available, misoprostol might be a suitable first-line treatment to stop excessive bleeding.

If medical and non-medical interventions fail to stop the bleeding, the intrauterine balloon tamponade is the least invasive and quickest of the surgical procedures. In Dhaka, Bangladesh, the balloon tamponade was used in 23 women with uterine atony. In all cases, the bleeding ceased within 15 min and there was no need for any further intervention (Akhter *et al.*, 2003). Although the technique shows promise and is recommended as a first-line surgical intervention in resource-poor settings, more research is needed to determine the efficacy of the procedure.

Puerperal sepsis

Between 8 and 12% of all maternal deaths in developing countries are due to puerperal sep-

Table 8.1. Interventions to treat postpartum haemorrhage.

Medical interventions	Oxytocin
	Ergometrine
	Prostaglandins (e.g. misoprostol)
Non-medical interventions	Uterine massage
	Non-surgical uterine compression (e.g. bimanual)
Surgical interventions	Balloon or condom tamponade
	Compression sutures
	Artery ligation (uterine, hypogastric)
	Uterine artery embolization
	Hysterectomy

sis (Khan *et al.*, 2006). Treatment is relatively straightforward, but postnatal supervision of women is key to ensuring a timely diagnosis as it is usually more than 24 h after delivery before the symptoms and signs (fever and/or offensive vaginal discharge) appear. The risk of sepsis is increased in cases of prolonged and/or obstructed labour. Findings from a number of new research studies on obstetric infection are pending, including identification of high-priority pathogens and promising diagnostic tools (M. Gravett, Seattle, 2010, personal communication) and infection control strategies within different developing country health systems (Hussein *et al.*, 2011).

Prevention

HYGIENE   The primary means of preventing infection and sepsis is through high standards of hygiene by medical and midwifery practitioners, including hand washing, use of gloves and gowns, sterilization of equipment and correct disposal of soiled linen. The most important element of this is hand hygiene. Evidence suggests and WHO recommends that antiseptic alcoholic hand rubs are a more effective alternative to hand washing with soap and water (Widmer, 2000; Kampf *et al.*, 2009; WHO, 2009a), yet such hand rubs are not widely available in developing country locations (Mehta *et al.*, 2011).

The use of a clean delivery kit (combined with education on hygiene for mothers) can reduce the incidence of sepsis according to a 2007 trial in Tanzania: 1.1% of women using a clean delivery kit developed sepsis compared to 3.6% of those who did not (Winani *et al.*, 2007). The contents of kits vary, but typically include a 1 m² plastic sheet, pictorial instructions, clean razor blade, string to tie the umbilical cord, and a bar of soap. A systematic review on use of birth kits showed increased likelihood of improved hand hygiene (Hundley *et al.*, 2011).

Routine vaginal cleansing with chlorhexidine during labour has also been suggested as a method of reducing the incidence of maternal and neonatal sepsis and two non-randomized trials in Malawi and Egypt showed some success. However, results from a randomized controlled trial in South Africa, published in 2009, show that chlorhexidine intravaginal and neonatal wipes did not prevent neonatal sepsis

and had no effect on serious maternal postpartum sepsis (Cutland *et al.*, 2009).

PROPHYLACTIC ANTIBIOTICS   A systematic review has shown that routine prophylactic antibiotics for all women undergoing Caesarean section reduced the risk of fever and of wound, womb and urinary tract infections in mothers (Smaill and Gyte, 2010). There is currently insufficient evidence to determine whether prophylactic antibiotics should also be routine for operative vaginal delivery, i.e. forceps and vacuum (Liabsuetrakul *et al.*, 2004). However, evidence suggests that antibiotic prophylaxis during the second or third trimester of pregnancy should be considered for high risk women (Thinkhamrop *et al.*, 2002). Given the number of women living with HIV/AIDS, questions remain on whether affected women should receive prophylactic antibiotics and, if so, what regimes are optimal (Sebitloane *et al.*, 2007).

ISOLATION AND BARRIER MIDWIFERY CARE   Isolation and barrier midwifery care should be practised to prevent the spread of infection to other women. Women with sepsis should be cared for in a separate room or a corner of the ward and, when treating infected women, extra care should be exercised in: hand hygiene; the use of dedicated gloves, gowns and equipment; and careful disposal of soiled dressings and linen. If possible, a nurse/midwife should be specifically allocated to the care of the infected woman.

Treatment

Without antibiotic treatment of the infection, sepsis will cause death (Stade *et al.*, 2004). For the general treatment of sepsis, the WHO recommends a regime of ampicillin (2 g IV every 6 h), gentamicin (5 mg/kg body weight IV every 24 h) and metronidazole (500 mg IV every 8 h) until the woman is fever-free for 48 h. For endometritis, a systematic review found that intravenous gentamicin plus clindamycin was more effective than other antibiotic regimes (French and Smail, 2004).

Rehydration (oral or IV) for women with sepsis is also key. Where the cause of sepsis is suspected to be retained placental fragments, a digital examination should be performed and any fragments removed, using forceps or a large curette if necessary. In severe cases, a laparotomy or hysterectomy may become necessary.

Pre-eclampsia and eclampsia

Pre-eclampsia is a multisystem disorder that complicates around 3% of pregnancies. Eclampsia is a much less common condition, complicating 0.05–1% of pregnancies in the developing world, but carrying a much higher risk of death for the mother. It is estimated that these two conditions together kill around 40,000 women each year, mainly in the developing world (Villar *et al.*, 2003), and accounting for 9–26% of direct maternal deaths in low and middle income countries (Khan *et al.*, 2006). Effective primary prevention is not possible because the causes are still unknown. However, with early detection and appropriate management of pre-eclampsia, the outcome for mothers and their babies can be greatly improved.

Prevention

ANTENATAL CARE   Several studies have shown that the risk of developing eclampsia is elevated in women without access to antenatal care (Abi Said *et al.*, 1995; MacKay *et al.*, 2001). The essential antenatal activities for detecting pre-eclampsia are routine blood pressure monitoring and testing urine for traces of protein after 20 weeks of gestation. These interventions have been implemented in developing country settings using a variety of simple strategies (MacGillivray *et al.*, 2004; McCaw-Binns *et al.*, 2004).

In 2001, WHO published the results of a large multicentre randomized controlled trial that compared the standard model of antenatal care with a new model that involves fewer clinic visits, emphasizing actions known to be effective in improving maternal and neonatal outcomes, including detection of pre-eclampsia. A minimum of four visits is recommended for an uncomplicated pregnancy. The results of the WHO trial suggest that the reduced number of visits did not result in more adverse maternal or perinatal outcomes

than with the traditional model and may reduce cost (Villar *et al.*, 2001).

CALCIUM SUPPLEMENTATION AND ASPIRIN   A systematic review involving 12 trials and 15,206 women concluded that calcium supplementation during pregnancy reduces the risk of pre-eclampsia by 48% (95% CI 0.33–0.69) and that the greatest benefit is for high risk women and women with low baseline calcium intake (Hofmeyr *et al.*, 2006). While not as effective as calcium, there is some evidence that low dose aspirin has some effectiveness as a preventive measure (Ruano *et al.*, 2005; Askie *et al.*, 2007).

MAGNESIUM SULPHATE   Strong evidence of the effectiveness of magnesium sulphate for women with eclampsia has been available since 1995 (Eclampsia Trial Collaborative Group, 1995). The results of the Magpie Trial, published in 2002, provide convincing evidence that magnesium sulphate is also effective for the *prevention* of eclampsia (Magpie Trial Collaborative Group, 2002). However, the drug is still not on the essential medicines list in many developing countries (Aaeserud *et al.*, 2005), while less effective and higher risk drugs such as diazepam and phenytoin are still widely used.

Unfortunately, the translation of this evidence into practice has been slow (Box 8.1). One promising solution is a simple flow-controlled pump (SpringFusor, Go Medical Industries, Subiaco, Australia) for safe and simpler administration of the drug. This technology is currently the subject of a trial by Gynuity Health Projects (2011) to explore the safety and feasibility of its use in health-care facilities without an intensive care unit.

The best regimen for magnesium sulphate administration is unclear. Some evidence suggests that a purely intramuscular route can be safely used in places where skills and equipment for intravenous use are not available (Begum *et al.*, 2001). Two studies from Bangladesh have suggested that a loading dose of magnesium sulphate alone may be sufficient for the majority of women with pre-eclampsia (Begum *et al.*, 2002; Shamsuddin

---

Box 8.1. Making magnesium sulphate available.

There is strong evidence for the use of magnesium sulphate for the prevention and treatment of eclampsia. In developed countries, magnesium sulphate has been the standard treatment for 20 years – so how do we account for the failure to use it in many developing countries?

Lack of relevant knowledge

Magpie Trial collaborators interviewed by Aaserud *et al.* (2005) expressed a view that 'few clinicians or policy makers in their settings were aware of the concept of evidence-based medicine, would read the Magpie Trial report, or be able to interpret the findings'. Respondents from South Africa and Asia also expressed concern regarding lack of knowledge on how to administer magnesium sulphate and the need for training. Sevene *et al.*'s (2005) study in Mozambique suggested lack of knowledge among clinicians as a major barrier, resulting in lack of requests for the drug and its unavailability. In Zimbabwe, blame for the drug's lack of availability was accorded to a lack of knowledge on the part of both the policy makers and clinicians.

Not registered for use

For health-care professionals to have access to magnesium sulphate its inclusion on the national essential medicines list is vital. Although the drug is on WHO's Model Essential Medicines List, a survey found that it was not licensed for the treatment of pre-eclampsia in 7 out of 13 low-income countries (Aaserud *et al.*, 2005). In Mozambique, lack of access was the result of a complex and ineffi-cient system of drug approval, acquisition and distribution. In Zimbabwe, magnesium sulphate had not been registered for use. One reason offered is that the low cost of the drug removes any incentive on the part of manufacturers to maximize its use (Sevene *et al.*, 2005).

Lack of guidelines

Aaserud *et al.*'s (2005) survey revealed that in 8 out of 13 low and lower-middle income countries national clinical guidelines for pre-eclampsia were absent, leading to a failure to provide magnesium sulfate when necessary. Those based in Latin America expressed a different concern: overuse of mag-nesium sulphate in situations not supported by recent evidence, indicating a failure to disseminate best practice guidelines effectively. In Mozambique, the study by Sevene *et al.* (2005) revealed obstetri-cians' frustration with the failure to ensure that guidelines were put into practice nationally.

Political barriers

Barriers identified included lack of political will, insufficiently involved or poorly informed policy makers and lack of prioritization of eclampsia/pre-eclampsia (Aaserud *et al.*, 2005). Concern was also expressed that clinicians have limited ability to influence the policy-making process, a reflection in part of the weakness of professional associations in much of the developing world.

---

et al., 2005). These findings need to be con-firmed by additional research.

Treatment by timely delivery

Ultimately, delivery is the only effective treat-ment for pre-eclampsia/eclampsia and is rec-ommended for:

- All women with preeclampsia at >37 weeks gestation.
- All women with severe pre-eclampsia, within 24 h of the onset of the symptoms, regardless of gestational age.

- All women with eclampsia, within 12 h of the onset of convulsions, regardless of gestational age (WHO, 2008).

If the cervix (the neck of the womb) is favour-able (soft, thin and partly dilated), induction of labour and vaginal delivery should be possible. If the cervix is unfavourable, deliv-ery should be by Caesarean section (WHO, 2008), although this introduces other life-threatening risks for the mother and new-born, including haemorrhage, anaesthetic complications and prematurity. Some groups suggest that use of misoprostol to induce labour is one possible way to effect vaginal delivery (Lapaire *et al.*, 2007).

Obstructed and prolonged labour

Between 4 and 13% of maternal deaths worldwide are believed to be the result of obstructed labour (Khan *et al.*, 2006). Furthermore, obstructed labour often leaves those who survive with a fistula, or an anatomical communication between the birth canal, the urethra and/or the rectum resulting in urine or faeces leakage or both. It is estimated that 2–3 million women around the world are currently living with untreated obstetric fistula, which results in health complications of different degrees of severity, great social stigmatization and often isolation. Every year another 50,000 to 100,000 more women join their ranks (WHO, 2006b).

Some cases of obstructed labour will unavoidably end in death unless the woman receives a Caesarean section but in other cases obstructed labour can be avoided by timely detection of prolonged labour and effective management and treatment. Unfortunately, trials of means to predict when obstructed labour might occur, for example by x-ray assessment or measuring maternal height and shoe size, have had mixed results and suggest they are not wholly reliable indicators (Liselele *et al.*, 2000; Pattinson, 2000; Rozenholc *et al.*, 2007).

Prevention

PARTOGRAPH   Key to timely identification of prolonged labour and prevention of obstructed labour and fistula formation is use of the partograph. The partograph is a simple graphic depiction of the progress of labour with a number of simple indicators. It typically includes 'action' and 'alert' lines to ensure the timely diagnosis of prolonged labour. Its use is recommended by WHO, with evidence from a large trial in Indonesia, Malaysia and Thailand showing a reduction in prolonged labour, operative vaginal deliveries by forceps and Caesarean section rates (WHO, 1994, 1996). However, a systematic review found inconclusive evidence to support the use of the partograph although it noted that two studies from low income countries did show a reduction in Caesarean rates with its use (Lavender *et al.*, 2008). Further research to establish its efficacy is required and WHO continues to recommend its use.

AUGMENTATION OF LABOUR   Standard measures to prevent prolonged labour include amniotomy (rupturing of membranes surrounding the fetus) and intravenous oxytocin where indicated. A systematic review concluded that 'a policy of early routine augmentation for mild delays in labour progress resulted in a modest reduction of the Caesarean section rate compared with expectant management' (Wei *et al.*, 2009).

Treatment

INSTRUMENTAL VAGINAL DELIVERY   Forceps extraction and vacuum extraction are internationally accepted assisted methods for a timely, safe vaginal delivery. Use of vacuum extraction is associated with lower risk of severe maternal injury (OR 0.41, 95% CI 0.33–0.50) when compared to forceps delivery. Serious injury to the newborn was not common (Johanson and Menon, 1999). WHO recommends that training of relevant personnel is important to ensure that vacuum extraction is the first choice for instrument-aided vaginal delivery (Althabe, 2002).

CAESAREAN SECTION   In a proportion of cases of obstructed labour the only way to save the mother's and the fetus's lives is to perform a Caesarean section. There are relatively complex health system requirements to perform this surgical procedure safely, especially in low resource settings. A number of adaptations can increase the ease with which the procedure can be performed. These include simplified surgical ('Joel-Cohen based') techniques, which have been shown to have a number of advantages including reduced blood loss, operating time, use of pain killers and fever (Hofmeyr *et al.*, 2008). Training appropriate personnel in these techniques is crucial – experience in Mozambique suggests that not only obstetricians but also assistant medical officers can be trained to safely use these techniques (Pereira *et al.*, 1996).

SYMPHYSIOTOMY Symphysiotomy is an alternative surgical procedure that can facilitate a vaginal birth by means of a simple technique to separate the pelvic bones and enlarge their capacity. Little used in high income countries, it has received renewed attention in the past decade because of its potential benefits in low resource settings where Caesarean sections are not available. A review of 5000 cases concluded that symphysiotomy was safe for the mother and life-saving for the newborn (Björklund, 2002). The WHO Integrated Management of Pregnancy and Childbirth manual recommends its use in certain situations (WHO, 2000).

Obstetric fistula

Following a prolonged or obstructed labour, an indwelling bladder catheter can prevent the formation of fistula. If a fistula does form, a careful regimen, including continuation of the indwelling bladder catheter, twice daily cleansing of the perineum and vagina and gentle excising of any necrotic tissue can result in spontaneous closure of around 15–20% of select, simple or small fistula. For other fistulas reparative surgery is the only treatment. Increasing access to this surgery requires addressing a widespread lack of trained staff and necessary facilities as well as the social, economic and cultural factors that prevent women from seeking treatment. Dedicated national strategies for the prevention and treatment of obstetric fistula are recommended (WHO, 2006b). Universally accepted fistula classification and standardized training programmes are being developed (Elneil and Browning, 2009).

Unsafe abortion

Each year, 68,000 deaths occur as a result of unsafe abortion, which accounts for one in eight maternal deaths (WHO, 2004a). Despite the dramatically increased use of contraception over the past three decades, an estimated 40–50 million abortions still occur annually, almost half of which are performed in circumstances that are unsafe (Grimes *et al.*, 2006).

Contraception – reducing the need for unsafe abortion

From a physical and mental health perspective, the prevention of unwanted and unplanned pregnancies is a better option than termination and is more cost effective for the health system (Prata *et al.*, 2010). Contraception is more accepted than abortion in most cultures, is more widely available and has a number of health benefits for the woman and her children.

Contraceptive methods include natural and fertility based methods, hormonal contraceptives (including implants, injectables, special devices and pills) and surgical procedures. Emergency contraception is an important addition to the menu of choices. While current methods of emergency contraception are most effective if used as soon as possible after sexual intercourse and before ovulation, a recent study shows that ulipristal acetate provides women and health-care providers with an effective alternative for emergency contraception that can be used up to 5 days after unprotected sexual intercourse (Glasier *et al.*, 2010). Making contraception widely available, including marketing a single-dose regimen of emergency contraception for over-the-counter purchase, is a priority.

Family planning for women admitted to facilities with post-abortion complications is often overlooked, particularly for unmarried women and adolescents (Grimes *et al.*, 2006). To reduce the risk of future unwanted pregnancies it is important to integrate post-abortion care and family planning services. Post-abortion patients have been shown to choose and continue to use contraception at high rates (Billings and Benson, 2005; Ceylan *et al.*, 2009). One study in Zimbabwe showed a 50% reduction over 1 year in unintended pregnancies and repeat abortion in patients who received contraceptive counselling and provision at the time of treatment compared with post-abortion patients who did not receive such services (Johnson *et al.*, 2002).

Procedures for safe abortion

Where carefully performed, abortion is one of the safest procedures in contemporary clinical practice, with case fatality rates less than 1 death per 100,000 procedures. However, around 26% of the world's population live where abortion is prohibited altogether or allowed only to save the woman's life (Center for Reproductive Rights, 2006). Under clandestine and unsafe conditions, the estimated case fatality rate rises to 367 deaths per 100,000 unsafe abortions, over 300 times higher than that for safe legal abortion in developed nations (WHO, 2004a).

MEDICAL ABORTION There is increasing evidence that misoprostol is a safe, effective and acceptable method to achieve uterine evacuation for abortion and post-abortion care (Wedisinghe and Elsandabesee, 2010). Nurses and midwives can safely provide first-line post-abortion care services, including in outpatient settings, provided they receive appropriate training and support (Tsu and Coffey, 2009).

For first trimester induced pregnancy terminations, a combination of misoprostol and mifepristone is recommended. However, the cost and limited availability of mifepristone has led to the evaluation of misoprostol alone and in combination with methotrexate. As methotrexate is not expensive and is widely accessible, combined methotrexate regimens (oral or intramuscular methotrexate followed by misoprostol a few days later) may be a good option in locations where access to mifepristone is limited (Tsu and Coffey, 2009).

For second trimester abortions between 13 and 24 weeks, a recent study in South Africa found a single regimen of misoprostol alone was successful in 91% of 273 women (van Bogaert and Sedibe, 2007).

MANUAL VACUUM ASPIRATION (MVA) MVA is a simple cost-effective procedure involving the use of suction to remove tissue and blood through a cannula and into a syringe. It does not require general anaesthesia and does not need to be performed in an operating room.

The technique has been shown to be highly effective in removing retained products of conception from the uterus and has been repeatedly associated with a lower complication rate than the traditional techniques of dilatation and curettage (Association of Reproductive Health Professionals, 2011). In one district hospital in Kenya, where the treatment protocol was changed from dilatation and curettage under general anaesthesia to MVA using local anaesthesia, the average cost of treating a patient fell by 66% (Johnson *et al.*, 1992).

In recent years advances have been made in MVA technology. For example, the double-valve aspirator has been redesigned to improve ease of cleaning and allow for boiling or autoclaving, with very little increase in cost (Hyman and Castleman, 2005). There is also some evidence that mid-level providers such as midwives and nurses can be trained to use MVA, as well as doctors (Warriner *et al.*, 2006).

A recent study has shown that for incomplete abortions MVA is slightly more effective than oral misoprostol but may be less acceptable to women. Misoprostol is well suited for use in low-resource settings and should be promoted as an option for the treatment of incomplete abortion (Bique *et al.*, 2007).

Managing the complications of unsafe abortion

It is estimated that between 10% and 50% of all women who experience unsafe abortion need medical care for complications such as incomplete abortion, sepsis, haemorrhage and intra-abdominal injury (e.g. puncturing and tearing of the uterus) (Shaikh *et al.*, 2010). Components of emergency post-abortion care include: management of shock; control of bleeding; and treatment of sepsis and surgical procedures for intra-abdominal injuries. It is also vital that health-care providers are trained to recognize the signs and symptoms of abortion complications, as women may be reluctant to reveal their attempts at termination in contexts where abortion is legally restricted and/or stigmatized.

Implementing Clinical Interventions

Great progress has been made in identifying single safe and effective interventions for the major causes of maternal morbidity and mortality over the last decade. However, there are a number of issues to consider for effective implementation of these clinical interventions: the need to package interventions to address maternal health issues holistically, the health system context and the actual delivery or implementation of interventions.

Integrated care

Targeted cause-specific interventions alone will not solve the multiplicity of maternal health needs often present in individual women. In reality maternal health conditions do not exist in isolation. Frequently, pregnant women have compound needs and conditions and simply trying to act on one of them, as most targeted interventions have been designed to do, will not affect the overall outcome of safe childbirth sufficiently. It is important to consider what is required when co-morbidities exist and multiple needs are present simultaneously. Reviews of causes of maternal death have demonstrated that a large proportion of women die from a combination of complications that may also include underlying medical conditions such as HIV/AIDS, malaria, anaemia or other conditions typically correlated with pregnancy (Sloan et al., 2001; Graham and Hussein, 2003; Fottrell et al., 2007).

In addition, maternal health is part of broader sexual and reproductive health; programmes and individual services need to adopt a holistic approach in order to be effective. For instance, family planning is one of the best interventions to reduce maternal mortality (Ross and Blanc, 2009) but maternal health and family planning services are usually separated and often isolated within health-care facilities or systems. To accelerate the progress of improved maternal health, comprehensive programmes need to be delivered, with complex interventions that address women's holistic needs.

The health system

Addressing maternal health needs requires a functional health system and coordination among its multiple components. The WHO estimates that one-third of the world's population is without access to the essential medicines and other health commodities it needs (WHO, 2004b). In many countries, the supply and distribution of health commodities in the public sector are ad hoc, with unauthorized private distribution, counterfeit medicines and poor accountability mechanisms (DFID, 2004). Logistical systems comprising warehouses, transport equipment, transportation routes and inventory quantities are required for differing product requirements (short shelf-life, cold chain, limited suppliers), especially for remote communities. Integrated logistics systems improve efficiency and sustainability and have been adopted in Bolivia, Zambia and Mali, where several different essential health commodities can be stored, delivered and ordered together (Rao, 2008). Price competition in the market, promoting bulk procurement, negotiating equitable pricing for newer essential medicines, reducing mark ups through more efficient distribution and dispensation and encouraging local production of essential medicines have also been recommended to improve supply and distribution of maternal health commodities (Travis et al., 2004).

Lack of access is not only relevant to supplies and commodities but also relevant to safe effective and affordable interventions. This lack of access occurs for a number of reasons: because a product or intervention is unavailable or not offered because of a lack of trained health-care providers; because of gender-related issues that prevent women from seeking care without permission from relatives; because of broader issues such as lack of transportation; or simply because health services are unaffordable. The cost of life-saving care can be financially crippling, especially to the poorer members of society (see Witter and Ensor, Chapter 7 this volume). Shortages in health-care personnel are especially crucial in ensuring access to the essential clinical interventions necessary to make childbirth safe. It is estimated that over

800,000 additional doctors and nurses are required to address current demand (WHO, 2009b). There is a 100-fold difference in the ratio of nurses to population between some African nations and the USA (Buchan, 2006) and in sub-Saharan Africa two-thirds of countries have just one medical school and some countries have none (Narasimhan *et al.*, 2004). Absenteeism is another key concern. In small rural health posts in Bangladesh, levels of over 74% are reported (Chaudhury and Hammer, 2004). A survey of health clinics in Bangladesh, Ecuador, India, Indonesia, Peru and Uganda found 35% of health workers absent (Chaudhury *et al.*, 2005). The phenomenon of 'brain-drain' – health-care personnel from developing countries working in developed nations – has worsened (Stilwell *et al.*, 2004). Imbalances in skill-mix are also crucial. In Bolivia, Brazil and Peru, there are two to four times more physicians than nurses and in some of these settings there are concerns of over medicalization of delivery care with high Caesarean section rates. In contrast, nurses outnumber doctors by a factor of 10:1 in countries like Burundi, Ghana and Kenya (Buchan, 2006), requiring considerations regarding training for upgrading skills of non-physicians (see Mavalankar and Sankara Raman, Chapter 6 this volume).

The policy environment

Leadership and governance form one of the six health system building blocks, which are described as 'arguably the most complex but critical building block of any health system' (WHO, 2007). The policies set out by decision makers can thus be considered the first step to ensuring access to the package of life-saving interventions outlined above. Too often the government's national policy framework for the care and treatment of women during pregnancy and childbirth is inadequate, out of date or incomplete. The impact of higher-level factors such as political will, policy environment and international funding is also felt directly at the maternal and perinatal health level. For example, WHO estimates that for each US$1 million shortfall in support for

contraceptives there are an additional 360,000 unwanted pregnancies, 150,000 induced abortions, 800 maternal deaths and 11,000 infant deaths (WHO, 2010a). In some countries policy and institutional constraints predominate over resource limitations (Travis *et al.*, 2004). Broader political frameworks and environment beyond the field of health can also act as a significant barrier.

The gap between policy and practice was highlighted by a survey of 1037 experts in 49 developing countries. Policy was not perceived as a major barrier, with government policies towards pregnancy and delivery services rated as adequate at 72%. Yet the participant ratings dropped to 54% when asked about active implementation of policies and 48% when asked if government budgets for safe pregnancy, delivery and postpartum care were adequate (Bulatao and Ross, 2002). Comprehensive frameworks for how to approach a certain condition – as recommended by WHO in relation to fistula, for example – can be vital to ensure that the resources, personnel and facilities exist to provide the necessary treatment, while also demonstrating that crucial political will is present. WHO's *Model List of Essential Medicines*, updated every 2 years, is another example (WHO, 2009c). Yet national adoption of these evidence-based recommendations is often not timely or universal. Efficient and effective systems for setting and disseminating policies are also crucial and the case study on magnesium sulphate (Box 8.1) showed that policy is meaningless without an effective plan to put it into practice and that the problem often lies not with policies directly but with the extent to which government takes appropriate action to see that they are implemented.

Legal and cultural factors

Legal, facility-based and community-level barriers must also be addressed to improve access to maternal and perinatal health-care interventions. Laws and restrictions can deny women of reproductive age easy access to family planning services. For example, keeping oral contraceptive pills on prescription often means that social marketing of this contraceptive method is restricted – an important distribution and financing mechanism in low-resource settings (Prata, 2009).

Facility and provider-based barriers include practices that are not codified in law but which create unnecessary barriers. Examples include refusal to see adolescent patients without parental permission or provision of contraceptive services only on specific days of the week. At the provider level, personal biases and beliefs might result in use of non evidence-based clinical practices.

Community level barriers particular to maternal and perinatal health care include lack of awareness about the importance of early and regular antenatal care (Villar *et al.*, 2001), delay in seeking medical care if complications occur, lack of awareness about the severity of certain symptoms, and costs of transportation between home and a health facility (Shah *et al.*, 2009). In some parts of the world there are cultural challenges that prevent women from seeking health care without the permission of spouses or family members. Often women cannot be attended to by male health providers without their spouses present. In many communities there is distrust of the medical profession and a preference for traditional healers. There can be lack of understanding of how family planning methods work, misinformation regarding safety, side effects and impact on future fertility and religious, traditional or cultural values that act as obstacles (see Mumtaz and Levay, Chapter 12 this volume).

Knowledge for implementation

The successful introduction and adoption of effective interventions are a complex process that requires knowledge and information that only 'implementation research' or 'implementation science' can provide.

Implementation research is an emerging field that requires attention and investment, especially in maternal health. Implementation research is designed to be intervention-specific, aiming 'to develop strategies for available or new health interventions in order to improve access to, and the use of, these interventions by the populations in need … designed with the intention of creating outputs that can [also] be applicable beyond the local environment in which the research is done' (Remme *et al.*, 2010). This approach is exactly what is needed to apply the existing and new scientific evidence in maternal health. Lack of priority and inadequate funding have led to inadequate 'evidence-based methods for implementing evidence-based interventions' (Guldbransson, 2008), resulting in a gap between knowledge and implementation in the health field (Sanders and Haines, 2006).

In maternal health, implementation research is needed in order to fully understand the barriers to mainstreaming best practices and to recognize effective and feasible ways to overcome them. The process of implementation is complex as it often does not involve a single product but a range of decisions, actions, technologies and stakeholders. These issues raise complicated questions for evaluation (Ross *et al.*, 2005; Craig *et al.*, 2008) but which can be feasible to rigorously assess, as demonstrated by the simplified antenatal care package that Villar and colleagues (2001) developed and tested. Crucial factors include the role of sound research to fill gaps, the need to communicate the findings effectively to policy makers (Bhutta *et al.*, 2003) and the importance of context, environment and the systems therein (Cavagnero *et al.*, 2008).

Some fields that are closely related to maternal health, such as newborn and child health, have been more effective in terms of designing, implementing, evaluating and introducing essential intervention packages that have significantly improved the health of their target populations. An important lesson from the field of newborn health is the value of funding large scale implementation research. Great strides have been made by convening and engaging interested parties, designing a variety of interventions adapted to the context and the health systems followed by careful assessment of how these interventions fared through focused implementation research. The child health community, as noted through the Child Survival Partnership, has proactively encouraged donors to consider how best to work synergistically in their field. In this case widespread agreement was reached early on to set priorities and identify areas of research and programming. Donors then pooled funds in order to move the field ahead more efficiently, while centralizing decision making at the country level where there are one plan, one budget and one set of resources (Martines *et al.*, 2005). Only recently has the maternal health field begun to consider this and other kinds of priority setting and donor harmonization.

Conclusion

Critical life-saving technologies, especially for the five leading causes of maternal mortality, have now been tested and proven, yet the number of maternal deaths remains far too high.

First, it is important to gain more and better knowledge about the variables that prevent women from having access to life-saving interventions (the 'barriers') and identify and implement actions to overcome them. Second, it is critical to package single interventions into complex ones in order to address the multiple and often overlapping needs of pregnant women and the newborn. Third, there is also much that the field of maternal health can learn from related fields, such as child health, which have been more successful in reducing morbidity and mortality. Fourth, we also must support and learn from implementation research. The news about reduction in maternal mortality is compelling (Hogan *et al.*, 2010; WHO, 2010b) yet does not provide the knowledge base sorely needed. Implementation research will play a key role in helping us gain that knowledge.

To narrow the gap between policy and practice requires commitment to learning about and acting on the needs of entire systems. It is time to take a bold step from rhetoric to action.

Here are five suggestions for actions to improve the state of maternal health in your country:

1. Find a 'champion' within the Ministry of Health or other policy-making body who can advocate for and share messages on the importance of maternal health. Be in direct touch with this person frequently about key issues, emerging evidence for solutions and important audiences for this information within professional communities.

2. Review the national essential drugs list and check for oxytocin, misoprotol (or other prostaglandins), magnesium sulphate and key antibiotics for prevention of infection. If these drugs are not present, investigate how to facilitate getting them approved and available in your country.

3. Look into the accessibility of family planning. Is there a national-level strategy that makes commodities available to women and men everywhere? If there are gaps, consider how best to fill them.

4. Is there a national 'map' of where emergency obstetric care is available? Are referral systems in place to get women to these locations in a timely way? Find ways to obtain or summarize this information and begin to find solutions through the networks and champions identified.

5. If unsafe abortion is a major problem in your country, consider strategies for change. Is political action needed? Do women and providers know their rights under the current law? What will best help them to address the issue?

References

Aaserud, M., Lewin, S., Innvaer, S., Paulsen, E.J., Dahlgren, A.T., Trommald, M., Duley, L., Zwarenstein, M. and Oxman, A.D. (2005) Translating research into policy and practice in developing countries: a case study of magnesium sulphate for pre-eclampsia. *BMC Health Services Research* 5, 68.

Abdel-Aleem, H., Hofmeyr, G.J., Chokry, M. and El-Sonoosy, E. (2006) Uterine massage and postpartum blood loss. *International Journal of Gynaecology and Obstetrics* 93, 238–239.

Abi Said, D., Annegers, J.F., Combs Cantrell, D., Frankowski, R.F. and Willmore, L.J. (1995) Case-control study of the risk factors for eclampsia. *American Journal of Epidemiology* 142, 437–441.

Akhter, S., Begum, M.R., Kabir, Z., Rashid, M., Laila, T.R. and Zabeen, F. (2003) Use of a condom to control massive postpartum hemorrhage. Medscape. Available at: http://www.medscape.com/viewarticle/459894_print.

Althabe, F. (2002) *Vacuum Extraction Versus Forceps for Assisted Vaginal Delivery: RHL commentary*. The WHO Reproductive Health Library, World Health Organization, Geneva.

Askie, L.M., Duley, L., Henderson-Smart, D.J. and Stewart, L.A., PARIS Collaborative Group (2007) Antiplatelet agents for prevention of pre-eclampsia: a meta-analysis of individual patient data. *Lancet* 369(9575), 1791–1798.

Association of Reproductive Health Professionals (2011) Manual Vacuum Aspiration. A quick reference guide for clinicians. Association of Reproductive Health Professionals, Washington, DC. Available at: http://www.rhtp.org/abortion/documents/MVArefGuide.pdf (accessed 30 August 2011).

Begum, R., Begum, A., Johnson, R., Ali, M.N. and Akhter, S. (2001) A low dose ('Dhaka') magnesium sulphate regime for eclampsia. *Acta Obstetricia et Gynecologica Scandinavica* 80, 998–1002.

Begum, M.R., Begum, A. and Quadir, E. (2002) Loading dose versus standard regime of magnesium sulfate in the management of eclampsia: a randomized trial. *Journal of Obstetrics and Gynaecology Research* 28, 154–159.

Bhutta, Z.A., Darmstadt, G.L. and Ransom, E.I. (2003) Using evidence to save newborn lives. *Policy Perspectives on Newborn Health*, Population Reference Bureau, Washington, DC.

Billings, D.L. and Benson, J. (2005) Post-abortion care in Latin America: policy and service recommendations from a decade of operations research. *Health Policy and Planning* 20, 158–166.

Bique, C., Ustá, M., Debora, B., Chong, E., Westheimer, E. and Winikoff, B. (2007) Comparison of misoprostol and manual vacuum aspiration for the treatment of incomplete abortion. *International Journal of Gynecology and Obstetrics* 98, 222–226.

Björklund, K. (2002) Minimally invasive surgery for obstructed labour: a review of symphysiotomy during the twentieth century (including 5000 cases). *British Journal of Obstetrics and Gynaecology* 109, 236–248.

Blum, J., Winikoff, B., Raghavan, S., Dabash, R., Ramadan, M.C., Dilbaz, B., Dao, B., Durocher, J., Yalvac, S., Diop, A., Dzuba, I.G. and Ngoc, N.T. (2010) Treatment of post-partum haemorrhage with sublingual misoprostol versus oxytocin in women receiving prophylactic oxytocin: a double-blind, randomized, non-inferiority trial. *Lancet* 375, 217–223.

Buchan, J. (2006) The impact of global nursing migration on health services delivery. *Policy, Politics and Nursing Practice* 7, 16S.

Bulatao, R.A. and Ross, J.A. (2002) Rating maternal and neonatal health services in developing countries. *Bulletin of the World Health Organization* 80, 721–727.

Cavagnero, E., Daelmans, B., Gupta, N., Scherpbier, R. and Shankar, A. (2008) Assessment of the health system and policy environment as a critical complement to tracking intervention coverage for maternal, newborn, and child health. *Lancet* 371, 1284–1293.

Center for Reproductive Rights (2006) The world's abortion laws poster. Available at: http://bookstore.reproductiverights.org/worablaw20.html (accessed 5 July 2006).

Ceylan, A., Ertem, M., Saka, G. and Akdeniz, N. (2009) Post abortion family planning counseling as a tool to increase contraception use. *BMC Public Health* 9, 20.

Chaudhury, N. and Hammer, J.S. (2004) Ghost doctors: absenteeism in rural Bangladeshi health facilities. *The World Bank Economic Review* 18(3), 423–441.

Chaudhury, N., Hammer, J., Kremer, M., Muralidharan, K. and Rogers, F.H. (2005) Missing in action: teacher and health worker absence in developing countries. *Journal of Economic Perspectives* 20(1), 91–116.

Cotter, A.M., Ness, A. and Tolosa, J.E. (2001) Prophylactic oxytocin for the third stage of labour. *Cochrane Database of Systematic Reviews* 4, CD001808.

Craig, P., Dieppe, P., Macintyre, S., Michie, S., Nazareth, I. and Petticrew, M. (2008) Developing and evaluating complex interventions: the new Medical Research Council guidance. *British Medical Journal* 337, a1655.

Cutland, C.L., Madhi, S.A., Zell, E.R., Kuwanda, L., Laque, M., Groome, M., Gorwitz, R., Thigpen, M.C., Patel, R., Velaphi, S.C., Adrian, P., Klugman, K., Schuchat, A. and Schrag, S.J. (2009) Chlorhexidine maternal-vaginal and neonate body wipes in sepsis and vertical transmission of pathogenic bacteria in South Africa: a randomized, controlled trial. *Lancet* 374, 1909–1916.

DFID (2004) *Increasing Access to Essential Medicines in the Developing World: UK Government policy and plans*. Department for International Development, London.

Eclampsia Trial Collaborative Group (The) (1995) Which anticonvulsant for women with eclampsia? Evidence from the Collaborative Eclampsia Trial. *Lancet* 345, 1455–1463.

Elneil, S. and Browning, A. (2009) Obstetric fistula – a new way forward. *British Journal of Obstetrics and Gynaecology* 116 (Suppl. 1), 30–32.

Fottrell, E., Byass, P., Ouedraogo, T.W., Tamini, C., Gbangou, A., Sombié, I., Högberg, U., Witten, K.H., Bhattacharya, S., Desta, T., Deganus, S., Tornui, J., Fitzmaurice, A.E., Meda, N. and Graham, W.J. (2007) Revealing the burden of maternal mortality: a probabilistic model for determining pregnancy-related causes of death from verbal autopsies. *Population Health Metrics* 5, 1. Available at: http://www.pophealthmetrics.com/content/pdf/1478-7954-5-1.pdf (accessed 24 February 2010).

French, L. and Smaill, F.M. (2004) Antibiotic regimens for endometritis after delivery. *Cochrane Database of Systematic Reviews* 4, CD001067. DOI: 10.1002/14651858.CD001067.pub2.

Glasier, A.F., Cameron, S.T., Fine, P.M., Logan, S.J., Casale, W., Van Horn, J., Sogor, L., Blithe, D.L., Scherrer, B., Mathe, H., Jaspart, A., Ulmann, A. and Gainer, E. (2010) Ulipristal acetate versus levonorgestrel for emergency contraception: a randomised non-inferiority trial and meta-analysis. *Lancet* 375(9714), 555–562.

Graham, W. and Hussein, J. (2003) Measuring and Estimating Maternal Mortality in the Era of HIV/AIDS. Proceedings from Workshop on HIV/AIDS and Adult Mortality in Developing Countries, Population Division. Department of Economic and Social Affairs, United Nations Secretariat, New York, 8–13 September 2003. Available at: http://www.un.org/esa/population/publications/adultmort/GRAHAM_Paper8.pdf (accessed 24 February 2010).

Grimes, D.A., Benson, J., Singh, S., Romero, M., Ganatra, B., Okonofua, F.E. and Shah, I.H. (2006) Unsafe abortion: the preventable pandemic. *Lancet* 368, 1908–1919.

Guldbransson, K. (2008) From news to everyday use: The difficulty of implementation. In: *A Literature Review.* Swedish National Institute of Public Health, Ostersund, Sweden.

Gülmezoglu, A.M., Widmer, M., Merialdi, M., Qureshi, Z., Piaggio, G., Elbourne, D., Abdel-Aleem, H., Carroli, G., Hofmeyr, G.J., Lumbiganon, P., Derman, R., Okong, P., Goudar, S., Festin, M., Althabe, F. and Armbruster, D. (2009) Active management of the third stage of labour without controlled cord traction: a randomized non-inferiority controlled trial. *Reproductive Health* 6, 2.

Gynuity Health Projects (2011) Pre-eclampsia. Available at: http://gynuity.org/programs/pre-eclampsia/ (accessed 4 January 2011).

Hofmeyr, G.J., Atallah, Á.N. and Duley, L. (2006) Calcium supplementation during pregnancy for preventing hypertensive disorders and related problems. *Cochrane Database of Systematic Reviews* 3, CD001059.

Hofmeyr, G.J., Mathai, M., Shah, A.N. and Novikova, N. (2008) Techniques for Caesarean section. *Cochrane Database of Systematic Reviews* 1, CD004662. DOI: 10.1002/14651858.CD004662.pub2.

Hogan, M.C., Foreman, K.J., Naghavi, M., Ahn, S., Wang, M., Maketa, S., Lopez, A., Lozano, R. and Murray, C. (2010) Maternal mortality for 181 countries, 1980–2008: a systematic analysis of progress towards Millennium Development Goal 5. *Lancet* 375(9726), 1609–1623.

Hundley, V.A., Avan, B.I., Braunholtz, D. and Graham, W.J. (2011) Are birth kits a good idea? A systematic review of the evidence. *Midwifery*, 9 May, (E-pub ahead of print).

Hussein, J., Mavalankar, D.V., Sharma, S. and D'Ambruoso, L. (2011) A review of health system infection control measures in developing countries: what can be learned to reduce maternal mortality. *Globalization and Health* 7, 14.

Hyman, A.G. and Castleman, L. (2005) *Woman-Centered Abortion Care: Reference manual.* IPAS, Chapel Hill, North Carolina

Johanson, R. and Menon, V. (1999) Vacuum extraction versus forceps for assisted vaginal delivery. *Cochrane Database of Systematic Reviews* 2, CD000224. DOI: 10.1002/14651858.CD000224.

Johnson, B.R., Benson, J. and Hawkins, B.L. (1992) Reducing resource use and improving quality of care with MVA. *Advances in Abortion Care* 2(2), 1–6.

Johnson, B.R., Ndhlovu, S., Farr, S.L. and Chipato, T. (2002) Reducing unplanned pregnancy and abortion in Zimbabwe through post-abortion contraception. *Studies in Family Planning* 33, 195–202, 4–15.

Kampf, G., Loffler, H. and Gastmeier, P. (2009) Hand hygiene for the prevention of nosocomial infections. *Deutsches Ärzteblatt International* 106(40), 649–655.

Khan, K., Wojdyla, D., Say, L.A., Gülmezoglu, M. and Van Look, P. (2006) WHO analysis of causes of maternal death: a systematic review. *Lancet* 367, 1066–1074.

Lapaire, O., Zanetti-Dällenbach, R., Weber, P., Hösli, I., Holzgreve, W. and Surbek, D. (2007) Labor induction in preeclampsia: is misoprostol more effective than dinoprostone? *Journal of Perinatal Medicine* 35(3), 195–199.

Lavender, T., Hart, A. and Smyth, R.M.D. (2008) Effect of partogram use on outcomes for women in spontaneous labour at term. *Cochrane Database of Systematic Reviews* 4, CD005461. DOI:10.1002/14651858. CD005461.pub2.

Liabsuetrakul, T., Choobun, T., Peeyananjarassri, K. and Islam, Q.M. (2004) Antibiotic prophylaxis for operative vaginal delivery. *Cochrane Database of Systematic Reviews* 3, CD004455. DOI: 10.1002/14651858. CD004455.pub2.

Liselele, H.B., Boulvain, M., Tshibangu, K.C. and Meuris, S. (2000) Maternal height and external pelvimetry to predict cephalopelvic disproportion in nulliparous African women: a cohort study. *British Journal of Obstetrics and Gynaecology* 107, 947–952.

MacGillivray, I., McCaw-Binns, A.M., Ashley, D.E., Fedrick, A. and Golding, J. (2004) Strategies to prevent eclampsia in a developing country: II. Use of a maternal pictorial card. *International Journal of Gynecology and Obstetrics* 87(3), 295–300.

MacKay, A.P., Berg, C.J. and Atrash, H.K. (2001) Pregnancy-related mortality from pre-eclampsia and eclampsia. *Obstetrics and Gynecology* 97, 533–538.

Magpie Trial Collaborative Group (The) (2002) Do women with pre-eclampsia, and their babies, benefit from magnesium sulphate? The Magpie Trial: a randomized placebo-controlled trial. *Lancet* 359, 1877–1890.

Martines, J., Paul, V., Bhutta, Z., Koblinsky, M., Soucat, A., Walker, N., Bahl, R., Fogstad, H. and Costello, A. (for the Lancet Neonatal Survival Series Steering Team: series 4) (2005) Neonatal survival: a call for action. *Lancet* 365(9465), 1189–1197.

McCaw-Binns, A.M., Ashley, D.E., Knight, L.P., MacGillivray, I. and Golding, J. (2004) Strategies to prevent eclampsia in a developing country: I. Reorganization of maternity services. *International Journal of Gynecology and Obstetrics* 87(3), 286–294.

Mehta, R., Mavalankar, D.V., Ramani, K., Sharma, S. and Hussein, J. (2011) Infection control in delivery care units, Gujarat state, India: A needs assessment. *BMC Pregnancy Childbirth* 20(11), 37.

Narasimhan, V., Brown, H., Pablos-Mendez, A., Adams, O., Dussault, G., Elzinga, G., Nordstrom, A., Habte, D., Jacobs, M., Solimano, G., Sewankambo, N., Wibulpolprasert, S., Evans, T. and Chen, L. (2004) Responding to the global human resources crisis. *Lancet* 363(9419), 1469–1472.

PATH (2011) Resources for Oxytocin in the Uniject™ injection system. Available at: http://www.path.org/projects/uniject-oxytocin-resources.php (accessed 2 August 2011).

Pattinson, R.C. (2000) Pelvimetry for fetal cephalic presentations at term. *Cochrane Database of Systematic Reviews* 2, CD000161.

Pereira, C., Bugalho, A., Bergstrom, S., Vaz, F. and Cotiro, M. (1996) A comparative study of Caesarean deliveries by assistant medical officers and obstetricians in Mozambique. *British Journal of Obstetrics and Gynaecology* 103, 508–512.

Prata, N. (2009) Making family planning accessible in resource-poor settings. *Philosophical Transactions of the Royal Society B: Biological Sciences* 364, 3093–3099.

Prata, N., Sreenivas, A., Greig, F., Walsh, J. and Potts, M. (2010) Setting priorities for safe motherhood interventions in resource-scarce settings. *Health Policy* 94, 1–13.

Prendiville, W.J.P., Elbourne, D. and McDonald, S.J. (2000) Active versus expectant management in the third stage of labour. *Cochrane Database of Systematic Reviews* 3, CD000007.

Rao, R. (2008) *Commodity Security for Essential Medicines: Challenges and Opportunities.* USAID Deliver Project, Arlington, Virginia.

Remme, J.H.F., Taghreed, A., Becerra-Posada, F., D'Arcangues, C., Devlin, M., Gardner, C., Ghaffar, A., Hombach, J., Kengeya, J.F.K., Mbewu, A., Mbizvo, M., Mirza, Z., Pang, T., Ridley, R.G., Zicker, F. and Terry, R.F. (2010) Defining research to improve health systems. *PLoS Medicine* 7(11), e1001000.

Ross, J. and Blanc, A. (2009) The contribution of family planning to reducing maternal deaths. *Proceedings of International Conference on Family Planning: Research and Best Practices*, 17 November 2009, Kampala, Uganda.

Ross, L., Simkada, P. and Smith, W.C.S. (2005) Evaluating effectiveness of complex interventions aimed at reducing maternal mortality in developing countries. *Journal of Public Health* 27(4), 331–337.

Rozenholc, A., Ako, S., Leke, R. and Boulvain, M. (2007) The diagnostic accuracy of external pelvimetry and maternal height to predict dystocia in nulliparous women: a study in Cameroon. *British Journal of Obstetrics and Gynaecology* 114, 630–635.

Ruano, R., Fontes, R.S. and Zugaib, M. (2005) Prevention of preeclampsia with low-dose aspirin – a systematic review and meta-analysis of the main randomized controlled trials. *Clinics (São Paulo)* 60(5), 407–414.

Sanders, D. and Haines, A. (2006) Implementation research is needed to achieve international health goals. *PLoS Medicine* 3, 6, 0722.

Sebitloane, H.M., Moodley, J. and Esterhuizen, T.M. (2007) Prophylactic antibiotics for the prevention of postpartum infectious morbidity in women infected with human immunodeficiency virus: a randomized controlled trial. *American Journal of Obstetrics and Gynecology* 198(2), 189.e1-6.

Sevene, E., Lewin, S., Mariano, A., Woelk, G., Oxman, A.D., Matinhure, S., Cliff, J., Fernandes, B. and Daniels, K. (2005) System and market failures: the unavailability of magnesium sulphate for the treatment of eclampsia and pre-eclampsia in Mozambique and Zimbabwe. *British Medical Journal* 331(7519), 765–769.

Shah, N., Hossain, N., Shoaib, R., Hussain, A., Gillani, R. and Khan, N.H. (2009) Socio-demographic characteristics and the three delays of maternal mortality. *Journal of the College of Physicians and Surgeons – Pakistan* 19(2), 95–98.

Shaikh, Z., Abbassi, R.M., Rizwan, N. and Abbasi, S. (2010) Morbidity and mortality due to unsafe abortion. Pakistan. *International Journal of Gynaecology and Obstetrics* 110(1), 47–49.

Shamsuddin, L., Nahar, K., Nasrin, B., Nahar, S., Tamanna, S., Kabir, R.M., Alis, M.J. and Anwary, S.A. (2005) Use of parenteral magnesium sulphate in eclampsia and severe pre-eclampsia cases in a rural set up of Bangladesh. *Bangladesh Medical Research Council Bulletin* 31, 75–82.

Sloan, N.L., Langer, A., Hernández, B., Romero, M. and Winikoff, B. (2001) The etiology of maternal mortality in developing countries: what do verbal autopsies tell us? *Bulletin of the World Health Organization* 79(9), 805–810.

Smaill, F.M. and Gyte, G.M.L. (2010) Antibiotic prophylaxis versus no prophylaxis for preventing infection after cesarean section. *Cochrane Database of Systematic Reviews* 1, CD007482. DOI: 10.1002/14651858. CD007482.pub2.

Stade, B.C., Shah, V.S. and Ohlsson, A. (2004) Vaginal chlorhexidine during labour to prevent early-onset neonatal group B streptococcal infection. *Cochrane Database of Systematic Reviews* 3, CD003520. DOI: 10.1002/14651858.CD003520.pub2.

Stilwell, B., Diallo, K., Zurn, P., Vujicic, M., Adams, O. and Dal Poz, M. (2004) Migration of health-care workers from developing countries: strategic approaches to its management. *Bulletin of the World Health Organization* 82, 595–600.

Thinkhamrop, J., Hofmeyr, G.J., Adetoro, O. and Lumbiganon, P. (2002) Prophylactic antibiotic administration in pregnancy to prevent infectious morbidity and mortality. *Cochrane Database of Systematic Reviews* 4, CD002250. DOI: 10.1002/14651858.CD002250.

Travis, P., Bennett, S., Haines, A., Pang, T., Bhutta, Z., Hyder, A.A., Pielemeier, N., Mills, A. and Evans, T. (2004) Overcoming health-systems constraints to achieve the Millennium Development Goals. *Lancet* 364, 900–906.

Tsu, V.D. and Coffey, P.S. (2009) New and underutilised technologies to reduce maternal mortality and morbidity: what progress have we made since Bellagio 2003? *British Journal of Obstetrics and Gynaecology* 116, 247–256.

Tsu, V.D., Luu, H.T. and Mai, T.T. (2009) Does a novel prefilled injection device make postpartum oxytocin easier to administer? Results from midwives in Vietnam. *Midwifery* 25, 461–465.

van Bogaert, L.J. and Sedibe, T.M. (2007) Efficacy of a single misoprostol regimen in the first and second trimester termination of pregnancy. *Journal of Obstetrics and Gynaecology* 27, 510–512.

Villar, J., Ba'ageel, H., Piaggio, G., Lumbiganon, P., Beliazan, J.M., Farnot, U., Al-Mazrou, Y., Carroli, G., Pinol, A., Donner, A., Langer, A., Nigenda, G., Mugford, M., Fox-Rushby, J., Hutton, G., Bergsio, P., Bekketeig, L. and Berendes, H. for the WHO Antenatal Care Trial Research Group (2001) WHO antenatal care randomised trial for the evaluation of a new model of routine antenatal care. *Lancet* 357(9268), 1551–1564.

Villar, J., Say, L., Gulmezoglu, M., Merialdi, M., Lindheimer, M. and Betran, A.P. (2003) Eclampsia and pre-eclampsia: a worldwide health problem for 2000 years. In: Critgley, H.O.D., Poston, L. and Walker, J.J. (eds) *Pre-eclampsia*. RCOG Press, London, pp. 189–207.

Warriner, I.K., Meirik, O., Hoffman, M., Morroni, C., Harries, J., My Huong, N.T., Vy, N.D. and Seuc, A.H. (2006) Rates of complication in first-trimester manual vacuum aspiration abortion done by doctors and mid-level providers in South Africa and Vietnam: a randomized controlled equivalence trial. *Lancet* 368, 1965–1972.

Wedisinghe, L. and Elsandabesee, D. (2010) Flexible mifepristone and misoprostol administration interval for first-trimester medical termination. *Contraception* 81(4), 269–274.

Wei, S., Wo, B.L., Xu, H., Luo, Z.C., Roy, C. and Fraser, W.D. (2009) Early amniotomy and early oxytocin for prevention of, or therapy for, delay in first stage spontaneous labour compared with routine care. *Cochrane Database of Systematic Reviews* 2, CD006794. DOI: 10.1002/14651858.CD006794.pub2.

WHO (1994) *Preventing Prolonged Labour: A practical guide*. WHO, Geneva.

WHO (1996) *Mother-Baby Package: Implementing safe motherhood in countries: A practical guide*. WHO, Geneva.

WHO (2000) *Integrated Management of Pregnancy and Childbirth, Managing complications in pregnancy and childbirth: a guide for midwives and doctors*. WHO, Geneva.

WHO (2004a) *Unsafe Abortion: global and regional estimates of the incidence of unsafe abortion and associated mortality in 2000*, 4th edn. WHO, Geneva.

WHO (2004b) *The World Medicines Situation*. WHO, Geneva.

WHO (2005) Attending to 136 million births, every year. *The World Report 2005. Make every mother and child count*. WHO, Geneva, pp. 62–63.

WHO (2006a) *Prevention of Postpartum Hemorrhage by Active Management of the Third Stage of Labor*. Department of Making Pregnancy Safer, WHO, Geneva.

WHO (2006b) Lewis, G. and de Bernis, L. (eds) *Integrated Management of Pregnancy and Childbirth, Obstetric Fistula: Guiding principles for clinical management and programme development*. WHO, Geneva.

WHO (2007) Strengthening Health Systems to Improve Health Outcomes. WHO's Framework for Action. Available at: http://www.who.int/reproductivehealth/topics/countries/systems/en/ (accessed 24 February 2010).

WHO (2008) Managing Eclampsia. Midwifery education modules. Available at: http://www.who.int/making_pregnancy_safer/documents/5_9241546662/en/index.html (accessed 30 June 2010).

WHO (2009a) *WHO Guidelines on Hand Hygiene in Health Care. First global patient safety challenge - clean care is safer care*. WHO, Geneva.

WHO (2009b) *Report on the WHO/PEPFAR Planning Meeting on Scaling Up Nursing and Medical Education Geneva, 13–14 October 2009*. WHO, Geneva.

WHO (2009c) *WHO Model List of Essential Medicines*. WHO, Geneva.

WHO, UNICEF, UNFPA and World Bank (2010a) *Packages of Interventions for Family Planning, Safe Abortion Care, Maternal Newborn and Child Health*. WHO, Geneva.

WHO, UNICEF, UNFPA and World Bank (2010b) *Trends in Maternal Mortality: 1990 to 2008*. WHO, Geneva.

Widmer, A.F. (2000) Replace hand washing with use of a waterless alcohol hand rub? *Clinical Infectious Diseases* 31, 136–143.

Winani, S., Wood, S., Coffey, P., Chirwa, T., Mosha, F. and Changalucha, J. (2007) Use of a clean delivery kit and factors associated with cord infection and puerperal sepsis in Mwanza, Tanzania. *Journal of Midwifery and Women's Health* 52(1), 37–43.

Winikoff, B., Dabash, R., Durocher, J., Darwish, E., Nguyen, T.N., León, W., Raghavan, S., Medhat, I., Huynh, T.K., Barrera, G. and Blum, J. (2010) Treatment of post-partum haemorrhage with sublingual misoprostol versus oxytocin in women not exposed to oxytocin during labour: a double-blind, randomised, non-inferiority trial. *Lancet* 375, 210–216.

9 Medical Conditions in Pregnancy

Roger Webber,[1] Affette McCaw-Binns[2] and Julia Hussein[3]
[1]*Argyll, Scotland, UK;* [2]*University of the West Indies, Kingston, Jamaica;*
[3]*University of Aberdeen, Scotland, UK*

Summary

- Medical conditions can have a major effect on the woman before, during and after pregnancy, some of which have particular importance to her offspring. The conditions are often exacerbated by pregnancy.
- Infectious conditions are common in developing country settings, with antenatal care providing an opportunity for detection of many conditions:
  - Human immunodeficiency virus (HIV) infection affects a woman's chance of surviving pregnancy. The condition can be transmitted to her offspring.
  - Sexually transmissible infections cause infertility and damage to the fetus.
  - While the mother's immunity is compromised during pregnancy, she is at risk from varicella, influenza and malaria and may transmit congenital infections to the fetus – syphilis, genital herpes, rubella, toxoplasmosis, cytomegalovirus, listerosis and parvovirus B19.
- Chronic and non-communicable medical conditions may be identified for the first time in pregnancy and include:
  - Nutritional deficiencies such as anaemia, other micronutrients and caloric restrictions.
  - Circulatory disorders, such as heart disease, chronic hypertension.
  - Gestational, Type I or Type II diabetes.
  - Haematological conditions such as sickle cell anaemia and thalassaemia, which have implications for the long-term health of offspring if both parents carry the trait and for the health of the mother if she is homozygous for the condition
- The management of medical conditions in pregnancy can be categorized in the following stages:
  - Preconceptually, couples planning to have children should be educated about immunization, improving diet and general health.
  - Antenatal care provides the opportunity to diagnose, manage and treat HIV, sexually transmitted infections, anaemia and other pre-existing medical conditions such as sickle cell disease, thalassaemia, heart disease and diabetes, to limit the effect of these problems.
  - Childbirth can be stressful physiologically. Acute management of conditions such as anaemia, diabetes and heart conditions may be necessary. Hygienic practices and HIV prophylaxis are also important.
  - Postpartum management of infant feeding will reduce HIV transmission, and use of insecticide-treated nets by the mother and child will contribute to preventing the consequences of malaria. Long-term management of medical conditions after pregnancy and planning for the next pregnancy are necessary.

Introduction

Indirect maternal deaths are those due to previous existing disease or disease that developed during pregnancy and which was aggravated by the physiologic effects of pregnancy (AbouZahr, 2003). These include conditions like anaemia, hypertension or diabetes, as well as infectious conditions such as HIV and malaria. In developing countries almost 30% of maternal deaths are due to indirect causes (Khan *et al.*, 2006).

Maternal deaths are prone to misclassification and under reporting because the cause of death may be incorrectly reported and many pregnancies are missed or not recorded. Indirect maternal deaths are particularly prone to being reported as non-maternal. Late (up to 1 year after the end of pregnancy) maternal deaths are of relevance particularly because pregnancy can contribute to the general deterioration of a medical condition many weeks or months after the usual postpartum period of 42 days. Countries differ in the way indirect maternal deaths are classified, with many countries reporting no indirect deaths at all (AbouZahr, 2003). These deaths may be misclassified if pregnancy is not noted on the death certificate, as the ICD10 has different codes for the same condition, depending on whether it is pregnancy related or not. Yet we know that indirect deaths are increasingly important, as seen from maternal death reports from, for example, Jamaica (McCaw-Binns and Lewis-Bell, 2009) and Nepal (Pant *et al.*, 2008; Suvedi *et al.*, 2009).

There have been recent calls to pay more attention to indirect maternal deaths (Cross *et al.*, 2010). Anaemia accounts for 3.7% of maternal deaths in Africa and 12.8% in Asia, while HIV/AIDS causes 6.2% in Africa but less than 1% in Asia (Khan *et al.*, 2006). Although these are two clearly identified conditions, much less is known about the specific contributions of other diseases, with more than half of the causes of all indirect maternal deaths unknown or unclassified.

This chapter aims to provide a brief overview of the many different medical and infectious conditions of particular pertinence in pregnancy. Readers are directed to further literature relevant to the specific conditions. Some medical conditions such as anaemia are not clearly distinguished from obstetric ones and others can lead to or increase the risk of obstetric conditions (for example, malaria in the mother can lead to abortions or preterm or low birth-weight babies). Although there are specific strategies to manage medical conditions in pregnancy, these may need to be combined with obstetric interventions, which are discussed elsewhere (see Stanton and Lawn, Chapter 5 this volume, and Langer *et al.*, Chapter 8 this volume).

Infectious Conditions in Pregnancy

During pregnancy, to ensure that the mother's immune system does not treat the developing fetus as a foreign body, a physiological process of immune down-regulation occurs (suppression of the immune reaction in the mother's body). However, this process makes the mother more susceptible to infections such as malaria, varicella, influenza and tuberculosis. With any infection, the extra strain on her body coupled with her lowered immunity will increase her chance of developing more serious disease than usual. For example, hepatitis E, which normally occurs in epidemics with a low mortality rate, has an increased fatality rate of up to 20% if the pregnant woman is infected in the third trimester (Beniwal *et al.*, 2003).

Early pregnancy is also a dangerous time for the developing fetus. Certain infections such as rubella, toxoplasmosis and cytomegalovirus can cause severe damage, leading to disability or death of the developing infant. Mumps contracted during the first trimester is a cause of abortion but not of congenital abnormality. Figure 9.1 outlines a range of important communicable diseases that affect maternal and perinatal health and demonstrates the most appropriate time when preventive strategies can be effectively applied. Some, such as use of insecticide-treated bed nets, need to be used consistently across the life cycle, while childhood immunization is the most effective strategy to limit those childhood disorders that have deleterious effects on the fetus, especially if the mother is

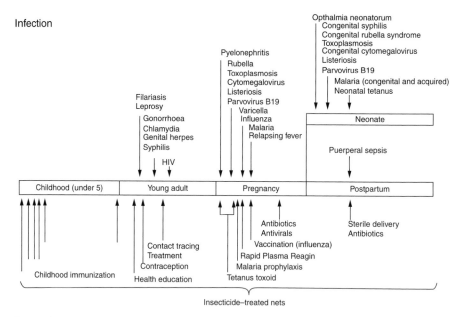

Infection

Preventive strategy

Fig. 9.1. Infectious conditions in pregnancy.

exposed in the first trimester. Health promotion outside pregnancy, as well as screening, contact tracing, treatment and contraceptive advice, including use of barrier methods, are the most effective strategies for reducing sexually transmitted infections and limiting mother to child transmission among HIV infected couples not desirous of having more children. During delivery, promoting clean delivery and limiting exposure of mother and the newborn will decrease risks to mother and baby in the postpartum period.

Human Immunodeficiency Virus (HIV)

The epidemiology of HIV/AIDS in women and children is discussed elsewhere (see McCaw-Binns and Hussein, Chapter 2 this volume). In developing countries HIV infection is mostly transmitted by sexual contact but can also be transmitted congenitally from mother to child during pregnancy, usually at birth by passage through an infected birth canal, and through breastfeeding. Other

persons are infected from blood products and body fluids of infected persons such as through blood transfusion. Efforts at guaranteeing a safe blood supply and proper handling of biological waste have reduced these sources of infection.

HIV infection progresses from a latent period of 2–4 weeks, when there is an acute febrile illness, into a dormant period of several months, after which symptoms of an opportunistic infection occur. Opportunistic infections range from persistent generalized lymphadenopathy (clinical stage 1), moderate unexplained weight loss and recurrent respiratory infections (clinical stage 2), chronic diarrhoea for longer than 1 month and unexplained anaemia (clinical stage 3) to HIV wasting syndrome and Kaposi's sarcoma (clinical stage 4). Any co-infections, for example, with tuberculosis or leishmaniasis, will progress and become more severe at this stage (WHO, 2005; Webber, 2009).

HIV infection is a serious disease in the woman in all stages of her life. Severity of the infection is measured by the CD4 level (the name given to a protein count to identify the level of infection), which determines her chance of surviving pregnancy and the likelihood of transmitting infection to her offspring.

Prevention

Effective HIV prevention requires a mix of behavioural, biomedical and structural intervention strategies. Primary prevention of HIV exposure is through health promotion activities aimed at delaying sexual debut: encouraging monogamous relationships and safe sexual practices. Interventions shown to reduce transmission of or acquiring HIV include consistent use of male and female condoms, reductions in concurrent and/or sequential sexual and needle-sharing partners, male circumcision and treatment with antiretroviral medications (Rotheram-Borus et al., 2009; Siegfried et al., 2009).

Scale-up of behavioural prevention programmes shown to be effective in reducing HIV transmission across a range of cultural settings is challenged by the consistent maintenance of effort required. Failures of HIV-prevention efficacy trials for HIV vaccines, treating herpes simplex 2 and other sexually transmitted infections and diaphragm and microbicide barriers highlight the need to continue to rely on behavioural strategies in the near future (Wilkinson et al., 2002).

COUNSELLING AND TESTING: SECONDARY PREVENTION HIV counselling and testing should be available at all special and general clinics. For known HIV-infected women, contraceptive advice should be provided to reduce unintended pregnancies and the number of HIV exposed and infected children. Pregnant mothers should be encouraged to be tested at antenatal clinic. If HIV positive on screening, the positive test should be confirmed using different antigens or confirmatory tests and her CD4 level determined.

Treatment and prevention of mother to child transmission (PMTCT)

An infected mother can pass on infection congenitally to her fetus or at the time of birth due to contamination by the mother's blood during delivery or for up to 2 years after if breast fed. Strategies to reduce mother to child transmission include:

1. Universal screening of all antenatal mothers.
2. Appropriate counselling of all HIV-positive mothers, providing appropriate antiretroviral treatment.
3. Ensuring prophylaxis before delivery and in the immediate puerperium.
4. Where appropriate, consider artificial feeding.

Good obstetric practice should be promoted to reduce unnecessary interference such as artificial rupture of the membranes and fetal scalp monitoring. There is no urgency to cut the umbilical cord, delaying this until it has stopped pulsating, or if the infant has taken its first breaths the placenta can even be delivered with the cord still intact. Gloves, syringes, needles, scissors and other instruments should be disposable or properly sterilized. All blood for transfusion should be screened. Caesarean section should not be encouraged in developing countries as a means to reduce the risk of HIV transmission, as the dangers in subsequent pregnancies are considerably increased, but is used as a strategy in developed countries.

An HIV mother should be advised on the risks to her and her infant during and after pregnancy and whether to breastfeed or artificially feed her child. Local circumstances will dictate policy and counsellors should weigh the relative risk of a child dying from diarrhoea due to contaminated bottles versus contracting HIV infection via breast milk in offering appropriate advice. Treatment must be accompanied by preventive methods as viral shedding can still occur and the importance of not missing any doses with the result of resistance developing must be explained.

The medical treatment goal for HIV-infected women, pregnant or not, is to maintain optimal health. If the CD4 level is less than 350, the mother should be given cotrimoxazole prophylaxis for opportunistic infection and started on long term antiretroviral therapy. If the CD4 level is greater than 350, she should be given prophylaxis with zidovudine (AZT) from 28 weeks until delivery and a single dose of nevirapine to take when she goes into labour. AZT and lamivudine should be given during the course of labour and continued for

7 days after delivery. Her CD4 level should also be checked to determine her risk of transmitting the virus due to breastfeeding. The infant should be given a single dose of nevirapine as soon after birth as possible and within the first 72 h and a course of AZT depending on how long its mother took AZT; if for less than 4 weeks then the infant should have a course of 4 weeks and if for 4 or more weeks then AZT should be given to the infant for 1 week. At 4 weeks the infant should be given cotrimoxazole/trimetho-prim prophylaxis (R. Gude Bukoba, Tanzania, 2009, personal communications). The risks of transmission to the infant during pregnancy and breastfeeding and of the mother dying are shown in Table 9.1 (Kuhn *et al.*, 2009).

Rapid progress is being made in the field of HIV, and updated guidance with signifi-cant changes has been recently introduced, with prophylaxis recommended to reduce the risk of breastfeeding and changes in the com-mencement of antiretroviral therapy in preg-nancy (Mepham *et al.*, 2010; WHO, 2010a). Many questions remain unanswered, for example, the effect of one or repeated courses of prophylaxis on progression of maternal HIV and the effectiveness of maternal com-pared to infant prophylaxis during breast-feeding (Mepham *et al.*, 2010).

Other sexually transmitted infections (STIs)

The common conditions encountered are gonorrhoea, chlamydial infection, syphilis, bacterial vaginosis, trichomoniasis and her-pes simplex. They are linked with adverse pregnancy outcomes such as miscarriage,

Table 9.1. CD4 levels in HIV infection and the risk of a mother passing on infection to her child during delivery or by breastfeeding and of dying as a result of her pregnancy (Kuhn *et al.*, 2009).

CD4 level	Transmission %	Breast feeding %	Maternal death %
>500	10	2	–
350–500	13	7.4	–
200–250	28	13	–
<200	44	21	55

perinatal death, low birth weight, prematurity and other specific neonatal morbidities; and infections of the cavity of the womb (endometri-tis) in the mother. Reported prevalence rates for these conditions during pregnancy in developing countries range from 1% to 20%, and can be as high as 50% for some conditions such as herpes simplex and bacterial vaginosis (Mullick *et al.*, 2005; WHO, 2011a).

The strategies for prevention and control of STIs are similar to those for HIV disease, except that it is possible to effect a cure with the non-HIV sexually transmitted infections. Control and prevention are mainly by:

- Health education.
- Family planning employing modern con-traceptives and dual protection using male and female condoms.
- Adequate diagnostic and treatment facili-ties and development of standard treat-ment protocols.
- Contact tracing.
- Routine testing of pregnant women.

Cheap, reliable screening tests are available for syphilis, trichomoniasis and bacterial vagi-nosis (and HIV), but even these are not often available in antenatal clinics in many develop-ing countries. In resource-poor settings, sexu-ally transmitted infection services can be based on syndromic management, which relies on management through the use of symptoms and treatment flow charts, although this method means that asymptomatic infec-tions will be missed (Mullick *et al.*, 2005).

Gonorrhoea

Neisseria gonorrhoeae is showing an increase in all parts of the world. It results in a urethral discharge in the male, but often goes undetec-ted in the female until resulting in pelvic inflammatory disease and subsequently ste-rility. Active infection while the mother is delivering can result in a severe conjunctivitis in the newborn (ophthalmia neonatorum). Diagnosis and adequate treatment require microbiological facilities and can be difficult in developing countries, yet treatment is straightforward with a single oral (cefixime) dose or intramuscular (ceftriaxone) injection (WHO, 2004a). Women with gonorrhoea often have chlamydia infection as well so treatment should be combined. Cases presenting should be encouraged to bring their partners (or provide information so they might be traced) for counselling and treatment.

Chlamydial infection

Infection with chlamydia may present as a cervical discharge or urethritis in the female but is usually asymptomatic and often indistinguishable from or present at the same time as gonorrhoea. Undiagnosed and untreated, it can lead to salpingitis and pelvic inflammatory disease, which can result in ectopic pregnancy and chronic pelvic pain. In pregnancy, *Chlamydia trachomatis* infection of the cervix can cause ophthalmia neonatorum and neonatal pneumonia. Treatment is with erthyromycin, azithromycin or amoxicillin (WHO, 2004a). As for gonorrhea, contact tracing is important.

Syphilis

The primary lesion of syphilis (the chancre, a painless ulcer with serous discharge) spontaneously heals after a few weeks, but 6 weeks to 6 months later signs of secondary syphilis are revealed. Should syphilis occur in early pregnancy, a miscarriage or stillbirth may result, while later in pregnancy the fetus is at risk of a range of abnormalities including deafness, abnormal bone formation and central nervous system involvement. Treatment is with intramuscular benzathine penicillin (Walker, 2001; WHO, 2004a).

Antenatal screening and treatment of syphilis are feasible and cost effective (Schmid, 2004). Non-treponemal tests such as RPR (rapid plasma reagin) and VDRL (venereal diseases research laboratory) are as effective and cheaper and easier to perform than treponemal tests; however, the former have low sensitivity and specificity. Confirmatory testing by a treponemal test like TPHA (Treponema pallidum haemoagglutination assay) has high sensitivity and specificity, but is expensive. In settings with limited resources and a high prevalence of syphilis, it is advisable to treat all pregnant women who test sero-positive on the non-treponemal tests (Peeling, 2004).

Bacterial vaginosis and trichomoniasis

Both these infections cause vaginal discharge but may be asymptomatic. They are a significant cause of prematurity and low birth weight. Antibiotic treatment (usually after the first trimester with metronidazole) improves outcomes in the case of bacterial vaginosis (Mullick *et al.*, 2005). In developing countries these common conditions are largely undetected and untreated as screening and management programmes are rarely available.

Herpes simplex

Infection with herpes simplex virus type 2 (HSV-2) produces painful vesicles on the genitalia, which can ulcerate. After apparent healing they recur at frequent intervals, often brought on by stress or menstruation. If the woman has a primary outbreak in late pregnancy this can cause fetal infection resulting in encephalitis, liver damage or lesions to the eye, mouth or skin. HSV-2 infection also carries an increased risk of the woman developing HIV infection. Acyclovir is used to treat the primary infection in pregnancy and famciclovir for recurrent infection (WHO, 2005).

Malaria

Women in malaria endemic regions may find that, despite previous and repeated infections which build immunity, pregnancy makes them susceptible to re-infection and associated complications. This is due to the combined immune suppression which occurs during the second half of pregnancy and the physiological mechanisms of malaria infection, which also depress the existing immunity to antigens related to the species of parasite, and together they unmask an infection. This is greater in the first pregnancy than subsequent ones, and the woman must be treated. Acute renal insufficiency as a complication of falciparum malaria is more likely in pregnant women and can often be confused with or superimposed on pre-eclampsia. Treatment should not be withheld because the mother is pregnant as her chance of dying is far greater than any risk to the developing fetus. For more details about malaria, see Warrell and Gilles (2002) and Webber (2009).

Epidemic malaria is an important cause of abortions and stillbirths, especially in communities with little immunity. Low birth weight is a feature of endemic malaria. Treatment contributes to reductions in preterm/low birth weight (Luntamo *et al.*, 2010) infants and infant deaths (Bardají *et al.*, 2011). The same benefit is seen when preventive methods are used (Tiono *et al.*, 2009).

Prevention

Prevention of malaria during pregnancy in highly endemic areas should include a combination of intermittent preventive treatment (IPT), insecticide-treated nets (ITN) and access to treatment facilities. IPT is with two doses of sulfadoxine-pyrimethamine given 1 month apart after quickening or one dose at 20–24 weeks and a second at 28–32 weeks (WHO, 2002). In other areas different IPT regimes maybe appropriate, such as chloroquine in areas where *Plasmodium vivax* is the predominant species and chloroquine resistance does not occur. This can be combined with proguanil. In other areas, mefloquine may be appropriate and local advice should be sought.

Pregnant women with HIV infection are more likely to have an increased prevalence and intensity of malarial infection, with the multigravida responding in a similar way to a primigravida (Reithinger *et al.*, 2009). They should have a course of prophylactic AZT plus sulfadoxine-pyrimethamine IPT unless on antiretroviral therapy, in which case cotrimoxazole prophylaxis will protect them against malaria.

The main method of preventing malaria is with an ITN, with added advantages of preventing other vector-borne infections such as filariasis and tick borne relapsing fever. Pregnant women and children, including newborns, should be given priority in the use of nets. Every effort should be made to reduce mosquito biting by using clothing that covers exposed parts of the body and by repellents. The newer, long-lasting insecticidal (polyester-based) nets have been found to be more effective and retain their knock-down power for up to 36 months (Kilian *et al.*, 2008).

Treatment

The development of widespread resistance to chloroquine makes treatment of malaria with this drug challenging, especially where infection is with *P. vivax*, *P. malariae* or *P. ovale*. Chloroquine resistant *P. vivax* is now found in Western Pacific islands and parts of northern South America.

Plasmodium falciparum is also resistant to chloroquine and many other antimalarials due to indiscriminate use, leaving the artemisinin group of compounds still effective. WHO recommends that they be used with other antimalarials as artemisinin combination therapies (WHO, 2010b). Unfortunately, cases of artemesinin-resistant malaria have now been reported from Cambodia (Dandorp *et al.*, 2009), so local advice needs to be taken on the treatment regime to be used. A recent systematic review concluded that existing antimalarial regimens in pregnancy still do not reach optimal efficacy rates, making the case for more evidence to be generated on malaria prevention and treatment in pregnancy (McGready *et al.*, 2010).

Respiratory tract infections

Tuberculosis

Pulmonary tuberculosis is the commonest manifestation of respiratory-tract infections in pregnancy, as with the non-pregnant population. It can be difficult to diagnose, as early symptoms such as lassitude and fatigue also often occur in pregnancy (Mnyani and McIntyre, 2010). The management of tuberculosis in pregnant women is similar to general management although streptomycin should be avoided as it is toxic to the fetus (WHO, 2010c). It is not clear to what extent tuberculosis affects pregnancy outcome as evidence is conflicting, although if treatment is started late in pregnancy prematurity and neonatal mortality have been noted to be higher. Co-infection with HIV in pregnancy remains a concern. The current recommendation is to start combination antiretroviral therapy after starting treatment for tuberculosis within 8 weeks, although antiretroviral therapy can aggravate tuberculosis (Mnyani and McIntyre, 2010).

Influenza

The recent H1N1 pandemic has emphasized the severity of influenza in pregnancy, with case fatality rates of over 20% in severely infected pregnant women and perinatal mortality almost six times that of uninfected women (CDC, 2011; Pierce *et al.*, 2011). Vaccinating pregnant women against influenza is an essential preventive measure. Of the two vaccines available currently, Pandemrix is recommended for pregnant women as it gives good levels of antibodies after a single dose. Frequent hand washing and reduction of contact are simple but essential control measures, as for many other infectious conditions.

TORCH infections

TORCH (toxoplasmosis, rubella, cytomegalovirus and herpes simplex) is a group of viral, bacterial and protozoal infections which are specially implicated in being passed from a pregnant mother to the fetus. They include other conditions such as hepatitis B, syphilis, chickenpox (varicella), listerosis, parvovirus B19, coxsackievirus and herpes simplex virus. Exposure to TORCH infection results in poor perinatal outcome. Many of the conditions have mild infective symptoms in the pregnant women, which may go unnoticed, but infants will be stillborn or suffer multiple organ defects (to the heart, brain, liver, eye), depending on the specific infection. Some conditions such as toxoplasmosis are transmitted by cats and can be controlled with hygiene and contact reduction. Immunization and vaccination programmes can control conditions such as rubella.

Neonatal tetanus

Neonatal tetanus remains a common condition in developing countries despite effective prevention by administration of tetanus toxoid (WHO, 2011b). It is often due to infection of the umbilical cord from unclean deliveries where the cord is cut with a non-sterile knife or when the stump is covered with an unsterile dressing. Some 5–10 days after birth the infant has difficulty in sucking, then rigidity of muscles and generalized convulsions develop, with high fatality rates.

Neonatal tetanus prevention begins in early pregnancy by ensuring the mother has been vaccinated. The WHO policy is to give all women a lifetime total of five doses of tetanus toxoid. This is preferable to waiting until the woman becomes pregnant because many of the women who do not attend antenatal clinic are more likely to have an unsterile delivery. The initial vaccination is given at first contact or as early as possible during pregnancy. The second is given 4 weeks later and the third 6–12 months after the previous dose or during the next pregnancy. Doses four and five are given at yearly intervals. If a woman has a certificate to show she was vaccinated as a child, she only needs two doses during the first pregnancy and one more before or during the second pregnancy.

Deliveries should be conducted using sterilized instruments and dressings. Mothers should be educated on the appropriate care of the umbilicus to reduce the risk of infection. Clean delivery kits (see Langer *et al.*, Chapter 8 this volume) have been used, although effects on maternal and perinatal outcome are not clear (Hundley *et al.*, 2011)

Puerperal sepsis is also an infectious condition of pregnancy and is discussed elsewhere (see Chapter 8 this volume).

Chronic and Non-Communicable Diseases in Pregnancy

With improved access to health care, many women with medical conditions survive into the child-bearing years and desire to have children. Among the conditions likely to be seen in developing countries are the chronic effects of infection (pyelonephritis and rheumatic fever) as well as other non-communicable diseases, including sickle cell disease, thalassaemia, cardiac conditions, gestational diabetes and, with increasing prevalence of obesity, Type II diabetes mellitus. In populations with a high prevalence of risk factors, it is advisable to include screening for these conditions as part of routine antenatal care.

Conditions of the urinary tract

Urinary tract infections in pregnancy range from a mild inconvenience in early pregnancy to severe renal disease; 75% of infections are due to *Escherichia coli*, the remainder to streptococci, staphylococci or the Proteus group of organisms. Early and adequate treatment with antibiotics will prevent the infection becoming chronic, which can result in damage to the kidneys, renal failure and hypertension. Renal failure may cause death several years after pregnancy and is often not included in any statistics on maternal mortality (Sandvik *et al.*, 2010).

The cardiovascular system

Pregnancy places added stress on the cardiovascular function of women, which can lead to life-threatening situations for both mother and baby in the case of any pre-existing cardiac condition. Rheumatic fever originates from a respiratory infection by Group A streptococcus. It is rare in developed countries but remains an important public health problem in developing countries. Chronic rheumatic heart disease can result from the acute infection, with permanent damage to the heart valves and function. Management of the condition may be medical or surgical and depends on the type and severity of the heart condition (WHO, 2004b).

Thalassaemias and sickle cell disease

Genetically transmitted disorders of the blood of importance in pregnancy include the thalassaemias and sickle cell disease. Both conditions are commoner in developing countries. The thalassaemias are common in parts of Africa, India and the Mediterranean and Southeast Asia, while sickle cell disease occurs mainly in Africa, India and in populations of African descent in the Americas (Prakash *et al.*, 1991; Piel *et al.*, 2010; Asnani *et al.*, 2011). Anaemia can result from both these conditions and can be acute and severe in cases. Women who carry the trait for these haemoglobinopathies should be counselled and partners invited for screening to determine the potential risk of passing the disease to the infant. Women who are homozygous for these conditions (indicating a severe form of the disease) should receive special management during pregnancy (de Montalembert, 2008).

Nutrition

Worldwide, 42% of pregnant women are anaemic, the most common form being iron deficiency anaemia, which increases the risk of death from haemorrhage (WHO, 2008). Malnutrition develops when the body lacks the vitamins, minerals and other nutrients needed to maintain healthy tissue and bodily function (McCafferty, 2009). Micronutrient deficiency, particularly iron and folate, and related supplementation are associated with improving pregnancy outcomes such as reducing low birth weight and small for gestational age and neural tube defects. Long-term benefits, such as improved growth at 2 years, were seen in children whose mothers received multiple micronutrient supplementation during pregnancy compared to standard iron–folate supplements (Huy *et al.*, 2009; Alwan *et al.*, 2011).

The growing prevalence of lifestyle-related conditions which contribute to the increased prevalence of obesity even in developing countries has contributed to a growing incidence of problems of obesity, diabetes mellitus, heart disease and hypertensive diseases. Women who are obese should have a careful medical history taken and be screened to ensure that these chronic conditions are not aggravated by the pregnancy.

Diabetes mellitus

Three types of diabetes can affect pregnancy: Type I, which is usually dependent on insulin therapy, Type II, the commonest form of which usually affects adults in later life, and gestational diabetes, which is first detected in pregnancy. Gestational diabetes has been described as a 'looming epidemic' in developing countries (Sadikot, 2009). Many countries with a high prevalence of Type II diabetes include developing nations, such as Bangladesh, Brazil, China, India, Indonesia and Pakistan. Diabetes is associated with a higher risk of hypertension in the mother and a myriad of fetal complications including stillbirths, abnormally large babies, congenital malformations and increased perinatal mortality. Gestational diabetes in the mother predisposes to the development of Type II diabetes in the mother later in life.

Mental health

Of the mental disorders of pregnancy, depression is one of the commonest. Prenatal depression is thought to be a precursor of postnatal depression and may be more common. Postnatal depression usually develops 4 weeks to 3 months after birth, but may occur later and may be seen in 10–15% of new mothers. It is associated with ambivalence towards the infant, low self esteem, general inability to cope and suicidal ideation. Women with a previous history or family history of depression, relationship problems, unplanned pregnancy and perinatal loss are at increased risk (Sit and Wisner, 2009).

Maternal Health Programme Strategies

If a patient gives a history of a chronic illness, she should be referred for evaluation by a physician who may be asked to co-manage her pregnancy. While women with chronic disorders may successfully complete the pregnancy, the long term management of their chronic condition, probably only diagnosed for the first time during pregnancy, should receive attention, with referral to a medical provider for continued care at the end of the puerperium. Data from developed (Berg *et al.*, 2001) and even developing countries suggest that the risk of death in this population (sometimes classified as pregnancy-associated deaths) remains elevated in the first year after delivery.

All pregnant women should be offered a minimum package of antenatal care, free of charge to all pregnant women to ensure universal access and utilization, which may be adapted to the epidemiological profile and disease burden in the community. Providers should be encouraged to allow women to carry their own obstetric case records, which include all the essential information on obstetric history, current pregnancy and general medical conditions, making the antenatal records available for the pregnant woman regardless of where she chooses to deliver. Key strategies pertinent to the different phases of pregnancy are listed in Table 9.2.

Conclusion

As efforts to reduce the leading direct causes of maternal death (haemorrhage, sepsis, eclampsia, obstructed labour and unsafe abortion) succeed, coupled with the increasing prevalence of lifestyle disorders, the relative and real importance of improving the management of the indirect causes of maternal death will increase. Unlike the direct causes, reducing the mortality in indirect conditions requires a set of different interventions from the obstetric and childbirth focused ones such as emergency obstetric care and provision of a skilled birth attendant. Although health programmes are implemented to combat communicable diseases and general medical conditions, they do not necessarily take account of the special needs of pregnant women.

The scale of the burden in pregnancy from medical conditions is mostly unknown in developing countries. Operational research is needed to determine how to design and best integrate these services into existing antenatal and post-delivery care, and community primary care programmes. Compared to long term obstetric morbidities such as obstetric fistula and uterine prolapse, less is known about the long term consequences of medical conditions that first arise in tandem with childbearing, such as chronic hypertension, cardiomyopathy, renal disease, diabetes mellitus and progression to HIV/AIDS, or about whether improved management of risk factors during pregnancy and the puerperium may reduce the development, severity and mortality from these disorders later in life.

Table 9.2. Strategies to manage medical disorders in pregnancy (Di Mario *et al.*, 2005; Powrie *et al.*, 2010).[a]

Period	Intervention
Pre-pregnancy	Measles/mumps/rubella and tetanus vaccination
	Family planning to prevent unwanted pregnancy, especially for high parity, older women and HIV-positive women
	Malaria prevention
	Improvements in general health and nutrition
	Folic acid supplementation to all women before conception and up to 12 weeks of gestation to avoid neural tube defects in the fetus
Antenatal	Iron/folate supplementation in populations with high prevalence of anaemia, including blood transfusion for severe anaemia
	Screening/counselling/treatment for HIV, other sexually transmitted infections and non-communicable diseases
	Tetanus vaccination
	Antimalarial prevention/treatment
	Access to specialist medical care, in case of disease progression
	Energy/protein supplementation in women at risk
	Smoking and alcohol consumption cessation
Intrapartum	Acute medical care for aggressive manifestation of condition during labour (e.g. cardiac failure, arrhythmias, diabetic control)
	Blood transfusion for severe anaemia
	Short course of antiretroviral drugs, and consider Caesarean section at 38 weeks for infected mothers to reduce vertical transmission of HIV
	Assessment of need for artificial feeding for newborn
Postnatal/neonatal and beyond	Awareness of specific diseases that can manifest postnatally in the mother, including mental conditions, sickle cell disease, chronic hypertension
	Continued care for women with medical conditions (e.g. HIV, tuberculosis, heart disease) or at high risk of developing them later in life or in subsequent pregnancy (e.g. hypertension, diabetes)
	Immunization and maternal education to recognize neonatal complications
	Exclusive breastfeeding/assessment of need for artificial feeding for newborn
	Assessment and management of congenital/inherited conditions in newborn
	Prevention of new conditions such as malaria, and immunization in newborn

[a]Additional obstetric and neonatal interventions will also be required for mothers and babies in women with medical conditions; these are listed elsewhere (see Stanton and Lawn, Chapter 5 this volume and Langer *et al.*, Chapter 8 this volume)

References

AbouZahr, C. (2003) Global burden of maternal death and disability. *British Medical Bulletin* 67, 1–11.

Alwan, N.A., Greenwood, D.C., Simpson, N.A., McArdle, H.J., Godfrey, K.M. and Cade, J.E. (2011) Dietary iron intake during early pregnancy and birth outcomes in a cohort of British women. *Human Reproduction* 26(4), 911–919.

Asnani, M.R., McCaw–Binns, A.M. and Reid, M.E. (2011) Excess risk of maternal death from sickle disease in Jamaica: 1998–2007. *PLoS ONE* 6(10): e26281.

Bardají, A., Sigauque, B., Sanz, S., Maixenchs, M., Ordi, J., Aponte, J.J., Mabunda, S., Alonso, P.L. and Menéndez, C. (2011) Impact of malaria at the end of pregnancy on infant mortality and morbidity. *Journal of Infectious Diseases* 203(5), 691–699.

Beniwal, M., Kumar, A., Kar, P., Jilani, N. and Sharma, J.B. (2003) Prevalence and severity of acute viral hepatitis and fulminant hepatitis during pregnancy: a prospective study from north India. *Indian Journal of Medical Microbiology* 21(3), 184–185.

Berg, C., Danel, I., Atrash, H., Zane, S. and Bartlett, L. (eds) (2001) *Strategies to Reduce Pregnancy Related Deaths: from identification and review to action.* Centers for Disease Control and Prevention, Atlanta, Georgia.

Centers for Disease Control and Prevention (CDC) (2011) Maternal and infant outcomes among severely ill pregnant and postpartum women with 2009 pandemic influenza A (H1N1) – United States, April 2009–August 2010. *MMWR Morbility and Mortality Weekly Report*, 9 September, 60(35), 1193–1196.

Cross, S., Bell, J.S. and Graham, W.J. (2010) What you count is what you target: the implications of maternal death classification for tracking progress towards reducing maternal mortality in developing countries. *Bulletin of the World Health Organization* 88(2), 147–153.

Dandorp, A.M., Norsten, F., Yi, P., Das, D., Phoya, A.P., Taming, J., Lwin, K.M., Ariey, F., Hanpithakong, W., Lee, S.J., Ringwald, P., Silamut, K., Imwong, M., Chotivanich, N., Lim, P., Herdman, T., An, S.S., Yeung, S., Singhasivan, P., Day, P.J., Lindegardh, N., Socheat, D. and White, N.J. (2009) Artemesinin resistance in *Plasmodium falciparum* malaria. *New England Journal of Medicine* 361, 455–467.

de Montalembert, M. (2008) Management of sickle cell disease. *British Medical Journal* 337, 626–630.

Di Mario, S., Basevi, V., Daya, L., Magnano, L. and Magrini, N. (2005) *What is the Effectiveness of Antenatal Care?* (Supplement) Copenhagen, WHO Regional Office for Europe Health Evidence Network, WHO, Geneva.

Hundley, V.A., Avan, B.I., Braunholtz, D. and Graham, W.J. (2011) Are birth kits a good idea? A systematic review of the evidence. *Midwifery*, 9 May [Epub ahead of print].

Huy, N.D., Le Hop, T., Shrimpton, R. and Hoa, C.V. (2009) An effectiveness trial of multiple micronutrient supplementation during pregnancy in Vietnam: impact on birthweight and on stunting in children at around 2 years of age. *Food and Nutrition Bulletin* 30(Suppl. 4), S506–S516.

Khan, K.S., Wojdyla, D., Say, L., Gülmezoglu, A.M. and Van Look, P.F.A. (2006) WHO analysis of causes of maternal death: a systematic review. *Lancet* 367, 1066–1074.

Kilian, A., Byamukama, W., Pigeon, O., Atieli, F., Duchon, S. and Phan, C. (2008) Long-term field performance of a polyester-based long-lasting insecticidal mosquito net in rural Uganda. *Malaria Journal* 7, 49.

Kuhn, L., Aldrovandi, G.M., Sinkala, M., Kankasa, C., Semrau, K., Kasonde, P., Mwiya, M., Tsai, W.Y. and Thea, D.M. (2009) Zambia Exclusive Breastfeeding Study (ZEBS). Differential effects of early weaning for HIV-free survival of children born to HIV-infected mothers by severity of maternal disease. *PloS One* 4(6), e6059.

Luntamo, M., Kulmala, T., Mbewe, B., Cheung, Y.B., Maleta, K. and Ashorn, P. (2010) Effect of repeated treatment of pregnant women with sulfadoxine-pyrimethamine and azithromycin on preterm delivery in Malawi: a randomized controlled trial. *American Journal of Tropical Medicine and Hygiene* 83(6), 1212–1220.

McCafferty, C. for UK All Parliamentary Group on Population, Development and Reproductive Health (2009) Better off dead? A report on maternal morbidity. Available at: http://www.appg-popdevrh.org.uk/.../AAPG_PDRH_ANN_REP_0102.pdf (accessed 11 November 2011)

McCaw-Binns, A. and Lewis-Bell, K. (2009) Small victories, new challenges: two decades of maternal mortality surveillance in Jamaica. *West Indian Medical Journal* 58(6), 518–532.

McGready, M., White, N.J. and Nosten, F. (2010) Parasitological efficacy of anitmalarials in the treatment and prevention of falciparum malaria in pregnancy 1998–2009: a systematic review. *BJOG: An International Journal of Obstetrics and Gynaecology* 118(2), 123–135.

Mepham, S.O., Bland, R.M. and Newell, M.-L. (2010) Prevention of mother to child transmission of HIV in resource rich and poor settings. *BJOG: An International Journal of Obstetrics and Gynaecology* 118(2), 202–218.

Mnyani, C.N. and McIntyre, J.A. (2010) Tuberculosis in pregnancy. *BJOG: An International Journal of Obstetrics and Gynaecology* 118(2), 226–231.

Mullick, S., Watson-Jones, D., Beksinska, M. and Mabey, D. (2005) Sexually transmitted infections in pregnancy: prevalence, impact on pregnancy outcomes, and approach to treatment in developing countries. *Sexually Transmitted Infections* 81, 294–302.

Pant, P.D., Suvedi, B.K., Pradhan, A., Hulton, L., Matthews, Z. and Maskey, M. (2008) *Investigating Improvements in Maternal Health in Nepal, Further Analysis of the 2006 NDHS*. ISA, Macro International Inc, Calverton, Maryland.

Peeling, R. (2004) Diagnostic tools for preventing and managing maternal and congenital syphilis: an overview. *Bulletin of the World Health Organization* 82, 439–446.

Piel, F.B., Patil, A.P., Howes, R.E., Nyangiri, O.A., Gething, P.W., Williams, T.N., Weatherall, D.J. and Hay, S.I. (2010) Global distribution of the sickle cell gene and geographical confirmation of the malaria hypothesis. *Nature Communications* 1, 104.

Pierce, M., Kurinczuk, J.J., Spark, P., Brocklehurst, P. and Knight, M.: UKOSS (2011) Perinatal outcomes after maternal 2009/H1N1 infection: national cohort study. *British Medical Journal* 14, 342. doi: 10.1136/bmj.d3214

Powrie, R.O., Greene, M.F. and Camann, W. (eds) (2010) *de Swiet's Medical Diseases in Obstetric Practice*. Wiley-Blackwell, Oxford, UK.

Prakash, A., Swain, S. and Seth, A. (1991) Maternal mortality in India: current status and strategies for reduction. *Indian Pediatrics* 28, 1395–4000.

Reithinger, R., Kamya, M.R., Whitty, C.J., Dorsey, G. and Vermund, S.H. (2009) Interaction of malaria and HIV in Africa. *British Medical Journal* 338, 1400–1401.

Rotheram-Borus, M.J., Swendeman, D. and Chovnick, G. (2009) The past, present, and future of HIV prevention: integrating behavioral, biomedical, and structural intervention strategies for the next generation of HIV prevention. *Annual Review of Clinical Psychology* 5, 143–167.

Sadikot, S.M. (2009) The epidemiology of diabetes in women and the looming epidemic of GDM in the Third World. In: Tsatsoulis, A., Wyckoff, J. and Brown, F.M. (eds) *Diabetes in Women: pathophysiology and therapy*. Humana Press, New Jersey, pp. 223–238.

Sandvik, M.K., Iversen, B.M., Irgens, L.M., Skjaerven, R., Leivestad, T., Søfteland, E. and Vikse, B.E. (2010) Are adverse pregnancy outcomes risk factors for development of end-stage renal disease in women with diabetes? *Nephrology, Dialysis, Transplantation* 25(11), 3600–3607.

Schmid, G. (2004) Economic and programmatic aspects of congenital syphilis prevention. *Bulletin of the World Health Organization* 82(6), 402–409.

Siegfried, N., Muller, M., Deeks, J.J. and Volmink, J. (2009) Male circumcision for prevention of heterosexual acquisition of HIV in men. *Cochrane Database Systematic Review: CD003362*. South African Cochrane Centre, South African Medical Research Council, PO Box 19070, Tygerberg, South Africa.

Sit, D.K. and Wisner, K.L. (2009) Identification of postpartum depression. *Clinical Obstetrics and Gynecology* 52(3), 456–468.

Suvedi, B.K., Pradhan, A., Barnett, S., Puri, M., Chitrakar, S.R., Poudel, P., Sharma, S. and Hulton, L. (2009) *Nepal Maternal Mortality and Morbidity Study 2008/2009: summary of preliminary findings*. Family Health Division, Department of Health Services, Ministry of Health, Government of Nepal, Kathmandu, Nepal.

Tiono, A.B., Ouedraogo, A., Bougouma, E.C., Diarra, A., Konaté, A.T., Nébié, I. and Sirima, S.B. (2009) Placental malaria and low birth weight in pregnant women living in a rural area of Burkina Faso following the use of three preventive treatment regimens. *Malaria Journal* 7(8), 224.

Walker, G.J.A. (2001) Antibiotics for syphilis diagnosed during pregnancy. *The Cochrane Database of Systematic Reviews* 3, CD001143.

Warrell, D. and Gilles, H. (2002) *Essential Malariology*, 4th edn. Hodder Arnold, London.

Webber, R. (2009) *Communicable Disease Epidemiology and Control*, 3rd edn. CAB International, Wallingford, UK.

WHO (2002) *Strategic Framework for Malaria Control during Pregnancy in the WHO Africa Region*. WHO, Geneva.

WHO (2004a) *Integrating Care for Reproductive Health, Sexually Transmitted and Other Reproductive Tract Infections; a guide to essential practice*. WHO, Geneva.

WHO (2004b) *Rheumatic Fever and Rheumatic Heart Disease: report of a WHO Expert Consultation*. WHO, Geneva.

WHO (2005) Interim WHO Clinical Staging of HIV/AIDS and HIV/AIDS Case Definition Surveillance. WHO, Geneva. Available at: http://www.who.int/hiv/pub/guidelines/casedefinitions/en/ (accessed 14 November 2011).

WHO (2008) Worldwide prevalence of anaemia report 1993–2005. Available at: http://www.who.int/vmnis/publications/anaemia_prevalence/en/index.html (accessed 14 November 2011).

WHO (2010a) *Antiretroviral Therapy for HIV Infection in Adults and Adolescents. Recommendations for a public health approach*, 2010 revision. WHO, Geneva.

WHO (2010b) *Guidelines for the Treatment of Malaria*, 2nd edn. WHO, Geneva.

WHO (2010c) *Treatment of Tuberculosis Guidelines*. WHO, Geneva.

WHO (2011a) Sexually transmitted infections. Available at: http://www.who.int/topics/sexually_transmitted_infections/en/ (accessed 4 August 2011).

WHO (2011b) Neonatal tetanus. Available at: http://www.who.int/immunization_monitoring/diseases/neonatal_tetanus/en/index.html (accessed 4 August 2011).

Wilkinson, D., Ramjee, G., Tholandi, M. and Rutherford, G. (2002) Nonoxynol-9 for preventing vaginal acquisition of sexually transmitted infections by women from men. *Cochrane Database Systematic Review*, CD003939. Division of Health Sciences, University of South Australia, Australia.

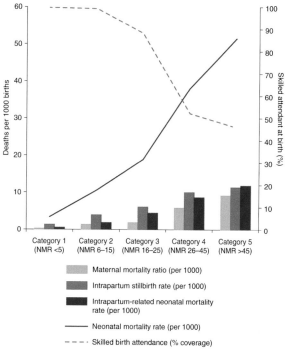

1

Category 1 (NMR <5) Category 2 (NMR 6–15) Category 3 (NMR 16–25) Category 4 (NMR 26–45) Category 5 (NMR >45)

☐ Maternal mortality ratio (per 1000)

▨ Intrapartum stillbirth rate (per 1000)

■ Intrapartum-related neonatal mortality rate (per 1000)

— Neonatal mortality rate (per 1000)

-- Skilled birth attendance (% coverage)

193 Countries organized in 5 neonatal mortality rate categories as markers of health system performance.
Note: the association between neonatal mortality and skilled attendance is ecological and cannot be assumed to be causal.
NMR, neonatal mortality rate.

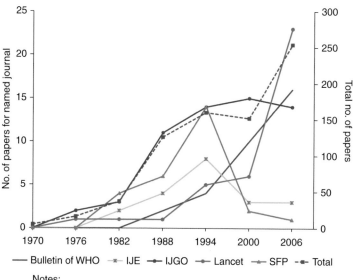

2

— Bulletin of WHO —✳— IJE —●— IJGO —✦— Lancet —▲— SFP —■— Total

Notes:
Total number of articles for each 6–year interval are plotted against the year at the start of the interval.
IJE *International Journal of Epidemiology*
SFP *Studies in Family Planning*
IJGO *International Journal of Gynaecology and Obstetrics*

Plate 1. Global relationship between maternal deaths, stillbirths and neonatal deaths and access to skilled care at birth (Lawn *et al.*, 2009b).

Plate 2. Trends in published articles from search on 'measuring maternal mortality in developing countries': 1970–2010.

3

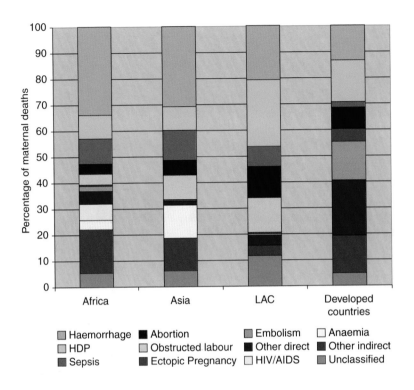

4

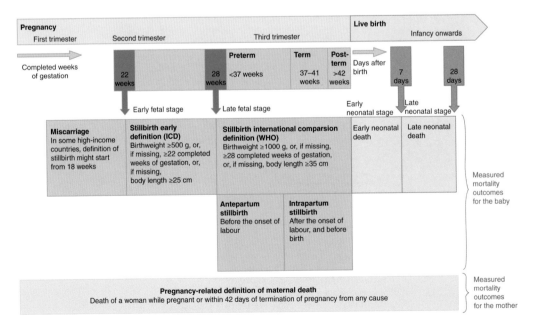

Plate 3. Percentage distribution of causes of maternal deaths by world region (Khan *et al.*, 2006).

Plate 4. Definitions of stillbirths, neonatal deaths and pregnancy-related deaths according to the International Classification of Diseases, 10th Revision (Lawn *et al.*, 2011).

5

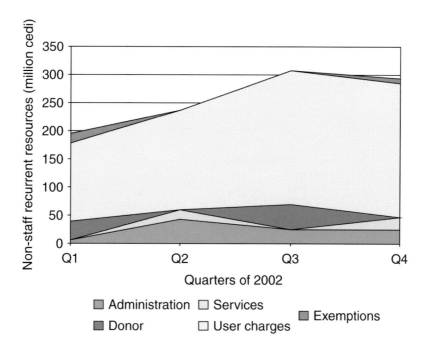

6

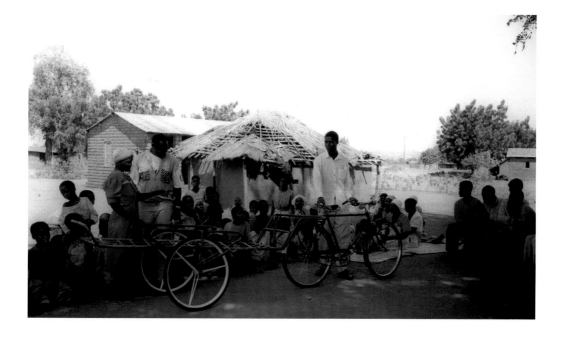

Plate 5. Recurrent revenue in one district hospital in Ghana, 2002.

Plate 6. Bicycle ambulance. Picture: Julia Hussein.

7

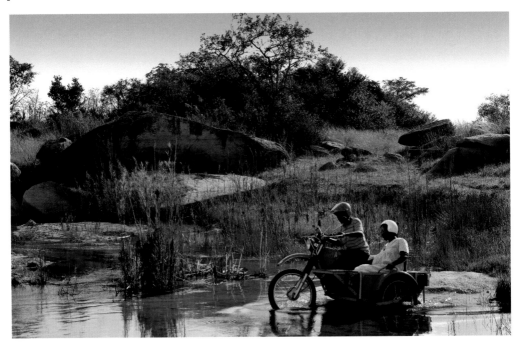

8

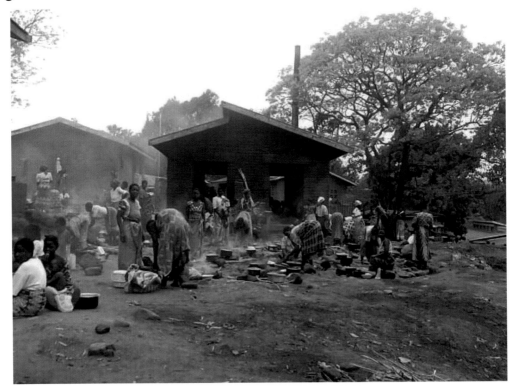

Plate 7. Motorcycle ambulance. Picture: Udo Thomas / Riders for Health.

Plate 8. Maternity waiting home. Picture: Paul Kwale Nkhoma Hospital Safe Motherhood Programme.

10 Improving the Availability of Services

Ann Phoya,[1] Dileep V. Mavalankar,[2] Parvathy Sankara Raman[2] and Julia Hussein[3]
[1]*Ministry of Health, Lilongwe, Malawi;*
[2]*Indian Institute of Public Health, Gandhinagar, India;*
[3]*University of Aberdeen, Scotland, UK*

Summary

- To ensure adequate coverage of care for maternal and perinatal health goals, maternity services (of good quality) must be made available.
- The availability of maternity services is dependent upon the health system and cannot be planned in isolation.
- Clear policies which draw upon principles of the primary health-care approach can guide identification of service availability needs.
- Geographical availability and distribution of health facilities influence the use of health services. Benchmarks for the catchment populations of different levels of maternity services vary across countries, but for emergency obstetric care a minimum of five facilities in a population of half a million is recommended.
- Once a network of maternity facilities has been established at the various levels of the health system, specification of the packages of interventions (for antenatal, delivery and postnatal care) that should be made available at each level is necessary.
- Human resources, physical infrastructure, drugs, equipment, transport and communications systems are the tangible health system elements that are crucial to service availability.
- Integrated services could contribute towards improving efficiency, but cannot be seen as a solution for lack of resource allocation to maternity services.

Introduction

As countries strive to identify the best ways to improve maternal and perinatal health, a focus on the 'coverage of care' has become a top priority. Coverage for maternity care can be defined as the proportion of women needing an intervention who receive it. It is a specific focus of the Countdown to 2015 initiative (http://www.countdown2015mnch.org), which tracks coverage for interventions needed to attain MDGs 4 and 5. Increases in coverage indicate that health policies and services are being implemented and are reaching pregnant women, although it is recognized that increasing coverage alone is not sufficient and has to be matched with improvements in quality and effectiveness (UNICEF, 2008).

Improvements in coverage cannot be achieved without ensuring that maternity services are available. National development programmes that aim to address issues of availability of maternity services should focus on strengthening health delivery systems at all levels, so this chapter is written in that context. A number of areas need to be addressed in order to have a functioning and effective health-care system that supports the improvement of service availability. Drawing from the experiences of two diverse settings – Malawi and India – some critical areas considered in this chapter include:

- Clear policy direction on maternal and perinatal health.
- Revitalizing the use of the primary health care approach for delivery of care.
- Improving geographical availability through strengthening the network of health facilities.
- Packaging interventions for different levels of the health-care system.
- Ensuring adequate resources (human resources, drugs, medical supplies, equipment) for each level of care.
- Integrating the delivery of different components of maternity care.

Institutionalization of the many elements to ensure a functioning health system that responds to the needs of pregnant women is a responsibility of all players in the health sector, including government agencies, profit and non-profit private institutions, non-government organizations, civil society, community groups and family members. The roles of these multiple players should be complementary and not competitive in nature, so that a coordinated approach to service delivery is made.

Overarching Policies and Approaches

Policy direction

In any country, policies that give direction for provision of social services such as health should be embedded in law or the national constitution. A constitution that spells out that provision of health care is one of the rights to be enjoyed by citizens, ensures that government, through its departments (such as ministries of health) or through local assemblies, will have strategic plans or policies that identify national health priorities and programmes and resources required to deliver

services and support the availability of services. Commitment to MDGs 4 and 5 should therefore be reflected in the national health sector plan to give direction to all stakeholders involved in health service delivery. Development of such policies, plans and programmes needs to be consultative in nature to allow for inclusion and fusion of ideas from a wide range of health sector players. Agreed-upon policies and programmes should be disseminated as widely as possible, especially to those at the operational and grassroots levels responsible for service delivery. Civil society plays a watchdog role to ensure that duty bearers of health policy and programmes fulfil their responsibilities. Policies should be flexible enough to allow for creativity and implementation of evidence-based interventions that may be generated as national plans and programmes are being operationalized.

An example of a concrete policy direction for provision of maternity services exists in Malawi where the constitution clearly states that government shall provide health care of an international standard for its people (Government of Malawi, 1996). This constitutional mandate has been translated into a 6-year national programme of work, which spells out an essential health package, including interventions related to maternal, newborn and child health. Resource mobilization strategies are also included in the programme of work to ensure availability of financial resources for the essential health package (Minstry of Health, 2010). To provide further policy direction for stakeholders and implementers, the Ministry of Health has developed a reproductive health strategic plan and road map for accelerating reduction of maternal and neonatal deaths in the country. As a result of this clear policy direction, all health sector players are aware of the commitment of the Government of Malawi to identification and implementation of interventions that would promote maternal health and reduce preventable maternal and perinatal deaths.

The primary health-care approach

The concept of primary health care adopted at the Alma Ata Conference in 1978 as a mechanism for achieving an acceptable level of health status is still valid today (WHO, 1978; Tarimo and Webster, 1997). Utilization of the primary health-care approach as a modality and an overarching strategy has proved fruitful in ensuring the availability of basic maternity services at most levels of the health system, but importantly in communities where people live. For example, the contraceptive prevalence rate has increased in many low income countries (UN, 2008), facilitated in part through door to door distribution of family planning methods by community volunteers in countries such as Bangladesh and Indonesia (Prata *et al.*, 2005). Increases in health facility delivery have also been documented in Asia, sub-Saharan Africa and Latin America (WHO, 2005). The advocacy functions of community leaders in Malawi illustrate how community members can exert considerable influence on uptake of maternity services (Kwataine, 2010).

The concept of the continuum of care describes the need to provide services for mothers and their children from before and during pregnancy to childbirth and the early days and years of life. In addition, it underscores the need to make services available to link the various levels from home to health facilities (PMNCH, 2011). Through application of primary health-care principles, countries can ensure that a range of promotive, preventive, curative and rehabilitative components for maternity care are available to urban and to rural poor populations. Recommitment to the primary health care concept will strengthen multisectoral collaboration, ensure coordination and improve accountability and performance of development partners – all in keeping with the revitalized calls to harmonize aid and reform the health sector (see Mavalankar and Sankara Raman, Chapter 6 this volume).

The Maternity Service Infrastructure

Geographical availability

Setting policy direction and recommitting to the primary health-care concept in itself will not ensure availability of maternity services. Health facilities are necessary for service delivery as not all services can be delivered under a tree or in the home of the mother. A health infrastructure network should be available in both urban and rural areas. Health facilities should specifically be targeting areas where the majority of vulnerable populations reside. In the community, women's homes can act as outlets for many promotive and preventive services. Dispensaries and primary health centres are situated within the community close to women's homes and act as the main community-level service delivery points. Despite experiencing fewer problems of geographical access, urban areas should also be serviced with primary health centres.

Table 10.1 provides a generic scheme of maternity (and related services) networks in Malawi. Broad similarities of primary, secondary and tertiary levels can be seen in other countries, even those like India (see Mavalankar and Sankara Raman, Chapter 6 this volume), which presents a very different setting from Malawi. Recommended catchment populations for the various types of facilities listed in Table 10.1 vary widely (across countries and also between recommended and operational norms) although a distance of 5 km from home to the nearest primary health facility is a commonly used benchmark (see Munjanja *et al.*, Chapter 11 this volume).

International guidelines have been developed for the availability and distribution of emergency obstetric care (EmOC) in particular and taken up in many countries throughout the world. It is recommended that there should be at a minimum five EmOC facilities including one comprehensive facility, for every 500,000 population (WHO *et al.*, 2009). In Malawi availability of EmOC is high at the comprehensive level – twice the minimum number of recommended comprehensive EmOC facilities exist (1.8 facilities per 500,000 population). Basic EmOC availability is more limited with only 2% of the recommended number of basic EmOC facilities – mainly because of the limited availability of particular functions (Table 10.2) such as manual vacuum aspiration and assisted delivery (Leigh *et al.*, 2008).

Table 10.1. Network of health infrastructure for delivery of maternity services, Malawi.

Type of facility	Services	Recommended personnel
Health post/Village clinic	Village health committee meetings Health promotion Outreach for antenatal care, postnatal care, HIV testing and counselling, family planning, distribution of insecticide-treated bed nets, immunizations, limited treatment of minor ailments, growth monitoring Community neonatal care and early breastfeeding support group activities Home visits and follow up of mothers and neonates Referral to dispensary level	Community health workers and volunteers, supported by dispensary and healthcentre personnel
Dispensary/Clinic	Health promotion Limited ambulatory care Support to community interventions	Nurses, midwives, clinicians and volunteers
Primary health centre	Health promotion Antenatal care, deliveries, postnatal care, immunizations, family planning, integrated management of childhood illness, distribution of insecticide-treated bed nets, basic EmOC, HIV testing and counselling, prevention of mother to child transmission, growth monitoring Outreach services to health posts Ambulatory care of common illnesses Home visits and follow up Referral to secondary facility	Nurses, midwives, clinical officers, medical assistants, community nurse, laboratory and pharmacy technicians, environmental health officer
Community/District hospital	As for primary health centre but also providing: Antiretroviral therapy for HIV Kangaroo care for neonates Comprehensive EmOC Support for primary health centres	General medical practitioners, clinical officers, nurses, midwives, pharmacy, laboratory, medical imaging, dental, ophthalmic technicians, environmental health officers
Tertiary/Teaching hospital	Full range of curative and rehabilitative services Teaching of health professionals Support for community and district hospital services	Health professionals with specialized skills in addition to above staff

Service facility location is important for its proper utilization (Fitzsimmons and Fitzsimmons, 1994). Facilities located away from the main habitations within towns and villages are inconvenient to reach and lead to low use and reluctance of health staff to reside in or near facilities. Special considerations in determining locations for maternity care include safe access during the night when childbirth and labour commonly occur and convenience of access for routine services such as antenatal care. Examples of unused facilities are common in many developing countries (Mavalankar *et al.*, 2004a). Health planning

Table 10.2. Recommended EmOC functions (WHO *et al.*, 2009).

Health centre, basic functions	Hospital, comprehensive functions
Intravenous/intramuscular:	Intravenous/intramuscular:
• Antibiotics (for infections)	• Antibiotics (for infections)
• Anticonvulsants (for pre-eclampsia/eclampsia)	• Anticonvulsants (for pre-eclampsia/eclampsia)
• Oxytocics (to improve uterine contractions in postpartum haemorrhage)	• Oxytocics (to improve uterine contractions in postpartum haemorrhage)
Manual removal of placenta for retained products of conception	Manual removal of placenta for retained products of conception
Manual vacuum aspiration for incomplete abortion	Manual vacuum aspiration for incomplete abortion
Assisted delivery with vacuum extraction	Assisted delivery with vacuum extraction
Neonatal resuscitation	Neonatal resuscitation
	Blood transfusion
	Surgical intervention with Caesarean section for obstructed labour

can be facilitated with new technologies such as geographic information systems (see Munjanja *et al.*, Chapter 11 this volume) to determine optimal locations for health facilities. Such techniques have been used to locate first referral units in Tamil Nadu and urban health centres in Gujarat, India (Ramani *et al.*, 2006; Padmanaban *et al.*, 2009).

The type of health facilities described in Table 10.1 can be operationalized by various health-sector partners. In Malawi, private-for-profit facilities tend to be located in urban areas, so consideration needs to be given to the availability of services run by the public sector in rural areas, but mechanisms to attract the private sector to operate in rural areas through public–private partnership arrangements are another option. In one strategy, the private sector can provide the structure and deliver the services and government buys and regulates services for the rural populations. (See Mavalankar and Sankara Raman, Chapter 6 this volume, for other examples.)

Packaging interventions for different levels of the health system

The packaging of interventions for different levels of the health-care system is also an important factor to be addressed when considering issues of availability. Once a network of facilities has been established, specification of the interventions that should be provided at each level is necessary, matched to the needs of pregnant women and the capabilities of the health staff.

At the community (village and dispensary) level, provision of health-related information for the promotion of maternal and neonatal health is necessary. Some of the health promotion interventions that can be undertaken at this level with support from community health workers include counselling for family planning and HIV, distribution of contraceptives and insecticide-treated bed nets, supporting exclusive breastfeeding and encouraging uptake of antenatal delivery and postnatal care. Community health workers can support mothers on nutrition, hygiene, cord care and help to take action when complications of pregnancy occur. They can also be trained to start antibiotic treatment to neonates with sepsis at community level before referral to a primary health centre. Village health committees play a part in creating demand, organizing community transport and participating to improve accountability and governance (see Afsana, Chapter 13 this volume).

For facility-based care, from the health centre to the teaching hospital, a number of international guidelines are available on effective packages of care. Of these, the EmOC package is clearly defined as basic and comprehensive functions (Table 10.2; WHO *et al.*, 2009).

For antenatal care, a reduced-visit package, specifying essential activities to be conducted during each of only four visits, was proposed after the conduct of a randomized controlled trial (Villar *et al.*, 2001). However, a systematic review subsequently raised the possibility that the reduced-visit programme may be associated with increased perinatal mortality compared to the standard higher number of visits (Dowswell *et al.*, 2010). Irrespective of the frequency of the visits, evidence-based interventions to be provided as part of antenatal care are nevertheless well accepted and described in detail in the WHO guidance for essential practice (WHO, 2011a).

Various postnatal care packages are also recommended, but consensus has not yet been reached on the content of care. There is broad agreement that postnatal care needs to address the management of life-threatening outcomes for the woman and her infant, routine preventive interventions for family planning, nutrition, communicable and non-communicable conditions and the special conditions and circumstances of the postnatal period for the mother and newborn. Further information is available in the WHO guidelines on pregnancy, childbirth, postpartum and newborn care (WHO, 2011a).

Ensuring Adequate Resources

Essential resources needed to make maternity services available include health personnel, physical infrastructure, drugs, equipment, transport and communications systems.

Human resources

The availability of services at each level of the health service network is dependent upon the skills of health workers, their availability and the legal requirements governing their practice. For maternity care, the global focus on the need for skilled care in pregnancy places the emphasis on the provider (see Achadi *et al.*, Chapter 14 this volume). Round the clock 24 h services are also important as many deliveries occur during the night or in the early hours of the morning. This situation requires special consideration

for staffing levels at each type of facility – even when workloads are not high, health workers cannot be expected to give round the clock services without sufficient periods of rest. With the existing critical shortage of health workers globally, strategies to provide an adequate skill mix and to promote task sharing are necessary (see Mavalankar and Sankara Raman, Chapter 6 this volume). In Malawi, non-physician clinical officers have performed Caesarean sections and other obstetric operative procedures for many years. The scope of midwives is also being expanded to include all basic EmOC functions, including neonatal resuscitation. Increasing use of community health workers has supplemented the available skill mix by performing essential tasks such as distributing contraceptives including injectables, providing immunizations, counselling and testing for HIV, initial treatment of neonatal sepsis and conducting microscopy to detect malaria. To ensure proper implementation of task sharing, proper training, creating an enabling legal environment, continuous supportive supervision and provision of job aids for the proper execution of the expanded roles are believed to help, although the effectiveness of such interventions are not yet well established (Rowe *et al.*, 2005).

Physical infrastructure

Poor infrastructure can lead to absent or poor-quality services, unmotivated health personnel, lack of privacy and acceptability to people, patient safety hazards and wastage of resources. Poor and rural populations often suffer the most as resources can be thinly spread out in rural areas and because poverty restricts the choices people can make for health care. There are substantial underinvestment and mismanagement as well as poor maintenance of infrastructure and equipment within the health systems of many countries, although it is a largely under-researched area (Mavalankar *et al.*, 2004a).

The common problems experienced with regard to physical infrastructure include:

- No buildings.
- Poor location of rural health centres or hospitals.
- Inferior quality of design and construction.
- Inadequate maintenance.
- Lack of availability of utilities such as water, electricity or fuel and telephones.

Old and dilapidated hospital and health-centre buildings, particularly in the public sector, are a characteristic of many resource-constrained developing countries. The continuous investment required for upgrading of facilities is not always available to governments. Monetary resources are not the only limitation. Other factors include poor political will to prioritize allocation of funds to ministries of health and lack of engineering skills and capacity to ensure proper repair and regular maintenance of the buildings. The problem tends to be worse in rural areas. In India, for example, there may not even be a building for peripheral health centres. It is reported that only 79,265 sub-centres (about half the total) have their own building. The remaining units operate out of rented private buildings or local, non-purpose-built government structures. Many district hospitals operate out of very small or old buildings, which need to be upgraded, renovated and, in many cases, rebuilt (Mavalankar *et al.*, 2004a; Sankara Raman *et al.*, 2010). Similar situations are found in many African and other countries, with lack of buildings in countries like Zambia (RHRC, 2001), Afghanistan, Liberia, Nepal and Tajikistan, which have suffered civil war or have internal resistance movements (McGinn, 2000; Sharma, 2010). Providing maternity services has some special infrastructure-related needs, which include a heightened need for privacy, infrastructure which allows disposal and cleaning of the body fluids emitted during childbirth and ability to accommodate the mother, newborn and a companion or chaperone.

The lack of simple utilities such as water, electricity, fuel and toilets has significant effects on service delivery. Storage of vaccines and other heat-sensitive supplies such as oxytocin (WHO, 1993) will clearly be affected. Sterilizing medical equipment is avoided or inadequately done, endangering the safety of the patients. Lack of water and sanitation makes infection control difficult, and lack of electricity hinders examination and treatment – particularly in childbirth and for gynaecological examinations in women. In India, a survey indicated that, out of 9688 primary health centres, only 23.5% have water, 66.4% have electricity and 52.3% have toilets (IIPS, 2003). In Malawi, similar problems exist and are not confined to rural areas (UN, undated).

Equipment

The availability of functioning equipment is essential for smooth health service delivery. Although national governments have increasingly invested in procuring equipment, in many low resource settings much medical equipment has been made available through international donors and other development agencies. This situation has led to some difficulties. Some equipment donated from developed countries can be too sophisticated to be maintained in developing countries. Mismatch between the equipment donated and the availability of skills for operation and maintenance of the equipment can occur (Cheng, 1995). Maternity care uses specialized equipment such as vacuum extractors, which need special maintenance (Hussein and Walker, 2010). Ultrasound scanning machines, neonatal resuscitation equipment and many other similar items can be seen lying idle in many health facilities in developing countries because of inadequate focus on maintenance needs (Mavalankar *et al.*, 2004b; Hambraeus, 2005). It has been estimated that nearly 40% of medical equipment in developing countries is out of service (Perry and Malkin, 2011).

The scarcity of medical equipment, even for the most basic items, remains a problem in many developing countries. For instance, in an infection control study in two states of Nigeria and in India, only two-thirds of maternity wards sampled had a thermometer available (Mehta *et al.*, 2011; Okonofua *et al.*, 2011). One obvious solution for medical equipment maintenance is to select equipment in keeping with conditions under which it will be used, by matching purchase protocols with rural conditions and skill availability. In some countries, the private sector can provide independent contractors who will maintain the equipment on an annual maintenance contract. In one district in the state of Rajasthan in India, the district health office has constituted a local mobile team for the simple maintenance of uncomplicated equipment such as operating tables, lights and medical furniture (Dwivedi *et al.*, 2002; Mavalankar *et al.*, 2004b). Such ideas could be used as examples for local problem solving. UN agencies have developed systems for maintenance of medical equipment (WHO, 2011b), but systematic action and scaling up of efforts is not yet visible in many countries.

Drugs, supplies and medical consumables

The availability of medical supplies is an essential part of all curative and preventive services. Approved treatment protocols for maternity care should guide the essential drugs and medical supplies that are to be made available at all service delivery points, although standardization across countries may not be always feasible or appropriate. Particular concerns for maternity care include lack of availability of essential drugs such as magnesium sulphate (see Langer *et al.*, Chapter 8 this volume), special gloves for obstetric care in high risk HIV settings (Tietjen *et al.*, 2003) and blood transfusions (Bates *et al.*, 2008).

As with infrastructure and equipment, improving the function of the health system is essential to improve the availability of drugs and supplies. The purchase of consumables can be highly politicized in many countries, with vested interests when bidding for and purchasing within government contracts. This leads to mismanagement, shortages, excesses and irrational purchases. UN agencies have developed procurement systems (UNICEF, 2011), but such externally driven measures can only be temporary and should not replace the need to build up national logistics systems that can provide rational procedures and system accountability.

Badly planned distribution, poor construction of storage facilities, lack of training of pharmacists and store keepers in modern inventory management procedures and underutilization of information technology also influence the availability of drugs and consumables. Budgets allocated for medicine and supplies can be inadequate. For example, in India the public health system allocates roughly Rs2–5 (US$0.02) per person per year for medicine and supplies at the primary health-centre level (D.V. Mavalankar, Ahmedabad, 2010, personal communication). Such inadequacies result in the unavailability of medicines in health facilities, proliferation of private pharmacies on the doorstep of hospitals and considerable additional costs to service users for purchase of medicines (Borghi *et al.*, 2008). Irrational prescribing practices by doctors and lack of official drug formularies – despite available guidance on best practice (WHO, 2008a) – compound these problems. Although there have been examples of supply chain improvement in developing countries (Box 10.1), the deep rooted vested interests in procurement, poor management capacity and lack of leadership continue to prevent replication of such successes.

Transport and communications

The range of maternity care services, from village to tertiary referral centres, necessitates linkages between levels in the form of a referral system. Transport and communications are only one element of a referral system, but their availability is required for support and supervision of health personnel and for the transportation of patients requiring health care available only at higher service levels – the latter being of especial importance in maternity care because of the rapidity with which complications can occur and progress in pregnant women and the newborn. A full discussion of transport, communications and referral systems is provided elsewhere (see Munjanja *et al.*, Chapter 11 this volume).

Box 10.1. Making medical supplies available: the Tamil Nadu Medical Services Corporation.

There have been laudable efforts in Tamil Nadu, India to reorganize logistics for medical supplies in the form of a semi-government medical supplies corporation, called the Tamil Nadu Medical Services Corporation (TNMSC), which became functional in January 1995. This has helped in a radical reform of purchase and distribution in Tamil Nadu.

TNMSC serves as an apex body for the purchase, storage and distribution of medicines, consumables and surgical instruments for various government medical institutions in the state. It also renders other services, such as supplying equipment to hospitals and maintaining medical scanning centres on the premises of selected government hospitals. The TNMSC also maintains the website of the Ministry of Health and Family Welfare, where the public can interact with doctors and other medical staff through health chats. A managing director looks after the day-to-day administration of the corporation. Professionals from academic faculties of medicine, pharmacology and related health sciences are employed on deputation to provide technical know-how. The Corporation is responsible for ensuring that all facilities have a regular supply of medicines and consumables. This has been achieved through a system of accountability, where streamlined procedures, adequate technical expertise, quality assurance and procurement and tendering rules work in an organized way for efficient system functioning.

After 15 years, no other state in India has set up such an efficient and transparent medical supply system. Some national reform efforts – providing additional flexible funds for drugs and cost-recovery mechanisms through patient welfare societies – have been developed, which may help improve the supply of medicines (Padmanaban *et al.*, 2009).

Integrating Service Delivery

The WHO defines integrated service delivery as 'the management and delivery of health services so that clients receive a continuum of preventive and curative services, according to their needs over time and across different levels of the health system' (WHO, 2008b). Integration of services is one of the tools recommended for use in many settings to improve the availability of health services, including those targeting women and children, especially in the light of the concept of continuum of care, which forms the underlying basis of global strategies to reduce maternal and child mortality (PMNCH, 2011).

Understanding of what is meant by integrated services varies (WHO, 2008b). At policy level, integration is seen as a way to organize services so that one management team can have responsibility for providing and supervising care for a predefined population. At the operational or clinic level, integration is viewed as a supermarket approach where a health unit provides a variety of services, though not necessarily in the same station or room. For example, a primary health facility can provide a wide range of services (family planning, HIV counselling and treatment, abortion care, maternal, newborn and child care) on the same day and/or by the same health worker but using different spaces or rooms. Others see integration of services as those which work across different sectors such as activities in schools to deliver health promotion services.

Integrated services bring resources together to increase efficiency and access to services. The advantages of integration are many – it can promote efficient use of resources by minimizing the number of user–provider contacts, while at the same time offering a range of services. Demands on the user's time and other resources needed to make contact with the health service can be minimized, with the potential for increasing user-friendliness and therefore uptake. Integrated services could minimize the duplication of resources needed for training, equipment, supervisory tools, quality guidelines, performance indicators and incentives. Arguments against integration have also been put forward. On the basis that it is easier to deliver a narrow range of services of good quality, there are fears that providing a broad range of integrated services can jeopardize quality. Some believe that certain conditions of epidemic proportions (e.g. HIV/AIDS) merit special, focused services. Integration may also mean that the achievement of short, time-bound targets cannot be demonstrated (WHO, 2008b).

The debate about whether integration can improve service availability (and quality) continues. A recent systematic review found that the integration of some reproductive health and maternal and child health services decreased utilization and user satisfaction, but called for more rigorous studies to investigate this finding further (Dudley and Garner, 2011). In any case, there should be awareness that integration can take many different forms and may need to be tailored to different needs, and certainly cannot replace the lack of resources for maternity care (WHO, 2008b).

Conclusion

A discussion of the availability of maternity services in isolation only tells part of the story of the many components needed to ensure appropriate uptake of good quality care. Nevertheless, improving availability alone is a complex process requiring consideration of a range of health system factors. Improving coverage of maternity care – a key global priority today – cannot be done without addressing issues of service availability, yet once services are available they will also need to be made accessible, acceptable and effective before the goal of maternal and perinatal health can be reached.

References

Bates, I., Chapotera, G.K., McKew, S. and van den Broek, N. (2008) Maternal mortality in sub-Saharan Africa: the contribution of ineffective blood transfusion services. *British Journal of Obstetrics and Gynaecology* 115(11), 1331–1339.

Borghi, J., Tagmatarchi Storeng, K. and Filippi, V. (2008) Overview of the costs of obstetric care and the economic and social consequences for households. In: Richard, F., Witter, S. and De Brouwere, V. (eds) Reducing financial barriers to obstetric care in low income countries *Studies in Health Services Organisation and Policy* 24, 21–46.

Cheng, M. (1995) An international strategy in medical equipment maintenance. *Journal of Clinical Engineering* 20(1), 66–69.

Dowswell, T., Carroli, G., Duley, L., Gates, S., Gülmezoglu, A.M., Khan-Neelofur, D. and Piaggio, G.G.P (2010) Alternative versus standard packages of antenatal care for low-risk pregnancy. *Cochrane Database of Systematic Reviews* 10, CD000934. DOI:10.1002/14651858.CD000934. pub2.

Dudley, L. and Garner, P. (2011) Strategies for integrating primary health services in low- and middle-income countries at the point of delivery. *Cochrane Database of Systematic Reviews* 6(7), CD003318.

Dwivedi, H., Mavalankar, D.V., Abreu, E. and Srinivasan, V. (2002) Planning and implementing a program of renovations of emergency obstetric care facilities: experiences in Rajasthan, India. *International Journal of Gynecology and Obstetrics* 78, 283–291.

Fitzsimmons, J.A. and Fitzsimmons, M.J. (1994) Service facility location. In: *Service Management for Competitive Advantage*. McGraw-Hill, New York, pp. 130–147.

Government of Malawi (1996) Constitution of the Republic of Malawi Chapter III. Available at: http://www. icrc.org/ihl-nat.nsf/.../Constitution%20Malawi%20-%20EN.pdf (accessed 13 August 2011).

Hambraeus, A. (2005) Lowbury Lecture: Infection control from a global perspective. *Journal of Hospital Infection* 64(3), 217–223.

Hussein, J. and Walker, L. (2010) Puerperal sepsis in low and middle income settings: past, present and future. In: Kehoe, S., Neilson, J.P. and Norman, J.E. (eds) *Maternal and Infant Deaths: chasing millennium development goals 4 & 5*. RCOG Press, London, pp. 131–147.

IIPS International Institute of Population Sciences (2003) Facility Survey. Available at: http://www.rchiips.org/pdf/rch2/National_Facility_Report_RCH-II.pdf (accessed 12 October 2010).

Kwataine, I. (2010) Maternal Health in Malawi Proceedings of the Women Deliver Conference 2010, Washington, DC. Available at: http://www.womendeliver.org/knowledge-center/publications/women-deliver-100/women-deliver-100-51-75/ (accessed 23 August 2011).

Leigh, B., Mwale, T.G., Lazaro, D. and Lunguz, J. (2008) Emergency obstetric care: how do we stand in Malawi? *International Journal of Gynecology and Obstetrics* 101(1), 107–111.

Mavalankar, D.V., Ramani, K.V., Patel, A. and Raman, P. (2004a) Building infrastructure to reach and care for the poor: trends, obstacles and strategies to overcome them: working paper. Indian Institute for Management, Ahmedabad, India.

Mavalankar, D.V., Raman, P., Dwivedi, H. and Jain, M.L. (2004b) Managing equipment for emergency obstetric care in rural hospitals. *International Journal of Obstetrics and Gynaecology* 87, 88–97.

McGinn, T. (2000) Reproductive health of war-affected populations: what do we know? *International Family Planning Perspectives* 26(4), 174–180.

Mehta, R., Mavalankar, D.V., Ramani, K.V., Sharma, S. and Hussein, J. (2011) Infection control in delivery care units, Gujarat state, India: a needs assessment. *BMC Pregnancy and Childbirth* 11, 37.

Ministry of Health (2010) *Evaluation Report of Programme of Work.* Ministry of Health, Malawi.

Okonofua, F.E., Okpokunu, E., Aigbogun, O., Nwandu, C., Mokwenye, C. and Hussein, J. (2011) *An Assessment of Infection Control Practices in Delivery Care Units in Edo State, Nigeria.* Report to the MacArthur Foundation, Chicago, Illinois.

Padmanaban, P., Raman, P. and Mavalankar, D.V. (2009) Innovations and challenges in reducing maternal mortality in Tamil Nadu, India. *Journal of Health Population and Nutrition* 29, 202–219.

Perry, L. and Malkin, R. (2011) Effectiveness of medical equipment donations to improve health systems: how much medical equipment is broken in the developing world? *Medical and Biological Engineering and Computing* 49(7), 719–722.

PMNCH Partnership for Maternal, Newborn and Child Health (2011) The continuum of care. Available at: http://www.who.int/pmnch/about/continuum_of_care/en/index.html (accessed 23 August 2011).

Prata, N., Vahidnia, F., Potts, M. and Dries-Daffner, I. (2005) Revisiting community-based distribution programs: are they still needed? *Contraception* 72(6), 402–407.

Ramani, K.V., Mavalankar, D.V., Patel, A. and Mehandiratta, S. (2006) A GIS approach to plan and deliver healthcare services to urban poor: a public private partnership model for Ahmedabad City, India. *International Journal of Pharmaceutical and Healthcare Marketing* 1(2), 159–173.

RHRC Reproductive Health for Refugees Consortium (2001) Assessment of Reproductive Health for Refugees in Zambia. Women's Commission for Refugee Women and Children, New York. Available at: http://www.rhrc.org/resources/wc_zambia_09_01.pdf (accessed 20 October 2010).

Rowe, A., de Savigny, D., Lanata, C.F. and Victora, C.G. (2005) How can we achieve and maintain high-quality performance of health workers in low-resource settings? *Lancet* 366(9490), 1026–1035.

Sankara Raman, P., Sharma, B., Mavalankar, D.V. and Upadhyaya, M. (2010) *Operationalization of First Referral Units in Gujarat: midwifery and maternal health in India: situation analysis and lessons from the field. Monograph 1,* Centre for Management of Health Systems, New Delhi.

Sharma, S.P. (2010) Politics and corruption mar health care in Nepal. *Lancet* 375(9731), 2063–2064.

Tarimo, E. and Webster, E.G. (1997) *Primary Health Care Concepts and Challenges in a Changing World: Alma-Ata revisited.* WHO, Geneva.

Tietjen, L., Bossemeyer, D. and McIntosh, N. (2003) Infection Prevention Guidelines for Healthcare Facilities with Limited Resources, Chapters 7 and 25. JHPIEGO Corporation, Baltimore, pp. 7-7 and 25-9. Available at: http://www.reproline.jhu.edu/english/4morerh/4ip/IP_manual/ipmanual.htm (accessed 23 August 2011).

UN (2008) *World Contraceptive Use 2007.* Department of Economic and Social Affairs, Population Division, United Nations, Geneva.

UN (undated) UN Habitat United Nations Malawi. Available at: http://www.unmalawi.org/agencies/unhabitat.html (accessed 23 August 2011).

UNICEF (2008) *Countdown to 2015: tracking progress in maternal, newborn and child survival. The 2008 report.* UNICEF, New York.

UNICEF (2011) Procurement services. Available at: http://www.unicef.org/supply/index_procurement_services.html (accessed 23 August 2011).

Villar, J., Ba'aqeel, H., Piaggio, G., Lumbiganon, P., Belizán, J.M., Farnot, U., Al-Mazrou, Y., Carroli, G., Pinol, A., Donner, A., Langer, A., Nigenda, G., Mugford, M., Fox-Rushby, J., Hutton, G., Bergsjø, P., Bakketeig, L., Berendes, H., Garcia, J. and the WHO Antenatal Care Trial Research Group (2001) WHO antenatal care randomised trial for the evaluation of a new model of routine antenatal care. *Lancet* 357(9268), 1551–1564.

WHO (1978) The Alma-Ata declaration. Available at: http://www.who.int/hpr/NPH/docs/declaration_almaata.pdf (accessed 23 August 2011).

WHO (1993) *Stability of Injectable Oxytocics in Tropical Climates.* WHO, Geneva.

WHO (2005) *The World Health Report: make every mother and child count.* WHO, Geneva.

WHO (2008a) WHO Model Formulary (eds: Stuart, M., Kouimtzi, M.and Hill, S.R.). WHO, Geneva. Available
   at: http://www.who.int/selection_medicines/list/WMF2008.pdf (accessed 18 June 2010).
WHO (2008b) Integrated health services what and why Technical Brief No 1. WHO, Geneva. Available at:
   http://www.who.int/healthsystems/service_delivery_techbrief1.pdf (accessed 23 August 2011).
WHO (2010) *WHO Technical Consultation on Postpartum and Postnatal Care.* Department of Making
   Pregnancy Safer, WHO, Geneva.
WHO (2011a) Making Pregnancy Safer. IMPAC. Available at: http://www.who.int/making_pregnancy_safer/
   documents/impac/en/index.html (accessed 23 August 2011).
WHO (2011b) Medical equipment maintenance programme overview. WHO Medical device technical
   series.   Available   at: http://www.whqlibdoc.who.int/publications/2011/9789241501538_eng.pdf
   (accessed 23 August 2011).
WHO, UNFPA, UNICEF and AMDD (2009) *Monitoring Emergency Obstetric Care: a handbook.* WHO,
   Geneva.

11 Geographical Access, Transport and Referral Systems

Stephen P. Munjanja, Tsitsi Magure and Gwendoline Kandawasvika
University of Zimbabwe, Harare, Zimbabwe

Summary

- Poor access to emergency obstetric care is due to one of three delays: deciding to seek care, reaching a health facility and receiving appropriate treatment.
- Poor geographical access in itself is not the cause of the second delay, but the delay results from failure to bridge it with adequate referral interventions and systems.
- Geographical access can be defined using several dimensions, including distribution and density of services, distance and time.
- Poor physical access to health services contributes to urban–rural inequities in the utilization of services and in health outcomes. It also compounds the problem of availability of human resources for health in rural areas.
- Geographical access is mainly a problem of rural populations, especially the poor.
- The two-tiered model of primary health care and hospital-level care makes referral and referral systems essential. Referral can be hampered and delays caused by a poorly functioning system.
- Solutions to overcome the problems of physical access include communication, transport, educational, financial, infrastructural and technological interventions.
- The effects and the effectiveness of many of these interventions are poorly understood and more evidence is needed to aid decision making, especially for low resource settings.

Introduction

A major contributor to the high maternal and perinatal mortality and morbidity in developing countries is the poor access to life-saving obstetric care when complications arise. Such poor access may be due to a variety of causes: personal or cultural barriers, failure to reach facilities in time and inadequate care at health facilities. Three delays have been described in order to conceptualize the problems of obstetric care in the developing world (Thaddeus and Maine, 1994). The three delays are:

- Delay in deciding to seek care.
- Delay in reaching a health facility.
- Delay in getting appropriate treatment.

Delays in the decision to seek care usually occur at the household level and include problems related to recognition of the complication and its nature as a life-threatening condition or an emergency. The distances involved in reaching care, the costs of care and perceptions regarding the quality of care available are also known to be key factors that affect women's decision making.

After the decision to seek care has been made, the second delay is concerned with the delay in arrival at the health facility. This delay is affected by the distribution and location of health facilities (and health professionals) that are equipped to deal with emergency obstetric and neonatal care, as well as the availability and costs of transportation and communication systems to reach facilities. The second delay is most common and severe in rural areas, where health professionals may not be available, transport and communication systems are limited and road conditions are changeable, depending on the season.

The third delay occurs after the facility is reached. Here, delays in various aspects of care can be due to poor procedures for triaging obstetric emergencies, staff shortages, staff attitudes and skills, a lack of functioning equipment or unreliable drug and blood supplies. Inadequate management structures and poor links between the primary, secondary and tertiary referral systems also cause delays in reaching an appropriate level of care.

The factors influencing all three delays are entwined and play a part in limiting women's access to health services. The second delay is directly linked to problems of geographical access. In many developing countries, utilization of health services is decreased by poor geographical access (Say and Raine, 2007; Gabrysch and Campbell, 2009) and the delay in reaching care is responsible for maternal and perinatal deaths in a significant proportion of cases globally (Ronsmans and Graham, 2006). This chapter focuses on issues relevant to geographical access in developing countries, discussing its definitions, the impact of poor access on maternal and perinatal outcomes and the interventions that have been attempted to improve access.

Definition of Geographical Access

There is no agreed definition of geographical or physical access because the time taken to transport a woman to a facility will depend on distance, terrain, quality of roads, season of the year and type of transport. There are three possible ways to define the concept. The first has been an attempt by UN agencies to define access to emergency obstetric care (EmOC) (UNICEF, 1997). The minimum desirable level of access to EmOC is defined as the availability of four basic and one comprehensive EmOC facility for every population of 500,000 people. The appropriateness of this definition depends on population density and the relative proportions of rural to urban populations. In a sparsely populated rural area, if there was only one basic EmOC facility for 125,000 people, some would have to walk very far to reach it. In contrast, in most urban areas in developing countries, this criterion can be relaxed (provided the services available can still cope with utilization levels) because the high population density enhances geographical proximity. The use of the UN criteria may pose difficulties if applied to all population densities. In fact, at least three different criteria are needed, for low, average and high density populations. Another problem with the use of the UN indicators of EmOC access is that it fails to discriminate between high and low maternal mortality settings. For example, in a study comparing indicators for EmOC in Zambia and Sri Lanka, both countries exceeded the recommended benchmarks and had similar EmOC facility density, yet they performed very differently in terms of maternal health outcomes (Gabrysch *et al.*, 2011b).

The next possible definition might use distance as a criterion. Several studies have used the distance of 5 km to determine whether rural women are more, or less, likely to use obstetric services (van den Broek *et al.*, 2003; Gage and Guirlene Calixte, 2006; Yanagisawa and Wakai, 2008). The choice of 5 km is not explained in the papers, but there are two probable reasons for the arbitrary selection of this distance: (i) distance is described in multiples of 5 km in most papers; and (ii) many rural women in labour will walk to the facility or be carried on a stretcher or hammock by people who are walking. They or their carriers are unlikely to attempt a distance of more than 5 km. The problem with using distance as a measure of geographical access is that it may not take into account other physical factors. Mountainous terrain or flood-prone areas can make some areas difficult to reach during certain times of the year, so a health facility that is 'nearby' during the dry or warm season may become inaccessible during monsoons or during winter, irrespective of its distance. The availability of transportation is another factor that changes the value of distance as a good indicator of geographical access. A health facility 20 km away may be easier to reach than one which is closer if, for example, the further facility is located in a busy market town, well connected by transport, and poorly maintained roads slow transit time.

A third method of defining geographical access is to describe it by the time by which a woman should reach an EmOC facility. The estimated average time from onset of complications to death for the leading causes of maternal mortality ranges from 2 h (in postpartum haemorrhage) and 6 days (in the case of infections). The implication is that it is not safe for women to be more than 2 h away from EmOC, since death can result from postpartum haemorrhage within this period (Maine, 1991). The updated guidelines for monitoring EmOC add that women should be within 2–3 h travel time to a facility that can offer life-saving treatment (WHO et al., 2009). However, travel time is not necessarily a static measure and it is possible that a facility could be 2 h away during the day but not at night because of the way transportation systems are organized. A facility may be 2 h away but not used because personal safety of travellers could be compromised by using that specific route.

In summary, although there are limitations to all definitions, geographical access is probably best defined by the time taken to reach a facility rather than by distance. The period of highest risk for pregnant women is around the time of delivery and this is when they should be within 2 h of life-saving care. For practical purposes, good geographical access in the context of care for the pregnant mother and her baby can be defined as the ability to reach an EmOC facility within 2 h after 37 weeks gestation and up to the first 3 days after delivery. This definition focuses on the period of greatest danger to pregnant women, the unborn baby and newborns and

avoids the need to make access available within 2 h throughout pregnancy, which is generally an unrealistic aim.

Impact of Poor Geographical Access

Urban–rural differentials in outcomes

At the national level, the most obvious result of poor geographical access is the difference in outcomes between urban and rural women. In low income countries, rural women usually have worse outcomes and this is partly due to poor access to high quality EmOC (Ronsmans et al., 2003; Hunger et al., 2007). Whereas it can be difficult to separate the effects of distance alone from poverty, education and other factors, it has been demonstrated that geographical access can act independently to reduce utilization of services (Hounton et al., 2008; Malqvist et al., 2010). Many developing country governments simply do not have the resources to make facilities as readily available in rural areas as they are in urban settings. Compounding the problem, there is little demand from rural women for equal access to EmOC since most of them have received less education than their urban counterparts.

Utilization of antenatal care

Utilization of antenatal services is reduced by increased distance to the health facility, as evidenced by a number of studies. In Kwale district, Kenya, women living further than 5 km from a dispensary were less likely to attend for antenatal care (OR 0.29; 95% CI 0.22–0.39) (Brown et al., 2008). In Haiti, the availability of a health centre within 5 km significantly increased the odds of receiving antenatal care in a timely manner and of attending for care on four or more occasions (Gage and Guirlene Calixte, 2006).

Women are able to travel further for antenatal visits than they can during labour. In Matebeland North Province, Zimbabwe, 63% of the clients who were within 10 km of health facilities (2 h walk) considered that they had adequate access to antenatal care (Sikosana, 1994). In Malawi, despite living an average of 5 km from the health centre, over 90% of women attended antenatal clinics with a mean of five visits (van den Broek et al., 2003). A study in Nepal noted that antenatal services were well utilized despite problems of geographical access, but mothers were less likely to access good quality delivery or postnatal care (Tuladhar et al., 2009). Clearly, however, the mere establishment of antenatal services is insufficient to increase their utilization and other factors are important, including women's satisfaction, autonomy and gender role in the decision to seek care (Bilenko et al., 2007; Simkhada et al., 2008).

Utilization of health facilities for labour and delivery

Poor geographical access has its greatest influence on the potential of women to reach a health facility during labour. Once a woman is in labour, there is a limit to how far she can travel if she has to walk or be carried by others. The situation is compounded if there are complications or if the woman needs emergency care.

In Nepal, a distance of more than 1 h to the maternity hospital was significantly associated with an increased risk of home delivery by almost eight-fold (Wagle et al., 2004). In many varied low income settings, poor geographical access has consistently been found to be associated with decreased use of health facilities for labour and delivery (Stekelenburg et al., 2004; Gage, 2007; Say and Raine, 2007; Yanagisawa and Wakai, 2008; Gabrysch and Campbell, 2009; Gabrysch et al., 2011a). In the countries described in these studies, the percentages of women delivering at home ranged between 50% and 84%. In contrast, unplanned home deliveries in high or middle income countries are very few at less than 1% (de Almeida et al., 2005; Scott and Esen, 2005; Homer et al., 2011). In the Netherlands, the arrival of a woman in labour at the facility is considered delayed if travel time is longer than 20 min (Ravelli et al., 2011).

The risks of complications occurring during childbirth make access during this time crucial. However, as interventions can be costly, it is even more important than with antenatal care to ensure that socio-economic factors and quality of services are addressed at the same time. Several studies in various settings including Nepal, Guatemala and Vietnam have demonstrated that improving proximity to biomedical services is unlikely to have a dramatic impact on utilization in the absence of additional changes addressing quality, social, cultural and economic factors (Glei et al., 2003; Duong et al., 2004; Tuladhar et al., 2005).

Maternal and perinatal outcomes

Poor access to maternity care can lead to higher morbidity and mortality. Obstetric fistula – development of an abnormal passage between the bowel or urinary tract and the birth canal – is the classic complication which arises from delayed treatment of obstructed labour. Although clinical factors such as young age, primigravida and short stature are the leading associated factors for obstetric fistula, a long distance to travel has also been shown to be a significant contributory factor (Muleta, 2004; Melah et al., 2007). Women have also been shown to be at higher risk of maternal death due to poor geographical access in South Africa, West Africa, Burkina Faso and Zimbabwe (Fawcus et al., 1996; Ronsmans et al., 2003; Moodley, 2004; Bell et al., 2008). In Pakistan an analysis of 104 consecutive maternal deaths showed that 74% of women experienced the second delay, and the most frequently stated reason for this was long distance, which was mentioned in 39.7% of cases (Shah et al., 2009).

Perinatal outcomes are also affected by poor geographical access, although this has not been studied as much as maternal outcomes. Mothers living furthest away from a health facility had an increased risk of neonatal mortality in northern Vietnam (OR 1.96, 95% CI 1.40–2.75) (Malqvist et al., 2010). The perinatal outcome most susceptible to delay in treatment is stillbirth. Obstetric emergencies can have catastrophic consequences for the unborn fetus within a short period of time. Although a serious postpartum haemorrhage can lead to death of a woman in less than 2 h, the unborn fetus may succumb much earlier (Maine, 1991; AbouZahr, 1998). If women are seen rapidly during an emergency obstetric event and effective action is taken, such as expediting delivery, intrauterine deaths could be averted or the baby delivered in a better condition. It is thus no surprise that sub-Saharan Africa has the highest intrapartum-related neonatal mortality and stillbirth rates, with a stillbirth rate of 32.2 per thousand in 2006 (Stanton *et al.*, 2006; Lawn *et al.*, 2009), with one of the main contributing factors being poor geographical access.

Impact on health providers

Most of the papers published on geographical access concentrate on the pregnant women and their babies. In remote facilities, health workers suffer from intellectual and social isolation and fear of mishandling complications and may fail or be unable to transfer women with complications on time. Although research evidence from developing countries is limited, transferable lessons can be drawn from other remote and rural settings. In British Columbia, Canada, health providers identified elements of personal risk they perceived as resulting from offering intrapartum care in communities without access to backup services such as Caesarean section. Maternity care was felt to be unique because things could change quickly. Emotional tensions were felt and social risks such as negative attitudes from community members feared (Kornelsen and Grzybowski, 2008). These social risks may be one reason why it is difficult to recruit or retain health providers in rural areas.

Contextual Factors

Population distribution

In many low income settings, most people live in rural areas, which is mainly where the problem of geographical access occurs. In urban areas, even in poor countries, most women can reach a facility within 1 h, so the problems of access tend to be related to decision making and getting appropriate treatment, rather than being a geographical or physical nature – although there may be some exceptions, such as heavy traffic in congested cities. The proportion of people living in rural areas is decreasing in developing countries, and in some parts of the world this transition is occurring rapidly. Sub-Saharan Africa is experiencing the slowest rate of this transition (UN Population Division, 2008), which means the problem of geographical access will persist there for a long time.

Infrastructure of health services in developing countries

In developing countries administrative authority is usually devolved by central government to regions (or provinces) and then to districts. The district is the smallest administrative sub-division of authority, with powers to implement government programmes in education, agriculture, health, etc. In sub-Saharan Africa, a district will range in population between 75,000 and 500,000 people, although districts may have higher populations in regions of South Asia.

Implementation of health programmes uses the district administrative infrastructure. The primary health-care model has been adopted by most developing countries to allow the majority of the population to access preventative services. In any district there are several primary health-care facilities which refer patients to the district hospital, resulting broadly in a two-tiered model of obstetric care. The model of obstetric care recommended by WHO comprises the basic and the comprehensive EmOC levels, partly based on the type of facilities on the ground in the district. The primary health centres serve as or can be upgraded to basic facilities, whilst the district hospital is the comprehensive level (see Phoya *et al.*, Chapter 10 this volume). Recommendations by WHO for implementation and monitoring of maternal and newborn health programmes is based on the district model (WHO, 1996b, 2006; WHO *et al.*, 2009).

The district model is well entrenched and, for better or worse, efforts to improve geographical access will have to be based on its structure. It is a compromise between providing primary health care for a lot of people and making sophisticated care available to the estimated 15% of women who develop complications. The problem is that even in rural areas of high population density the primary health centres which serve as basic EmOC units may be more than 2 h away (by walking) from many women's homes. In many countries the district health team does not assume any responsibility for the movement of women from homes to the primary health centre beyond providing childbirth preparedness advice during antenatal care.

The referral system

The two-tiered model of obstetric care, which results from poverty of resources and considerations of efficient functioning of the health system, makes referral between tiers necessary. The process of referral is the responsibility of the district health team.

Expedient referral, although dependent on many other factors within the health system, is often made difficult by poor geographical access between the basic and comprehensive levels. The principal requirements of a referral system have been summarized recently, and formalized communications and transport arrangements are among them (Murray and Pearson, 2006). Until recently, communication between basic and comprehensive EmOC facilities was through either poorly maintained telephone landlines or unreliable radio systems. The advent of mobile telephones is already bringing about a revolution for communication for referral in developing countries, especially as coverage is progressing rapidly (Krasovec, 2004).

The minimum transport requirement in any district is a motor car ambulance dedicated to obstetric and neonatal emergencies only, but it is rare to find a district with such a

facility in low income settings. After a woman has successfully reached a basic EmOC facility, she may find herself trapped there, at the mercy of a health system that is unable to transfer her in a timely manner. In some countries this has given rise to by-passing, in which women with means avoid the lower level facilities and go direct to the district hospital as self-referrals (Jahn *et al.*, 1998; Low *et al.*, 2001).

Interventions that Overcome Barriers to Geographical Access

This section will describe interventions that have been attempted or have been implemented in order to improve geographical access or reduce its harmful impact. There have been very few randomized controlled trials done with distance or geographical access as the sole parameter under study – for obvious reasons such a study would be technically difficult and pose ethical challenges. Most studies are descriptive or are about composite interventions in which access was one of several.

Communication

Communication is vital in managing complications of pregnancy and is even more important in areas of poor geographical access. Unfortunately, these are the same areas that experience poor communication facilities, although the situation is already changing rapidly with mobile phone technology.

Communication needs to be addressed at the community level and at health facilities to:

- Summon transport or call for help.
- Seek advice and initiate first aid or stabilization.
- Arrange prompt referral and allow the receiving facility to prepare for the emergency.
- Allow reassuring communication between a woman far from home and her family (Holmes and Kennedy, 2010).

In most developing countries the mainstay technologies for communication were fixed landline telephones and two-way radio. Communication was only available to the woman after she reached a primary facility for the purpose of referral. Landline facilities do not reach every facility and their overhead cables are subject to weather storms, falling trees and theft.

There have been more reports about the use of two-way radio, since it allows the primary facility, referral facility and ambulance to communicate (Musoke, 2002; Krasovec, 2004; Santos *et al.*, 2006; UNFPA, 2011). In these reports use of two-way radio decreased referral times significantly, in the case of Mali from up to a day to just a few hours (UNFPA, 2011).

The rapid expansion of mobile phone usage, its low cost and its widespread availability will soon make other forms of communication redundant. The growth of mobile phone ownership is quite high in the developing world because the market has not yet been saturated. For the year 2010, in Asia and the Pacific there were 70 subscriptions per 100 people, in Africa the figure was nearly 30 per 100 people (International Communication Union, 2010). Health services in many countries have also started supplying handsets and mobile numbers to facilities. This combination of extended use by the public and by the health services will allow women to communicate with facilities from home. It will also enable primary centres to contact the referral facilities and health facilities to keep track of ambulances. Innovative uses for mobile technologies in health (mHealth) are increasing all the time – with consultations, sharing of case notes with referral facilities, feedback and follow-up reported (WHO, 2011). A potential role in referral for mobile telephones is to allow electronic funds to be confirmed with or transferred to drivers of private cars in the absence of cash. Women can also be sent funds by relatives for transport and user fees. Communications technology has opened opportunities for new partnerships between public and private providers of health at global level (see http://www.mhealthalliance.org) and within countries (Box 11.1).

Transport

In urban areas, public and private transport is usually available and sufficiently affordable by women seeking health care. City authorities and municipalities usually have ambulance services, although in sub-Saharan Africa they are usually oversubscribed (Nkyekyer, 2000; Thomson, 2005) and private taxis are widely used as they are cheaper and quicker. Obstetric flying squads, which send ambulances with health personnel to attend and transport women with complications, have been used in a few developing countries such as Pakistan but have not been scaled up, probably due to a mixture of difficulties in linking with communications systems and shortages

---

Box 11.1. Emergency referral in India: a public–private partnership.

GVK EMRI (Emergency Management and Research Institute: http://www.emri.in) is a not-for-profit professional organization operating in a public–private partnership mode to supply emergency referral services in India. It handles medical as well as police and fire emergencies through their '108 Emergency service' line. This is a free service which utilizes the expanding telephone and communications systems in India. The group has a fleet of nearly 3000 ambulances across the states of Andhra Pradesh, Gujarat, Uttarakhand, Goa, Tamil Nadu, Karnataka, Assam, Meghalaya, Madhya Pradesh, Himachal Pradesh and Chhattisgarh, responding to an estimated 30 million emergencies annually in both rural and urban environments. The organization has arrangements with over 6800 hospitals, which provide initial stabilization of patients, free of cost for the first 24 h.

The 108 Emergency Response operates round the clock through a call centre and a toll-free number accessible from landline or mobile telephone. Medical advisers are on hand at the call centre to provide expert advice. Calls for emergency transfer of pregnant women make up a significant proportion of their work.

of human resources (Andina and Fikree, 1995). In the urban setting, poverty and belief systems (see Mumtaz and Levay, Chapter 12 this volume) rather than physical access may be predominant barriers.

It is in the rural areas that transport interventions are crucial. There have been several recent reviews on the subject (Krasovec, 2004; Babinard and Roberts, 2006; Holmes and Kennedy, 2010; Hussein *et al.*, 2011). The range of physical transport options includes: pick-up trucks; taxis; buses; reconditioned vehicles; tractors; motorcycles; tricycles; bicycles; bicycles/tractors/tricycles with trailers; motorboats; canoes; wheelbarrows; animal-drawn carts; home-made stretchers; rickshaws; aircraft and trains.

Non-motorized options do not have the potential to transport a woman needing emergency care in good time. There are very few reports on non-motorized means of transport, but there have been publications on bicycles and tricycles (Plate 6) (Lungu *et al.*, 2001; Schmid *et al.*, 2001; Bossyns *et al.*, 2005). This mode of transport has not become more widely used because of its limitations. There is a limit to the distance that a rider can carry a woman, probably no more than 20 km. The rough terrain may make use of the bicycles/tricycles difficult or impossible, and the wear and tear on them as a result can be considerable. In extreme weather conditions, such as heat or rain, they may be very uncomfortable for both the rider and the passenger. And, lastly, the family cannot accompany the woman.

Motorcycle ambulances (Plate 7) have been tried in a few settings and the experience of Malawi has been reported (Hofman *et al.*, 2008). In that study, motorcycle ambulances were placed at three remote rural health centres and their effectiveness was compared with that of a four-wheel-drive car ambulance at the district hospital. The median referral delay in the centres using the motorcycle ambulances was reduced by 2–4.5 h (35–76%). The purchase price of a motorcycle was 19 times cheaper than a car ambulance and annual operating costs were 24 times cheaper. Currently, on land the motorcycle ambulance is the only way that large numbers of women can be moved at a relatively affordable cost from primary facilities to district hospitals.

Health ministries have been slow to try them in sub-Saharan countries, however. Even though they are more comfortable than tricycles, they are seen as 'backward' by some administrators.

Car ambulances, private cars and taxis would be the most effective method of transferring women, but the problem is availability and affordability. Public sector ambulances stationed at district hospitals are extremely busy and not dedicated to obstetric emergencies only. Vehicles often get put into service for other non-emergency messenger services once available. The positive reports on the impact of using car ambulances are few. In Sri Lanka, the government equipped every district hospital with between three and five ambulances, which greatly reduced the delay in transporting women (Pathmanathan *et al.*, 2003). In Sierra Leone, a collaboration between the Prevention of Maternal Mortality Network and the Ministry of Health studied the use of a four-wheel-drive vehicle at the referral hospital (Samai and Sengeh, 1997). Referrals for serious obstetric complications increased from 0.9 to 2.6 per month and average referral time was just over 3 h.

Due to the cost of running a public sector ambulance service in rural areas, women and their families have to depend on private transport using either their own funds or financing schemes. Holmes and Kennedy (2010) presented a detailed description of the initiatives in a wide variety of developing country settings and concluded that community-based schemes have demonstrated some potential to overcome financial barriers to reaching EmOC. These included emergency loan funds, insurance and prepayment schemes. Challenges included the generation of sufficient funds, particularly in small communities, and sustainability. Government programmes have introduced, sometimes in partnership with non-government organizations or the private sector, cost-sharing initiatives: vouchers and entitlement cards, and cash transfers and reimbursements (see Witter and Ensor, Chapter 7 this volume). Attention to management, transparency and regulations to ensure rationalization is recommended to ensure the success of the initiatives.

The most feasible transport arrangements for many low income settings would be a motorcycle ambulance at all primary centres attending to pregnant women, complemented by a car ambulance at the referral centre. The motorcycle ambulance would perform two tasks: taking women from the community to the primary facility, and then transferring them to a referral facility when the need arose. The car ambulance would then be reserved for collecting women from primary facilities more than 30 km away or for situations in which the woman might deliver in transit.

Childbirth and emergency preparedness

Pregnant women are now routinely offered birth and complication readiness advice, usually in the third trimester, regardless of where they live. However, this is much more relevant to women living in areas of poor geographical access. Birth preparedness and complication readiness are meant to improve the access to skilled providers and consist of the following: knowledge of labour symptoms; knowledge of danger signs; plan for where to give birth; plan for a birth attendant; plan for transportation; and plan for saving money (Moran et al., 2006). These interventions aim to overcome the delays in decision making while simultaneously addressing planning to improve geographical access.

However, the results of providing this advice have been mixed. In Koupela district, Burkina Faso, a survey of 180 women who had given birth was done after a district-based service delivery system had been implemented by Jhpiego, an international non-profit health organization. Of these women, 46.1% had a plan for transportation and 83.3% had a plan to save money. Women with these plans were more likely to give birth with a skilled provider ($p=0.07$ and $p=0.03$, respectively). Controlling for education, parity, age, average distance to the health facility and number of antenatal visits, planning to save money was associated with giving birth with the assistance of a skilled provider ($p=0.05$). Most women saved money for delivery but

had less concrete plans for delivery care (Moran et al., 2006). In Ile-Ife, Nigeria, 400 women attending the antenatal clinic were asked about their birth preparedness and complication readiness plans. By the study criteria, 61% had made adequate preparations for delivery while only 4.8% were ready for complications (Onayade et al., 2010).

Other studies have failed to demonstrate the effectiveness of birth preparedness, which did not change key maternal health indicators such as skilled attendance and use of EmOC, although it positively influenced knowledge and some intermediate health outcomes such as household practices and use of other health services in Siraha district, Nepal (McPherson et al., 2006). At Kenyatta Hospital in Kenya, education and counselling on different aspects of birth and complications were not consistently provided during antenatal care. A survey found that knowledge of danger signs in pregnancy was low (Mutiso et al., 2008).

It is not clear from most of the studies how far the women were on average from the facilities, what the actual plans for transportation were and the modes of transport for those who were delivered by a skilled attendant.

Maternity waiting homes

A maternity waiting home (Plate 8) is a facility within easy reach of a hospital or health centre that provides EmOC. Women use the waiting homes at the end of their pregnancy, while awaiting labour. Once labour starts, women move to the health facility, so that they may be assisted by a skilled birth attendant (WHO, 1991). Maternity waiting homes evolved initially as a means of getting women living in remote areas closer to a health facility. Later, women at high risk, such as primigravidae, grand multiparae, women with a previous Caesarean section or a previous history of complications were encouraged to stay at the waiting homes. A review was conducted by the WHO in 1996 (WHO, 1996a). This showed that in different countries the infrastructure of the waiting homes, the clientele accommodated and the services offered varied greatly. That review concluded that waiting homes can be viewed as one possible option for areas with poor geographical access and should be considered as part of a comprehensive safe motherhood programme. There is insufficient evidence on which to base recommendations about the effectiveness of waiting homes and well-controlled trials are needed (van Lonkhuijzen *et al.*, 2009). Six retrospective population cohort studies have described the effectiveness of maternity waiting homes in decreasing maternal deaths and stillbirths (Millard *et al.*, 1991; Chandramohan *et al.*, 1994, 1995; Tumwine and Dungare, 1996; Spaans *et al.*, 1998; van Lonkhuijzen *et al.*, 2003). Three provided information on stillbirths (Millard *et al.*, 1991; Chandramohan *et al.*, 1995; Tumwine and Dungare, 1996). A recent meta analysis combined the findings of these three studies and found a significant reduction in the stillbirth rate (OR 0.52 95% CI 0.34, 0.80) (Hussein *et al.*, 2011).

The maternity waiting home is the only intervention which addresses both the first and second delay simultaneously. If women return to the waiting home after delivery for 2–3 days postnatally, neonatal problems can also be managed at the facility. It is potentially one of the more cost-effective solutions to poor geographical access, particularly in sub-Saharan Africa, but will need adequate assessment of effectiveness.

Community-based interventions

Community-based interventions aim to prevent maternal and newborn illness and death and to improve neonatal outcomes. The expected outcome is to ameliorate the harmful effects of poor geographical access. The packages include some or all of the activities listed in Box 11.2.

There have been a number of systematic reviews of community-based interventions in the past 4 years. Some have looked at the effect of community-level interventions as a whole (including referral components, but with many others) to reduce maternal mortality. Five cluster randomized controlled trials (RCTs) were included in one study (Kidney *et al.*, 2009), with two trials showing a combined reduction in maternal mortality reaching statistical significance (OR 0.62 95% CI 0.39, 0.98). Kidney and colleagues (2009) concluded that community-level interventions to improve perinatal care can bring about a reduction in maternal mortality. A larger systematic review, which looked at 18 studies covering a wide range of intervention packages (Lassi *et al.*, 2010), did not show any reduction of maternal mortality (RR 0.77, 95% CI 0.59–1.02). However, reductions in maternal morbidity (RR 0.75, 95% CI 0.61–0.92), neonatal mortality (RR 0.76, 95% CI 0.68–0.84), stillbirths (RR 0.84 05% CI 0.74–0.97) and perinatal mortality (RR 0.80, 95% CI 0.71–0.91) were noted. The conclusion of the review was that there is encouraging evidence of the value of integrating maternal and newborn care in community settings through a range of interventions which can be delivered through community health workers and health promotion groups.

A few systematic reviews have looked at the specific effect of interventions on referral. Sibley *et al.* (2009) revisited traditional

---

Box 11.2. Elements of community-based referral packages.

- Health education for women and their families, especially on danger signs.
- Birth preparedness and complication readiness.
- Transport arrangements.
- Generation of funds for transport.
- Referral advice.
- Training of community health workers and traditional birth attendants on first aid, danger signs, good practices and referral.
- Upgrading of local health facilities in EmOC.

birth attendant training for improving health behaviours and pregnancy outcomes. Results were mixed, with one study included in the review reporting lower perinatal deaths (adjusted OR 0.70, 95% CI 0.59–0.83) and stillbirths in the intervention group (adjusted OR 0.69, 95% CI 0.57, 0.83) (Jokhio et al., 2005), while another study showed no differences in perinatal outcome. Similarly, in one study, referral rates were significantly higher in trained traditional birth attendants (adjusted OR 1.50, 95% CI 1.18–1.90, $P < 0.001$) but another study reported no differences in the number of monthly referrals. The effectiveness of primary-level referral systems for emergency maternity care in developing countries has recently been systematically reviewed (Hussein et al., 2011). Nineteen papers from 14 studies, which included RCTs, controlled before-after studies and interrupted time series, were included. In several South Asian settings, the organization of communities to generate funds for transport, implemented as part of other community mobilization activities, reduced neonatal deaths significantly (OR 0.69, 95% CI 0.53, 0.90). Conclusions were limited by difficulties in isolating the effects of the multiple components and factors related to the design of some studies. The review recommended the continued inclusion of referral interventions within maternal and newborn health programmes as part of wider health system improvement, and suggested that practices in research, monitoring and evaluation of these interventions be improved.

Geographical information systems

Geographical information systems (GIS) are an emerging technology in the analysis of health from a geographical or location context. They are potentially powerful assessment tools for the investigation of health-care access, health outcomes and the possible resulting health disparities (Graves, 2008). The technology captures geographical data and can analyse, manage and display relevant information for various purposes. The technology has already been used in both developed and developing country settings to map diseases and infectious outbreaks, calculate distances from health centres, conduct surveys and aid in decision making (Kohli et al., 1995; WHO and UNEP, 2011). In reproductive health, GIS was used to integrate health facility and demographic health survey data to ascertain the value of distance to health services as a proxy variable for access to family planning services (Heard et al., 2004). In maternal and perinatal health, one of the most significant uses of this technology would be to find out which women in a district suffer from the poorest geographical access and where new facilities should be built. Mortality and morbidity data can be linked to the assessment to provide the best potential to save lives. GIS data could be used to inform the building or upgrading of facilities and infrastructure.

Conclusion

Poor geographical access is a major determinant of maternal and perinatal mortality and morbidity. This is mainly a problem of rural areas in low income countries. Poor geographical access in itself is not the cause of the second delay, but the delay results from failure to bridge it with communications, transport and adequate referral systems. In high income countries pregnant women may live quite far from facilities but do not suffer unfavourable outcomes (Box 11.3). The economic potential of each country to deal with access and physical obstacles differs, so in resource poor settings decision making regarding referral needs will be aided through the generation of reliable evidence describing the relationship between geographical access and pregnancy outcomes and evidence which rigorously assesses the impact of interventions to improve access. New technologies should be exploited for their potential to resolve problems of communications and transport especially for the rural poor, but underlying the success of any referral intervention is its reliance on an efficiently functioning health system.

Box 11.3. Selected experiences from high income countries.

High income countries have largely solved the problem of geographical access. Good communication and excellent transport systems allow women to reach services within an acceptable time period. In countries such as Australia, the USA and Canada and in Europe pregnant women may live quite far from facilities in remote locations but do not suffer unfavourable outcomes. There is little difference in maternal or perinatal outcomes between women living in urban or rural areas (Baird *et al.*, 1996; Schmidt *et al.*, 2002; Hughes *et al.*, 2008; Pilkington *et al.*, 2008; Homer *et al.*, 2011).

A report from California, USA on 2,620,096 births conducted between 1998 and 2002 showed that rural obstetric services had favourable neonatal and maternal safety profiles. Maternal death rates were not different (Hughes *et al.*, 2008). The good outcomes for rural women in isolated circumstances in the USA and Canada are the result of regionalization of perinatal care combined with efficient telecommunication and transport systems (Nesbitt, 1996; Larson *et al.*, 1997; Kornelsen and Grzybowski, 2005). However, even in these settings there are problems with providing rural services, such as the resources required to maintain the performance of a facility (Heaphy and Bernard, 2000), the viability of primary facilities which have high referral rates (Iglesias *et al.*, 2005) and the fact that subgroups of women may still actually experience poor outcomes due to poor geographical access (Hulme and Blegen, 1999).

In Europe, the use of hospital-based Obstetric Flying Squads shortens the time it takes for women to access emergency care. Travel time is measured in minutes rather than hours (Hauspy *et al.*, 2001; Pilkington *et al.*, 2008; Ravelli *et al.*, 2011). The flying squad members are staff of the nearest maternity unit. In the UK, one health authority assessed the potential benefits of using paramedics as primary responders for domiciliary obstetric and gynaecological emergencies. It was found that targets for response times were met and the mean response time for providing appropriate skilled help was halved compared to the previous arrangements. Medical staff depletion in the delivery unit was minimized (Hibbard *et al.*, 1993).

Reports of the use of maternity waiting homes in high income countries are few as they are largely unnecessary in those settings. Islands with small populations may have to transfer women to larger islands, as in the Seychelles, or to the mainland, as in Scotland. In Australia, the use of a Cairns Base Hospital for late pregnancy care and delivery by women from the distant communities of Cape York has been described. The women were transferred at 36 weeks, which resulted in a mean stay of 24 days before birth (range 0–86 days). Referring at 36 weeks was concluded to be medically appropriate although there were some detrimental social, cultural and financial consequences (Arnold *et al.*, 2009).

Almost all industrialized countries have air transport facilities for geographically distant communities. Reports have described the successful air transport of women (Jony and Baskett, 2007) and neonates (Lang *et al.*, 2007). However, these experiences are hardly relevant to developing countries because of the costs involved.

References

AbouZahr, C. (1998) *Antepartum and Postpartum Haemorrhage*, 1st edn. Harvard School of Public Health on behalf of WHO and the World Bank, Boston and Geneva.

Andina, M.M. and Fikree, F. (1995) Pakistan: the Faisalabad Obstetric Flying Squad. *World Health Statistics Quarterly* 48(1), 50–54.

Arnold, J.L., de Costa, C.M. and Howat, P.W. (2009) Timing of transfer for pregnant women from Queensland Cape York communities to Cairns for birthing. *Medical Journal of Australia* 190, 594–596.

Babinard, J. and Roberts, P. (2006) Maternal and child mortality development goals: What can the transport sector do? *Transport Papers. TP-12.* The World Bank, Washington.

Baird, A.G., Jewell, D. and Walker, J.J. (1996) Management of labour in an isolated rural maternity hospital. *British Medical Journal* 312, 223–226.

Bell, J.S., Ouedraogo, M., Ganaba, R., Sombie, I., Byass, P., Bagley, R.F., Filippi, V., Fitzmaurice, A.E. and Graham, W.J. (2008) The epidemiology of pregnancy outcomes in rural Burkina Faso. *Tropical Medicine and International Health* 13 (Suppl. 1), 31–43.

Bilenko, N., Hammel, R. and Belmaker, I. (2007) Utilization of antenatal care services by a semi-nomadic Bedouin Arab population: Evaluation of the impact of a local Maternal and Child Health Clinic. *Maternal and Child Health Journal* 11, 425–430.

Bossyns, P., Abache, R., Abdoulaye, M.S. and Lerberghe, W.V. (2005) Unaffordable or cost-effective? Introducing an emergency referral system in rural Niger. *Tropical Medicine and International Health* 10, 879–887.

Brown, C.A., Sohani, S.B., Khan, K., Lilford, R. and Mukhwana, W. (2008) Antenatal care and perinatal outcomes in Kwale district, Kenya. *BMC Pregnancy Childbirth* 8, 2.

Chandramohan, D., Cutts, F. and Chandra, R. (1994) Effects of a maternity waiting home on adverse maternal outcomes and the validity of antenatal risk screening. *International Journal of Gynaecology and Obstetrics* 46, 279–284.

Chandramohan, D., Cutts, F. and Millard, P. (1995) The effect of stay in a maternity waiting home on perinatal mortality in rural Zimbabwe. *Journal of Tropical Medicine and Hygiene* 98, 261–267.

de Almeida, M.F., Alencar, G.P., Novaes, M.H., Franca, I., Siqueira, A.A., Schoeps, D., Campbell, O. and Rodrigues, L. (2005) Accidental home deliveries in southern São Paulo, Brazil. *Revista de Saude Publica* 39, 366–375.

Duong, D.V., Binns, C.W. and Lee, A.H. (2004) Utilization of delivery services at the primary health care level in rural Vietnam. *Social Science and Medicine* 59, 2585–2595.

Fawcus, S., Mbizvo, M., Lindmark, G. and Nystrom, L. (1996) A community-based investigation of avoidable factors for maternal mortality in Zimbabwe. *Studies in Family Planning* 27, 319–327.

Gabrysch, S. and Campbell, O.M. (2009) Still too far to walk: Literature review of the determinants of delivery service use. *BMC Pregnancy Childbirth* 9, 34.

Gabrysch, S., Cousens, S., Cox, J. and Campbell, O.M. (2011a) The influence of distance and level of care on delivery place in rural Zambia: A study of linked national data in a geographical information system. *PLoS Medicine* 8, e1000394.

Gabrysch, S., Zanger, P., Seneviratne, H.R., Mbewe, R. and Campbell, O.M. (2011b) Tracking progress towards safe motherhood: Meeting the benchmark yet missing the goal? An appeal for better use of health-system output indicators with evidence from Zambia and Sri Lanka. *Tropical Medicine and International Health* 16, 627–639.

Gage, A.J. (2007) Barriers to the utilization of maternal health care in rural Mali. *Social Science and Medicine* 65, 1666–1682.

Gage, A.J. and Guirlene Calixte, M. (2006) Effects of the physical accessibility of maternal health services on their use in rural Haiti. *Population Studies (Cambridge)* 60, 271–288.

Glei, D.A., Goldman, N. and Rodriguez, G. (2003) Utilization of care during pregnancy in rural Guatemala: Does obstetrical need matter? *Social Science and Medicine* 57, 2447–2463.

Graves, B.A. (2008) Integrative literature review: A review of literature related to geographical information systems, healthcare access, and health outcomes. *Perspectives in Health Information Management* 5, 11.

Hauspy, J., Jacquemyn, Y., Van Reempts, P., Buytaert, P. and Van Vliet, J. (2001) Intrauterine versus postnatal transport of the preterm infant: A short-distance experience. *Early Human Development* 63, 1–7.

Heaphy, P.E. and Bernard, S.L. (2000) Maternal complications of normal deliveries: Variation among rural hospitals. *Journal of Rural Health* 16, 139–147.

Heard, N.J., Larsen, U. and Hozumi, D. (2004) Investigating access to reproductive health services using GIS: Proximity to services and the use of modern contraceptives in Malawi. *African Journal of Reproductive Health* 8(2), 164–179.

Hibbard, B.M., Dawson, A., Boyce, J., Oliver, M., Goodall, K., Organ, P. and Rookes, N. (1993) A paramedic based emergency domiciliary obstetric service: The South Glamorgan experience. *British Journal of Obstetrics and Gynaecology* 100, 618–622.

Hofman, J.J., Dzimadzi, C., Lungu, K., Ratsma, E.Y. and Hussein, J. (2008) Motorcycle ambulances for referral of obstetric emergencies in rural Malawi: Do they reduce delay and what do they cost? *International Journal of Gynaecology and Obstetrics* 102, 191–197.

Holmes, W. and Kennedy, E. (2010) *Reaching Emergency Obstetric Care: Overcoming the 'Second Delay'.* Burnet Institute on behalf of Compass, the Women's and Children's Knowledge Hub, Melbourne.

Homer, C.S., Biggs, J., Vaughan, G. and Sullivan, E.A. (2011) Mapping maternity services in Australia: location, classification and services. *Australian Health Review* 35, 222–229.

Hounton, S., Chapman, G., Mente, J., De Brouwerer, V., Ensor, T., Sombie, I., Meda, N. and Ronsmans, C. (2008) Accessibility and utilisation of delivery care within a Skilled Care Initiative in rural Burkina Faso. *Tropical Medicine and International Health* 13, 44–52.

Hughes, S., Zweifler, J.A., Garza, A. and Stanich, M.A. (2008) Trends in rural and urban deliveries and vaginal births: California 1998–2002. *Journal of Rural Health* 24, 416–422.

Hulme, P.A. and Blegen, M.A. (1999) Residential status and birth outcomes: Is the rural/urban distinction adequate? *Public Health Nursing* 16, 176–181.

Hunger, C., Kulker, R., Kitundu, H., Massawe, S. and Jahn, A. (2007) Assessing unmet obstetric need in Mtwara Region, Tanzania. *Tropical Medicine and International Health* 12, 1239–1247.

Hussein, J., Kanguru, L., Astin, M. and Munjanja, S. (2011) The effectiveness of primary level referral systems for emergency maternity care in developing countries: A systematic review. Available at: http://www.dfid.gov.uk/r4d/SystematicReviewNew.asp (accessed 27 July 2011).

Iglesias, S., Bott, N., Ellehoj, E., Yee, J., Jennissen, B., Bunnah, T. and Schopflocher, D. (2005) Outcomes of maternity care services in Alberta, 1999 and 2000: A population-based analysis. *Journal of Obstetrics and Gynaecology of Canada* 27, 855–863.

International Communication Union (2010) The World in 2010: ICT facts and figures. Available at: http://www.itu.int/ITU-D/ict/material/FactsFigures2010.pdf (accessed 25 July 2011).

Jahn, A., Kowalewski, M. and Kimatta, S.S. (1998) Obstetric care in Southern Tanzania: Does it reach those in need? *Tropical Medicine and International Health* 3, 926–932.

Jokhio, A.H., Winter, H.R. and Cheng, K.K. (2005) An intervention involving traditional birth attendants and perinatal and maternal mortality in Pakistan. *New England Journal of Medicine* 352, 2091–2099.

Jony, L. and Baskett, T.F. (2007) Emergency air transport of obstetric patients. *Journal of Obstetrics and Gynaecology of Canada* 29, 406–408.

Kidney, E., Winter, H.R., Khan, K.S., Gulmezoglu, A.M., Meads, C.A., Deeks, J.J. and Macarthur, C. (2009) Systematic review of effect of community-level interventions to reduce maternal mortality. *BMC Pregnancy and Childbirth* 9, 2.

Kohli, S., Sahlen, K., Sivertun, A., Lofman, O., Trell, E. and Wigertz, O. (1995) Distance from the Primary Health Center: A GIS method to study geographical access to health care. *Journal of Medical Systems* 19, 425–436.

Kornelsen, J. and Grzybowski, S. (2005) Is local maternity care an optional service in rural communities? *Journal of Obstetrics and Gynaecology of Canada* 27, 329–331.

Kornelsen, J.A. and Grzybowski, S.W. (2008) Obstetric services in small rural communities: What are the risks to care providers? *Rural Remote Health* 8, 943.

Krasovec, K. (2004) Auxiliary technologies related to transport and communication for obstetric emergencies. *International Journal of Gynaecology and Obstetrics* 85 (Suppl. 1), S14–S23.

Lang, A., Brun, H., Kaaresen, P.I. and Klingenberg, C. (2007) A population based 10-year study of neonatal air transport in North Norway. *Acta Paediatrica* 96, 995–999.

Larson, E.E., Hart, L.G. and Rosenblatt, R.A. (1997) Is non-metropolitan residence a risk factor for poor birth outcome in the US? *Social Science and Medicine* 45, 171–188.

Lassi, Z.S., Haider, B.A. and Bhutta, Z.A. (2010) Community-based intervention packages for reducing maternal and neonatal morbidity and mortality and improving neonatal outcomes. *Cochrane Database of Systematic Reviews* CD007754.

Lawn, J.E., Lee, A.C., Kinney, M., Sibley, L., Carlo, W.A., Paul, V.K., Pattinson, R. and Darmstadt, G.L. (2009) Two million intrapartum-related stillbirths and neonatal deaths: Where, why, and what can be done? *International Journal of Gynaecology and Obstetrics* 107(Suppl. 1), S5–S18.

Low, A., De Couvere, D., Shivute, N. and Brandt, L.J. (2001) Patient referral patterns in Namibia: Identification of the potential to improve the health care system. *International Journal of Health Planning and Management* 16, 243–257.

Lungu, K., Kamfosa, V., Hussein, J. and Ashwood-Smith, H. (2001) Are bicycle ambulances and community transport plans effective in strengthening obstetric referral systems in Southern Malawi? *Malawi Medical Journal* 12, 16–18.

Maine, D. (1991) *Safe Motherhood Programs: Options and issues.* Centre for Population and Family Health, School of Public Health, Columbia University, New York.

Malqvist, M., Sohel, N., Do, T.T., Eriksson, L. and Persson, L.A. (2010) Distance decay in delivery care utilisation associated with neonatal mortality. A case referent study in northern Vietnam. *BMC Public Health* 10, 762.

McPherson, R.A., Khadka, N., Moore, J.M. and Sharma, M. (2006) Are birth-preparedness programmes effective? Results from a field trial in Siraha district, Nepal. *Journal of Health Population and Nutrition* 24, 479–488.

Melah, G.S., Massa, A.A., Yahaya, U.R., Bukar, M., Kizaya, D.D. and El-Nafaty, A.U. (2007) Risk factors for obstetric fistulae in north-eastern Nigeria. *Journal of Obstetrics and Gynaecology* 27, 819–823.

Millard, P., Bailey, J. and Hanson, J. (1991) Antenatal village stay and pregnancy outcome in rural Zimbabwe. *Central African Journal of Medicine* 37, 1–4.

Moodley, J. (2004) Maternal deaths associated with hypertensive disorders of pregnancy: A population-based study. *Hypertension and Pregnancy* 23, 247–256.

Moran, A.C., Sangli, G., Dineen, R., Rawlins, B., Yameogo, M. and Baya, B. (2006) Birth-preparedness for maternal health: Findings from Koupela District, Burkina Faso. *Journal of Health Population and Nutrition* 24, 489–497.

Muleta, M. (2004) Socio-demographic profile and obstetric experience of fistula patients managed at the Addis Ababa Fistula Hospital. *Ethiopian Medical Journal* 42, 9–16.

Murray, S.F. and Pearson, S.C. (2006) Maternity referral systems in developing countries: current knowledge and future research needs. *Social Science and Medicine* 62, 2205–2215.

Musoke, M.G.N. (2002) Maternal health in rural Uganda. Leveraging traditional and modern knowledge systems. *IK Notes No. 40.* The World Bank, Washington, DC.

Mutiso, S.M., Qureshi, Z. and Kinuthia, J. (2008) Birth preparedness among antenatal clients. *East African Medical Journal* 85, 275–283.

Nesbitt, T.S. (1996) Rural maternity care: New models of access. *Birth* 23, 161–165.

Nkyekyer, K. (2000) Peripartum referrals to Korle Bu teaching hospital, Ghana: A descriptive study. *Tropical Medicine and International Health* 5, 811–817.

Onayade, A.A., Akanbi, O.O., Okunola, H.A., Oyeniyi, C.F., Togun, O.O. and Sule, S.S. (2010) Birth preparedness and emergency readiness plans of antenatal clinic attendees in Ile-Ife, Nigeria. *Nigerian Postgraduate Medical Journal* 17, 30–39.

Pathmanathan, I., Liljestrand, J., Martins, J.M., Rajapaksa, L.C., Lissner, C. and De Silva, A. (2003) Investing in maternal health: Learning from Malaysia and Sri Lanka. *Health Nutrition and Population Series.* The World Bank: Human Development Network, Washington.

Pilkington, H., Blondel, B., Carayol, M., Breart, G. and Zeitlin, J. (2008) Impact of maternity unit closures on access to obstetrical care: The French experience between 1998 and 2003. *Social Science and Medicine* 67, 1521–1529.

Ravelli, A.C., Jager, K.J., De Groot, M.H., Erwich, J.J., Rijninks-Van Driel, G.C., Tromp, M., Eskes, M., Abu-Hanna, A. and Mol, B.W. (2011) Travel time from home to hospital and adverse perinatal outcomes in women at term in the Netherlands. *BJOG: An International Journal of Obstetrics and Gynaecology* 118, 457–465.

Ronsmans, C. and Graham, W.J. (2006) Maternal mortality: Who, when, where, and why. *Lancet* 368, 1189–1200.

Ronsmans, C., Etard, J.F., Walraven, G., Hoj, L., Dumont, A., De Bernis, L. and Kodio, B. (2003) Maternal mortality and access to obstetric services in West Africa. *Tropical Medicine and International Health* 8, 940–948.

Samai, O. and Sengeh, P. (1997) Facilitating emergency obstetric care through transportation and communication, Bo, Sierra Leone. The Bo PMM Team. *International Journal of Gynaecology and Obstetrics* 59 (Suppl. 2), S157–S164.

Santos, C., Diante, D., Jr, Baptista, A., Matediane, E., Bique, C. and Bailey, P. (2006) Improving emergency obstetric care in Mozambique: The story of Sofala. *International Journal of Gynaecology and Obstetrics* 94, 190–201.

Say, L. and Raine, R. (2007) A systematic review of inequalities in the use of maternal health care in developing countries: Examining the scale of the problem and the importance of context. *Bulletin of the World Health Organization* 85, 812–819.

Schmid, T., Kanenda, O., Ahluwalia, I. and Kouletio, M. (2001) Transportation for maternal emergencies in Tanzania: Empowering communities through participatory problem solving. *American Journal of Public Health* 91, 1589–1590.

Schmidt, N., Abelsen, B. and Oian, P. (2002) Deliveries in maternity homes in Norway: Results from a 2-year prospective study. *Acta Obstetrica et Gynecologica Scandinavica* 81, 731–737.

Scott, T. and Esen, U.I. (2005) Unplanned out of hospital births: Who delivers the babies? *Irish Medical Journal* 98, 70–72.

Shah, N., Hossain, N., Shoaib, R., Hussain, A., Gillani, R. and Khan, N.H. (2009) Socio-demographic characteristics and the three delays of maternal mortality. *Journal of College of Physicians and Surgeons Pakistan* 19, 95–98.

Sibley, L.M., Sipe, T.A., Brown, C.M., Diallo, M.M., Mcnatt, K. and Habarta, N. (2009) Traditional birth attendant training for improving health behaviours and pregnancy outcomes. *Cochrane Database of Systematic Reviews* CD005460.

Sikosana, P.L. (1994) An evaluation of the quantity of antenatal care at rural health centres in Matebeleland North Province. *Central African Journal of Medicine* 40, 268–272.

Simkhada, B., Teijlingen, E.R., Porter, M. and Simkhada, P. (2008) Factors affecting the utilization of antenatal care in developing countries: Systematic review of the literature. *Journal of Advanced Nursing* 61, 244–260.

Spaans, W.A., Van Roosmalen, J. and Van Wiechen, C.M. (1998) A maternity waiting home experience in Zimbabwe. *International Journal of Gynaecology and Obstetrics* 61, 179–180.

Stanton, C., Lawn, J.E., Rahman, H., Wilczynska-Ketende, K. and Hill, K. (2006) Stillbirth rates: Delivering estimates in 190 countries. *Lancet* 367, 1487–1494.

Stekelenburg, J., Kyanamina, S., Mukelabai, M., Wolffers, I. and Van Roosmalen, J. (2004) Waiting too long: Low use of maternal health services in Kalabo, Zambia. *Tropical Medicine and International Health* 9, 390–398.

Thaddeus, S. and Maine, D. (1994) Too far to walk: Maternal mortality in context. *Social Science and Medicine* 38, 1091–1110.

Thomson, N. (2005) Emergency medical services in Zimbabwe. *Resuscitation* 65, 15–19.

Tuladhar, H., Dali, S.M. and Pradhanang, V. (2005) Complications of home delivery: A retrospective analysis. *Journal of Nepal Medical Association* 44, 87–91.

Tuladhar, H., Khanal, R., Kayastha, S., Shrestha, P. and Giri, A. (2009) Complications of home delivery: Our experience at Nepal Medical College Teaching Hospital. *Nepal Medical College Journal* 11, 164–169.

Tumwine, J.K. and Dungare, P.S. (1996) Maternity waiting shelters and pregnancy outcome: Experience from a rural area in Zimbabwe. *Annals of Tropical Paediatrics* 16, 55–59.

UNFPA (2011) *Maternal Mortality and Transport Services: Crisis, journeys and gender.* UNFPA, New York.

UNICEF (1997) *Guidelines for Monitoring the Availability and Use of Obstetric Services.* UNICEF/WHO/UNFPA, New York.

UN Population Division (2008) World Urbanization Prospects: The 2007 Revision Population Database. Available at: http://esa.un.org/unup/ (accessed 22 July 2011).

van den Broek, N.R., White, S.A., Ntonya, C., Ngwale, M., Cullinan, T.R., Molyneux, M.E. and Neilson, J.P. (2003) Reproductive health in rural Malawi: A population-based survey. *British Journal of Obstetrics and Gynaecology* 110, 902–908.

van Lonkhuijzen, L., Stegeman, M., Nyirongo, R. and Van Roosmalen, J. (2003) Use of maternity waiting home in rural Zambia. *African Journal of Reproductive Health* 7, 32–36.

van Lonkhuijzen, L., Stekelenburg, J. and Van Roosmalen, J. (2009) Maternity waiting facilities for improving maternal and neonatal outcome in low-resource countries. *Cochrane Database of Systematic Reviews* CD006759.

Wagle, R.R., Sabroe, S. and Nielsen, B.B. (2004) Socioeconomic and physical distance to the maternity hospital as predictors for place of delivery: An observation study from Nepal. *BMC Pregnancy Childbirth* 4, 8.

WHO (1991) *Essential Elements of Obstetric Care at First Referral Level.* WHO, Geneva.

WHO (1996a) *Maternity Waiting Homes.* WHO, Geneva.

WHO (1996b) *Mother–Baby Package: Implementing safe motherhood in countries.* WHO, Geneva.

WHO (2006) *Monitoring and Evaluation of Maternal and Newborn Health and Services at the District Level.* Department of Making Pregnancy Safer, Geneva.

WHO (2011) *mHealth: new horizons for health through mobile technologies: second global survey on eHealth.* WHO, Geneva.

WHO and UNEP (2011) The Health and environment linkages initiative. Available at: http://www.who.int/heli/tools/maps/en/index.html (accessed 27 July 2011).

WHO, UNFPA, UNICEF and AMDD (2009) *Monitoring Emergency Obstetric Care: A handbook.* WHO, Geneva.

Yanagisawa, S. and Wakai, S. (2008) Professional healthcare use for life-threatening obstetric conditions. *Journal of Obstetrics and Gynaecology* 28, 713–719.

12 Demand for Maternity Care: Beliefs, Behaviour and Social Access

Zubia Mumtaz and Adrienne Levay
University of Alberta, Edmonton, Canada

Summary

- Demand side interventions are necessary to increase use of maternity services.
- Factors that affect demand include knowledge of danger signs in pregnancy and childbirth; financial, geographical and social access to health care; quality of care and the gendered norms and values around maternal health-seeking behaviours.
- Three key concepts related to influencing the demand for care during pregnancy and childbirth are discussed in detail: providing culturally sensitive contextual knowledge; how health systems create social barriers to uptake of services; and the overarching influence of gender.
- Empowering people by providing culturally contextual knowledge that does not devalue local beliefs and practices is crucial to improve the acceptability of biomedical services.
- Communication and education approaches that focus on eliciting a dialogue between traditional understandings of health and biomedical priorities may produce a greater demand for services than the traditional unidirectional 'transmission-persuasion' approach.
- Societal values and norms are signalled and reinforced by the health system. The commonly reported neglect, abuse and exclusion within health-care systems may be a reflection of the experience of being poor and socially marginalized in that society.
- There are few published interventions aimed at reducing social barriers to health services. Existing initiatives include improving health worker attitudes and using rights based frameworks to develop client centred non-discriminatory service delivery systems.
- Aspects of the gender order that affect demand for maternity care include women's social and economic dependency on men, limited decision-making authority and restricted access to financial and material resources. For women living in unequal gender contexts, policies to create social change at the group level may be needed, rather than focusing on women's individual-level bargaining power.

Introduction

Increasingly, availability, access and uptake of maternity services are seen as a dynamic system of entitlement and obligation between people, communities, providers and governments (UNICEF, 2009). This approach assumes that, while governments are obliged to ensure that high quality services are available and accessible, users are also encouraged to articulate and advocate for what they need and expect in terms of services. In other words, a health-care system is the product of a balance between demand and supply. Ongoing and sustained interaction between these two parts of the system should lead to improved maternal and perinatal health.

The traditional focus on supply-side determinants has concentrated on delivery of essential services – improving quality of provider skills, protocols of treatments, availability of supplies and the health facility infrastructure (Campbell and Graham, 2006). While these interventions are necessary, they are insufficient to significantly increase uptake of maternity services or reduce maternal and perinatal mortality, particularly in countries with the highest burdens (WHO, 2010). One key reason is that women and their families have to make a number of decisions well before they arrive at a health facility. Whether, where and when to go for treatment involves making decisions that take into account complex interactions between the woman and her family's understanding of ill health and the causes of the illness, the type of treatment needed, knowledge of the types of services offered by different providers, acceptability of these services and social, financial and geographical barriers to health facilities. Gender values are interwoven throughout the entire process, from the values placed on seeking care for women to dynamics of decision making and women's degree of mobility and visibility.

This chapter reviews contemporary understandings of demand for maternity services and factors that promote or suppress demand. Interventions aimed at increasing demand are critically analysed. A conceptual framework to describe the factors that affect the creation or suppression of demand for services is presented. Three factors are discussed in detail: knowledge of danger signs in pregnancy and childbirth, social access to health systems and the gendered norms and values around maternal health-seeking behaviours.

Demand for Maternity Services

There have been many attempts to define 'demand for health care' but a standard definition remains elusive. Most definitions use an economic framework for health-care utilization, which defines demand-side determinants 'as factors that influence demand and operate at the individual, household and community level' (Ensor and Cooper, 2004).

The Thaddeus and Maine (1994) three delays model provides a convenient framework to locate and understand factors that influence demand for maternal health services. This model proposes that barriers to accessing care can be divided into three delays: the delay in the decision to seek care, the delay in reaching a health facility and the delay in obtaining appropriate care once the woman reaches a health facility. Based on this model, Fig. 12.1 provides a framework of determinants and factors affecting demand for maternity services.

The first delay occurs when there is an apparent 'failure' by the woman, her family or attendants to recognize the signs and symptoms of danger in pregnancy or childbirth. It has been assumed that, if people are educated about the signs and symptoms of danger and risk in pregnancy and childbirth, they will seek biomedical care, but this is an oversimplification. Other factors are interwoven in the decision-making process and in the second delay, i.e. reaching care. A large body of evidence has documented the financial costs of seeking care; these include the high direct costs of services as well as indirect consumer costs such as opportunity costs that occur when the patient and caregiver have to stop working in order to seek institutional care (see Witter and Ensor, Chapter 7 this volume). Geographical barriers (see Munjanja et al., Chapter 11 this volume) are experienced in the form of difficulties or discomforts endured when a transport infrastructure is absent or inadequate and over travel-related costs and opportunity costs of time spent travelling long distances (Porter, 2002; McCray, 2004). Social costs and delays are magnified in contexts where gendered norms promote women's seclusion (Mumtaz and Salway, 2005).

As part of the third delay of obtaining high quality appropriate care, demand for services will be affected by the expectation of at least a minimal level of quality of the services being sought. Staff availability and their levels of motivation and inter-personal behaviour and availability of drugs and even water and electricity in the facility are factors that determine

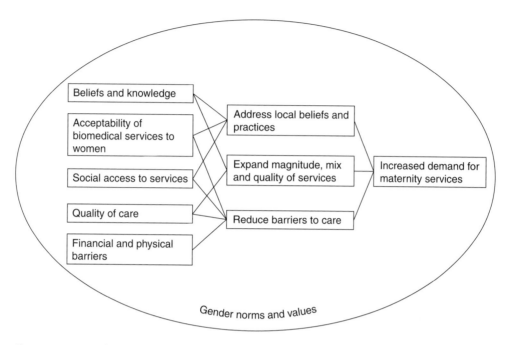

Fig. 12.1. Factors related to demand for maternity care.

quality of care. The choice of facilities available and their distribution are other important factors (see Phoya *et al.*, Chapter 10 this volume). Both the first and the third delays are influenced by social access. Social barriers occur with abusive and humiliating treatment by health-care providers. Health-care systems are core social institutions and, as such, they can replicate and reproduce the exclusion, marginalization and humiliation that are the experience of poor people (Freedman, 2005). Among poor women, those of a particular ethnicity or religion may face additional stigma or marginalization. The supposition underlying the links between the health system as a perpetuator of exclusion and abuse is that women who are treated poorly and are repeatedly excluded in a health-care setting will be less likely to demand health services.

Underlying and interwoven throughout all the determinants of demand for maternity care are the gender norms and values of a society. The link between gender norms and maternal health (and consequently perinatal health) operates at three levels: in the production of vulnerability to maternal ill health, in the financial, social and geographical access to

health services and around disadvantages within the health-care system. Poor maternal health is fundamentally a reflection of the social and gender norms that put women at high risk of reproductive health problems to begin with (Okojie, 1994). The same cluster of social and gender norms that operate to produce greater risks for women's reproductive health (social and economic dependency, limited decision-making authority and limited access to financial, material and knowledge resources) also appears to be associated with the lower likelihood of demanding, accessing and utilizing health services The paucity of maternal health services in terms of magnitude, type of services offered and acceptable quality are also a reflection of societal level and gendered ideologies that devalue women's health and consequently do not give women's health the necessary priority or resources (Simawa *et al.*, 2005).

Figure 12.1 shows that demand for biomedical services can potentially be created: by providing women, their families and communities culturally contextual knowledge that does not devalue local beliefs and practices; by reducing the financial, geographical, social and gendered barriers to seeking services; and by expanding the magnitude and mix of services and improving the quality of care. Three key concepts within this framework will be explored next: providing culturally sensitive contextual knowledge, how health systems create social barriers to uptake of services and the role of gender in increasing or decreasing demand for services.

Providing Culturally Contextual Knowledge

Central to the idea of individuals' rights to exert control over their reproductive and sexual health is that they have sufficient knowledge and information of the signs and symptoms of haemorrhage, hypertensive disorders, infection, obstructed labour and other complications of pregnancy and understand what action to take and where help can be found. This knowledge, with support, will enable pregnant women and their families to identify an obstetric emergency and make an informed decision to seek appropriate services. Implicit in this discourse and supported by a large body of evidence is the fact that women and men lack 'correct' knowledge and need to be educated (Thaddeus and Maine, 1994; Atkinson and Farias, 1995; White, 2002; Khan et al., 2005). Studies have presented data illustrating this 'lack' of knowledge. For example, in one district in Bangladesh, only 36.2% of women correctly identified retained placenta, obstructed labour (14.8%) or convulsions (35.6%) as potentially life-threatening conditions (Salam et al., 2009). Exit interviews with women attending an antenatal clinic in the Gambia showed that only 14.8% identified haemorrhage as a danger sign and prolonged labour was not recognized as a danger sign (Anya et al., 2008). Unsurprisingly, providing information to 'educate' women regarding signs and symptoms of danger is therefore a cornerstone of many maternal health programmes that aim to create a demand for and increase women's use of maternity services.

This discourse – located in the biomedical perspective – offers important information.

Medical science clearly provides effective treatment for the immediate causes of mortality. However, such restricted views fail to appreciate that pregnancy and childbirth are, in all societies in the world, embedded in explanatory models and illness theories imbued with values that are consistent with life representations of each particular social group. Each society has its own understanding of reproductive vulnerability, risk perception and pregnancy and childbirth management strategies. In Mozambique, for example, women's understanding of reproductive vulnerability and pregnancy management strategies is expressed as a cogent folk epidemiology that traces reproductive crises in terms of personalistic harm caused by witchcraft or sorcery. Some of the most serious reproductive problems – difficulty in conceiving, bleeding, threatened miscarriage, constant illness and all birth complications – were believed to be caused by human or spirit foes (Chapman, 2004). In Honduras, in 12 of the 55 cases of maternal mortality, witchcraft/sorcery was cited as the ultimate cause of death (Arps, 2009). In two diverse societies, in Nepal and in Morocco, childbirth is understood as a polluting condition and postpartum bleeding as a means of cleansing the body of contamination (Obermeyer, 2000; Matsuyama and Moji, 2008). In Nepal, there is no understanding of the difference between 'normal' and 'excessive' bleeding and most study participants felt 'the more the better'. Only when postpartum bleeding exceeded 6 or 7 days postpartum was it considered excessive. The causes of excessive bleeding are believed to be the consequence of heavy work, hot–cold imbalance, an attack by a *bokshi* (human witch) or entry of lower caste people into the womb (Matsuyama and Moji, 2008). In Cambodia, a small amount of postpartum bleeding is perceived to be dangerous, as the trapped blood might attract ghosts and spirits (White, 2002). In regions of Nigeria and Ghana, obstructed labour is thought to be a sign of woman's infidelity (Asowa-Omorodion, 1997; Wilkinson and Callister, 2010) and an unassisted home delivery raises the birthing mother's status for it reflects her fidelity (Bazzano *et al.*, 2008).

The standard biomedical discourse tends to view these local cultural 'traditions' as 'mistaken beliefs' that constitute the key barrier to uptake of biomedical maternity services (Dujardin *et al.*, 1995; Myer and Harrison, 2003). The cognitive gap between local explanatory models of risk in pregnancy and childbirth and the biomedical model is considerable (Berry, 2006). A large body of anthropological literature indicates that perceived need is the major predictor of whether one uses health services (Weiss, 1988; Thaddeus and Maine, 1994; Atkinson and Farias, 1995; Whiteford and Szelag, 2000; Harrison and Montgomery, 2001; White, 2002; Ensor and Cooper, 2004; Khan *et al.*, 2005; Norris, 2009). Perceived need, in turn, is said to be underpinned by the explanatory models people hold regarding functioning of the body, classifications and aetiologies of illness and the related remedies (Weiss, 1988; Atkinson and Farias, 1995; White, 2002; Norris, 2009). It was the logic of witchcraft and sorcery as the cause of their ill health that led women in Mozambique and Cameroon to seek care from the informal and church sector (Beninguisse and De Brouwere, 2004; Chapman, 2004). In Honduras, community members believe that the number and quality of doctors, nurses and health facilities had no impact on the incidence of maternal mortality since they offer no protection against sorcery, nor do they have the ability to neutralize its effects (Arps, 2009).

Most maternal health interventions have, however, disregarded these local understandings and explanatory models of ill health and instead focused on delivering 'health education' messages to women and other community members. In a language steeped in biomedical-scientific rationality, succinct messages are provided to persuade women and their husbands and mothers-in-law to adopt expert-prescribed behaviour regarding use of modern biomedical services. Grounded in the transmission–persuasion model of education and communication (Waisbord, 2001), this predominant pedagogical approach of message delivery is commonly referred to as 'health communication' or 'information, education and communication' (WHO, 1997) and more recently as 'behaviour change communication'.

It is essentially a top down and one way approach involving audiences, target groups and message delivery (Thomas, 1994). A basic assumption made in this directive method of message delivery is that if women and their families acquire the information on optimal maternal health practices they will adopt these practices. An accepted wisdom amongst maternal health programme planners, this approach has been the foundation for many large programmes that aim to reduce maternal and neonatal mortality.

There is, however, an emerging realization that the current directive approach to health education message delivery is having a limited impact on bringing about changes in health-seeking behaviours and practice, even if it does increase knowledge levels (Aboud, 2010). Although few rigorous evaluations of these communication interventions have been done, simple pre- and post-intervention surveys suggest the strategies are failing. In Pakistan, a study showed that, when asked to give spontaneous responses to simple dichotomous questions regarding recall of any of the 11 sponsored television dramas on pregnancy and childbirth, only 2% could do so. Furthermore, less than 15% of women could identify the key health message embedded within the dramas (Arjumand and Associates, 2009). In the southern areas of Nigeria, another study showed that 78% of women attending antenatal health information sessions failed to understand the information provided, despite their relatively high levels of education (Umoiyoho *et al.*, 2010).

If programmatic interventions aimed at increasing demand for maternity services are to be effective, there is a need to bridge the gap between local understandings of danger signs and those understood within the biomedical model. This requires taking into account local explanatory models and understandings of ill health. If women in South Asia and South-east Asia regard bleeding as desirable and cleansing (White, 2002; Matsumaya and Moji, 2008), it will probably be unproductive to educate them that bleeding is a sign of danger. To ensure recognition of dangers of postpartum haemorrhage, messages will have to acknowledge the cultural belief that bleeding is good before highlighting the dangers of postpartum haemorrhage. White (2002) suggests that one way to bridge the gap is to 'reload' local understandings of danger and risk in pregnancy with biomedical understandings rather than trying to change the local ways of thinking. For example, 'swelling (in the mother) from the baby' is considered normal in Cambodia. This idea can be altered by acknowledging that swelling in the legs and feet is normal but when accompanied by other symptoms and signs, such as dizziness and blurry vision, the swelling is dangerous.

A small body of emerging literature suggests that communication and education approaches that focus on eliciting a dialogue between traditional 'emic' understandings (explanations of belief/behaviour from within a culture, in contrast to supposedly 'objective' descriptions) of health and biomedical priorities may produce a greater demand for services than the unidirectional transmission–persuasion method. These approaches draw upon various concepts. In transformative learning (Mezirow, 1991), 'learners' actively and critically analyse both their own experience and alternative solutions in order to construct their own strategies to deal with everyday problems. Other approaches include empowerment education (Freire, 1970), adult learning (Mezirow, 1991) and community organizing for health (Minkler, 1998). These approaches tend to challenge communities to integrate the 'old' and the 'new' and increase community commitment and capacity to collectively solve problems (Aubel *et al.*, 2004). It is within these conceptual frameworks that women's groups are showing promise as a strategy for increasing demand for maternity services. For example, women's group meetings convened by a female facilitator in rural Nepal led to demonstrable increases in antenatal care, institutional delivery and skilled birth attendance (Manandhar *et al.*, 2004). Involving older women in women's groups in a maternal nutrition education programme in Senegal demonstrated significant improvements in the nutrition-related practices of younger women, during both pregnancy and later infant feeding (Aubel *et al.*, 2004).

Changing health behaviour is difficult but possible and doable (Aboud, 2010). Clearly the strategies currently employed – the education default, that teaching people with the help of culturally sensitive pictures, stories and songs will lead to behaviour change – are inadequate (Holford, 1995; Jewkes *et al.*, 2006). There is a need to explore alternative theoretical frameworks of behaviour change and even consider the possibility that the focus need not be on changing individual behaviours at all but on societal norms.

Last, a point of debate where maternal health education programmes are concerned is whether the reductionist focused messages located in the biomedical discourse contravene local understandings of ill health and may, therefore, be counterproductive (Dutta, 2010; Yeha and Dutta, 2010). These researchers believe that certain local practices and traditional discourses around understandings of health continue to exist because they are useful and functional. Furthermore, there is the issue of whether biomedical messages are challenging traditional authority structures around pregnancy and childbirth (Pigg, 1995; Wreford, 2005; Smid *et al.*, 2010). Others, however, believe that cultures are flexible and will not be destroyed by the introduction of new practices. However, there is almost unanimous agreement that change agents should come from within the local setting (Laverack and Labonte, 2000; Rosato *et al.*, 2008).

Social Access and the Health System

In the three delays model (Thaddeus and Maine, 1994), financial, geographical and social costs of seeking care emerge as important barriers to seeking maternal health services. The focus of this literature is primarily on individual characteristics of the women and their families – how the direct and indirect financial costs and difficulties of a poor transport infrastructure determine the calculus of seeking care. Far less attention has been given to how features of the health system may shape people's choices (Maine and Larsen, 2004). Even the first delay, the decision to seek care, is influenced by factors relating to the third delay. Doctors and other care providers in the nearest health facilities are often not there; health personnel demand bribes for tasks that are part of routine care; providers are abusive and treatment is unaffordable because the doctors prescribe expensive medications instead of generic drugs that might be available in the facilities (Jewkes *et al.*, 1998; Afsana, 2004). Yet the decision not to seek care is often regarded as the failure of the woman and her family to make the 'right' decision (Freedman *et al.*, 2005).

A health system is defined as 'all the activities whose primary purpose is to promote, restore or maintain health' (see Mavalankar and Sankara Raman, Chapter 6 this volume). The dominant discourse views them as mechanical structures that provide health care; tweaking one part of it will lead to changes in another part in a linear manner (Campbell and Graham, 2006; Bhutta *et al.*, 2008). Recent thinking challenges this approach and suggests that health systems are 'core social institutions, culturally embedded, politically contingent, and part of the very fabric of social and civic life' (Freedman, 2005). As complex socio-political institutions, health systems function at the interface between people and the power structures that shape their broader society. They therefore signal and reinforce societal values and norms and play a key role in people's experiences of power (Gilson, 2003; Freedman, 2005).

The commonly reported differential treatment of patients based on their perceived socio-economic status is but one example of how health systems may replicate societal norms and values. A growing body of research indicates that poverty is not just an individual state of lack of income or resources; it is relational and embedded within power hierarchies. The commonly reported neglect, abuse and exclusion within health-care systems may thus essentially be a reflection of the experience of being poor and socially marginalized in that society (Jewkes *et al.*, 1998; Afsana, 2004; Arps, 2009). In Nepal, utilization of emergency obstetric care varies by caste (Department of Community Medicine and Family Health, 2004). In Uganda, essential medicines that were supposed to be free

but were 'officially unavailable' could be arranged by staff if the patients had money to pay for them (McPake *et al.*, 1999). The fact that the odds of having a skilled birth attendant at delivery for women in the poorest quintile are 94% lower than for women in the highest wealth quintile provides empirical evidence of this discrimination (Ahmed *et al.*, 2010).

Societal values and norms are also signalled and enforced through the structuring, functioning and financing of the health system. Health systems in countries with the greatest burdens of maternal ill health are in profound crises (Freedman, 2005). Health providers routinely describe dehumanizing and demoralizing working conditions. Their salaries are well below living wages (Sundari, 1992; Mumtaz *et al.*, 2003). In Pakistan, 'status centric' norms and values of the wider feudal society translate into hierarchical management and abusive power structures within the health system. These values together with gender norms that devalue women's work for wages and their visibility in normatively male spaces (formal workplace) means that women health-care providers experienced a high degree of gendered harassment. This no doubt influenced the treatment of their patients, a fact that was recognized by the providers (Mumtaz *et al.*, 2003). It also led to a paucity of female health-care providers, a crucial determinant of demand in a context where gendered norms require women to be attended by only female health-care providers (Bhatti and Fikree, 2002; Mohana, 2005). In South Africa, nurses deployed violence against patients as a means of creating social distance to maintain their identity as middle class professionals that was distinct from their 'poor and dirty' patients (Jewkes *et al.*, 1998). Health system funding structures have traditionally benefited the better off more than the disadvantaged, especially for secondary and tertiary care, which accounts for most government health-care expenditures (Castro-Leal *et al.*, 2000; Afsana, 2004). In most South Asian countries, the health budget is 1–2% of the total compared to 30–50% for defence (Bhutta, 2002; Afsana, 2004). Corruption – under the table costs, pilfering of drugs and other resources – is common in a number of countries and is essentially a reflection of wider societal values (McPake *et al.*, 1999; Afsana, 2004).

It is reasonable to assume that these social barriers to health facilities are likely to dampen demand for maternity services. There is, however, a paucity of empirical evidence of a direct relationship between social barriers and demand. Varley (2010) shows how sectarian-based Shia–Sunni (two factions of Islam) tensions in northern Pakistan played a determinative role in Sunni women's choice of hospital to seek obstetric care. An interplay of Sunni women's religious, social and cultural identity, differential treatment in hospitals and the fact that their husbands or other male family members could not accompany them to hospitals located in Shia dominant areas, as Sunni men were the target of Shia attacks, greatly dampened demand for services (Varley, 2010).

There are few published interventions that are specifically aimed at reducing social barriers to health-care facilities. One such initiative was aimed at improving health-worker attitudes (Fonn and Xaba, 2001; Onyango-Ouma *et al.*, 2001). Tested in six African and one South American country, the intervention led to an improvement in patient experience with shorter waiting times, friendlier patient–provider interaction, more privacy and reduction in under-the-table payments (Onyango-Ouma *et al.*, 2001). However, the changes were not embraced or capitalized on by system-level management, resulting in minimal impact on health system functioning. There is also no evidence that demand for services increased. In Peru, a project sought to increase access, availability and utilization of emergency obstetric care (EmOC) services for approximately 48,000 pregnant women (Kayongo *et al.*, 2006). A rights-based framework was used to develop a client centred, culturally acceptable and non-discriminatory service delivery system. This included putting up signage in local languages to ease patient navigation of the system, use of special birthing chairs designed to match women's preferred birthing positions, increased privacy and encouraging presence of family members during childbirth. A number of interventions centred on improving staff management and their inter-personal relationships.

After 4 years, the use of emergency obstetric services for complications nearly trebled at 84% and numbers of maternal deaths dropped (Kayongo *et al.*, 2006). None the less, it is difficult to conclude the intervention increased demand as the total number of deliveries increased only by 117 (from 3002 at baseline to 3119 after 4 years).

According to Freedman (2005), social barriers to health care will only be reduced if health systems are structured within a human rights framework. Human rights activists have long understood the political arms of the state – prisons, judicial systems and police forces – to have the power to exclude, abuse and silence. But rarely have similar analyses been extended to health systems to understand how health systems, as a part of the very fabric of social and civic life, may be reproducing societal values of marginalization and exclusion of the poor. Within this framework, some areas that require further research include: ways of eliminating or at least reducing hierarchical power structures; developing gender sensitive policies to ensure retention of female staff and make their work experience more positive; and assessing possibilities of female-only staff in contexts where gendered norms require women to be attended by female health-care providers. Furthermore, strategies must be implemented in order to boost staff morale and improve salary structures and career paths. Some of these issues are complex and rooted in deep power structures that are not easy to alter. For example, poor staff attitudes and use of violence against patients are rooted in societal values that will not be altered overnight. The social distance between nurses and patients and hierarchical, abusive management structures rooted in feudal values will require more than lectures or sensitivity workshops; they require a paradigm shift in ways of thinking and doing 'power' (Jewkes *et al.*, 1998; Mumtaz *et al.*, 2003; Freedman, 2005).

The Influence of Gender

Contemporary maternal health scholarship recognizes the importance of gender ideologies, structures and processes in the creation of demand for maternity services (West and Zimmerman, 1987; Raikes *et al.*, 1992; Mumtaz and Salway, 2009). Largely the result of feminist critique, the discourse sees reproductive and maternal health as biomedical outcomes pertinent to the individual woman, although health outcomes and demand and supply of services are embedded in larger social, economic and political contexts. The International Conference on Population and Development in 1994 first endorsed this concept while MDG 3, the promotion of gender equality and empowerment (see McCaw-Binns and Hussein, Chapter 2 this volume), supported it further.

As a concept, gender has been interpreted in widely different ways in different disciplines; it is difficult to generalize and define it. In this chapter, gender is understood as a social construct, a set of criteria by which we all distinguish 'femaleness' from 'maleness', on top of the obvious biological differences (Doyal, 1998). Constituted variably in different historical and social contexts, gender has an astonishingly wide ranging and cross-cultural expression (DiStephano, 1990; Standing, 1991). One important consequence of gender is the justification of patterns of inequality between women and men. Gender systems are hierarchal and largely to the detriment of women. The gendered social order in most societies of the world creates structures, processes and relations that give men a greater capacity than women to mobilize a variety of human, social and material resources in pursuit of their own interests. For example, the gender order of most patriarchal societies constructs men as economic providers and women as dependants. This social norm is, in turn, the basis of a sexual division of labour, but it also ensures that employment opportunities, with its associated social and financial resources, favour men. Furthermore, this ideological construction is presented as biologically determined or divinely ordained, thus rationalizing the exclusion of women from main sources of power, privilege and prestige (Kabeer, 1994).

As stated previously, the gender order operates at three levels to affect demand for maternity services: in the production of

vulnerability to maternal ill health; in the creation of financial, social and geographical barriers; and in the creation of disadvantages once within the health-care system. Poor maternal health is first and foremost a reflection of the social and gendered norms that put women at high risk of reproductive health problems in the first place (Okojie, 1994). Most patriarchal societies are characterized by early and universal marriage. Early marriages, understood primarily as a strategy to control unmarried women's sexuality, lead to early initiation of sexual activity and early motherhood (Oppenheim Mason, 1987; Wall, 1998). The health problems of adolescent pregnancies are well documented: obstructed labour, obstetric fistulas, eclampsia and high maternal mortality rates (Wall, 1998). Preference for sons (a gendered preference) means women will continue to have children until they have the requisite number of sons. Not only are higher order pregnancies dangerous to women's health, but in Pakistan women who did not have a son were considered incomplete and not deserving of health resources (Winkvist and Akhtar, 2000). In contexts where the gender order is highly inequitable, women are more likely to suffer from poor nutrition and anaemia because limited food resources are directed to men (Winkvist and Akhtar, 2000). HIV infection, to which women are more susceptible because of unequal gender relations, makes women more susceptible to puerperal sepsis, postpartum haemorrhage and complications of Caesarean sections (Bicego *et al.*, 2002).

The same cluster of social and gender norms that operates to produce greater risks for women's reproductive health, such as women's social and economic dependency on men, their limited decision-making authority and restricted access to financial and material resources, also appears to be associated with lower demand for maternity services. Gendered norms in most patrilineal and patrilocal societies situate young women in a structurally weak position, possibly the weakest of any part of their lives. It is at this stage that women come closest to the ideal of feminine subordination and dependence (Winkvist and Akhtar, 2000). In diverse geographical societies, including Bangladesh,

Pakistan, Nepal, Nigeria and Senegal, the decision-making authority regarding a young woman's pregnancy and childbirth needs is located in older women and occasionally male family members who are older than the husband (Wall, 1998; Mumtaz and Salway, 2007; Brunson, 2010). In Pakistan, older women are considered *siyarni* (wise and experienced) and vested with the authority to make decisions around whether or not antenatal care should be sought, place of delivery and type of attendant at delivery, which are binding (Mumtaz and Salway, 2007). However, the older women's authority is characterized by a tension between a culturally ordained authority of the mother-in-law and the fact that this authority is subject to the quality of interpersonal relationships between the two women, which traditionally in the South Asian context often tends to be hostile rather than friendly. A hostile *saas–bahu* (mother-in-law/daughter-in-law) relationship can be a more important determinant of poor uptake of maternity services than any real or perceived need (Mumtaz, 2002; Allendorf, 2010). Moreover, gendered norms of masculinity in Nepal, Nigeria and Pakistan exclude men from their wife's pregnancy and childbirth experiences (Wall, 1998; Mumtaz and Salway, 2007). Consequently, most men have minimal knowledge of signs and symptoms of danger in pregnancy and subscribe to the notion of pregnancy as a normal physiological event (Mumtaz and Salway, 2007; Brunson, 2010). This has an important impact on reducing the demand for maternity services. In Bangladesh, if husbands were concerned about complications during childbirth, 33.6% of their wives were significantly more likely to seek care from a skilled birth attendant, compared to 21.7% of women whose husbands were not worried (Chowdhury et al., 2007).

One aspect of the gender order that has an impact on demand is the notion of women's seclusion (Mumtaz and Salway, 2005). Known as '*purdah*' in South Asia as well as a number of other societies, including the Hausa in northern Nigeria, women's seclusion is a key gendered institution that limits women's mobility, but it also consists of a complex set of rules that governs all interactions between women and men (Papanek, 1973; Donnan, 1988; Shaheed, 1989). Women's limited mobility has been postulated to be a major factor in affecting their ability to geographically access maternity services. It is not just the practical problem of traversing large geographical distances, but the social distance is equally, if not more, important in dampening demand (Mumtaz and Salway, 2005). In Pakistan, restrictions on women's movement are, normatively, even greater during pregnancy. Pregnancy, an obvious manifestation of sexual activity, is associated with '*sharam*' (shame). Pregnant women are expected to avoid public spaces, making travel to access antenatal care particularly problematic. Contravention of norms regarding such female seclusion carries heavy social costs that can include the overarching danger of loss of '*izzat*' (honour) by a simple accusation of sexual misdemeanour. Combined with poor transport infrastructure, these gendered values act as powerful deterrents to women's desire to travel, including travel to receive antenatal care (Mumtaz and Salway, 2005). When they do travel, women in Pakistan could possibly travel to health facilities only if somebody, preferably an older woman, accompanied them (Winkvist and Akhtar, 1997; Mumtaz and Salway, 2007). Accompanied mobility was also women's preferred behaviour, for it demonstrated that they were acting within the gender norm.

Another aspect of the gender order hypothesized to dampen demand for maternity care is women's limited access to financial resources. Since health care requires financial outlays, it is postulated that if women work for wages and have greater control over their incomes they will be able to direct some of this income towards health care for themselves. Empirical evidence in support of this assertion is limited. Research from Pakistan and Bangladesh suggests women's work for wages is poverty driven (Goetz and Gupta, 1996; Mumtaz, 2002). A majority of women who work for wages do so in low skilled, poorly paid conditions that do not alter their gendered position within their household or society, nor do their wages provide them with significant independent income. For some women, credit makes them worse off in terms of net income, while raising their hours of wage labour (Garikipati, 2008). Research from sub-Saharan Africa indicates that the higher the women's income, the lower men's contribution to the household and an increase in men's personal consumption (Van Staveren and Odebode, 2007). Women's work for wages and control over their income also had no bearing on women's use of antenatal care services in Pakistan (Mumtaz and Salway, 2007). Anthropological work from Pakistan shows that women's work for wages may, however, improve a household's overall socio-economic status, increasing the amount of disposable income that may possibly be directed for maternal health needs. There is also a large body of evidence demonstrating a link between household poverty and lower rates of utilization of antenatal care and skilled birth attendants (Mayhew *et al.*, 2008; NIPS, 2008). None the less, in Bangladesh, 37% of women in the upper household wealth quintile reported not using a skilled birth attendant, suggesting that factors other than financial resources remain an important determinant of demand for maternity services.

Most empirical analyses of the links between gender and demand for maternity services have focused on individual-level and household-level variables. While important, Price and Hawkins (2007) argue that a paradigm that focuses on the individual as the unit of analysis, detached from her/his social moorings, is a flawed paradigm in its understanding of human action. An emerging body of literature suggests that gendered structures of constraint acting at the societal level – the gendered norms, beliefs and practices around women and men's normative behaviours – can erode any bargaining power women may have acquired as a result of individual income, assets or education (Mumtaz and Salway, 2009; Mabsout and Van Staveren, 2010). West and Zimmerman (1987) explain the overwhelming influence of such societal institutions with the help of the concept of 'doing gender'. 'Doing gender' refers to the

often subtle social activities by women and men in their everyday life that express their femininity and masculinity, thereby reasserting their membership of their respective sex categories, female or male. It is in this context that women in Nepal refuse to go to a health facility during childbirth even if their marital families recommend them to do so (Brunson, 2010). This is done in order to demonstrate their fidelity to the gendered social script of being good wives and daughters-in-law and good women – women who are self-effacing and undemanding (Brunson, 2010).

Mullany *et al.* (2009) conducted a randomized controlled trial to assess the impact of husband's involvement in demand for postnatal care. The results showed that husband's involvement, as measured by his attendance at antenatal classes, led to higher maternal health knowledge levels and uptake of postpartum care, compared to women who attended the classes alone and those who did not attend the classes at all.

However, despite the recognition of the importance of gender around demand for health services in contemporary maternal health discourse, gender has received considerably less systematic attention than other aspects of maternal health, both in research and in policy (Horton, 2010).

Conclusion

Demand for maternity services is a multidimensional, highly textured issue. Consequently, there is no one universal solution that, if applied, will lead to an increase in demand for maternity care. The socioeconomic conditions, cultures, norms and values that affect demand for maternity care vary across different regions and therefore they require context-specific solutions (Campbell and Graham, 2006). Contemporary understandings of demand are beginning to provide insights on how to redress the balance between demand and supply, but solutions will need to have their foundations rooted in changing power structures that are not easy to alter.

References

Aboud, F. (2010) Virtual special issue introduction: Health behaviour change. *Social Science and Medicine* 71, 1897–1900.

Afsana, K. (2004) The tremendous cost of seeking hospital obstetric care in Bangladesh. *Reproductive Health Matters* 12(24), 171–180.

Ahmed, S., Creanga, A.A., Gillespie, D.G. and Tsui, A.O. (2010) Economic status, education and empowerment: Implications for maternal health service utilization in developing countries. *PLOS One* 5(6), doi: 10.1371/journal.pone.0011190.

Allendorf, K. (2010) The quality of family relationships and use of maternal health-care services in India. *Studies in Family Planning* 41(4), 263–276.

Anya, S.E., Hydara, A. and Jaiteh, L.E.S. (2008) Antenatal care in The Gambia: Missed opportunity for information, education and communication. *BMC Pregnancy and Childbirth* 8, 9.

Arjumand and Associates (2009) *PAIMAN Monitoring and Impact Evaluation for the Mass Media Products: Household survey report.* Islamabad, Pakistan.

Arps, S. (2009) Threats to safe motherhood in Honduran Miskito communities: Local perceptions of factors that contribute to maternal mortality. *Social Science and Medicine* 69, 579–586.

Asowa-Omorodion, F.I. (1997) Women's perceptions of the complications of pregnancy and childbirth in two Esan communities, Edo State, Nigeria. *Social Science and Medicine* 44(12), 1817–1824.

Atkinson, S.J. and Farias, M.F. (1995) Perceptions of risk during pregnancy amongst urban women in Northeast Brazil. *Social Science and Medicine* 41(11), 1577–1586.

Aubel, J., Touré, I. and Diagne, M. (2004) Senegalese grandmothers promote improved maternal nutrition practices: The guardians of tradition are not averse to change. *Social Science and Medicine* 59, 945–959.

Bazzano, A.N., Kirkwood, B., Tawiah-Agyemang, C., Osuwu-Agyei, S. and Adongo, P. (2008) Social costs of skilled attendance at birth in rural Ghana. *International Journal of Gynecology and Obstetrics* 102, 91–94.

Beninguisse, G. and De Brouwere, V. (2004) Tradition and modernity in Cameroon: The confrontation between social demand and biomedical logics of health services. *African Journal of Reproductive Health* 8(3), 152–175.

Berry, N. (2006) Kaqchikel midwives, home births, and emergency obstetric referrals in Guatemala: Contextualizing the choice to stay at home. *Social Science and Medicine* 62, 1958–1969.

Bhatti, L.I. and Fikree, F.F. (2002) Health-seeking behaviour of Karachi women with reproductive tract infections. *Social Science and Medicine* 54(1), 105–117.

Bhutta, Z.A. (2002) Thinking the unthinkable! Preparing for Armageddon in South Asia. *British Medical Journal* 15(324), 1405–1406.

Bhutta, Z.A., Ali, S., Cousens, S., Ali, T.M., Haider, B.A., Rizvi, A., Okong, P., Bhutta, S.Z. and Black, R.E. (2008) Interventions to address maternal, newborn, and child survival: What difference can integrated primary health care strategies make? *Lancet* 372, 972–989.

Bicego, G., Boerma, J.T. and Ronsmans, C. (2002) The effect of AIDS on maternal mortality in Malawi and Zimbabwe. *AIDS* 16(7), 1078–1081.

Brunson, J. (2010) Confronting maternal mortality, controlling birth in Nepal: The gendered politics of receiving biomedical care at birth. *Social Science and Medicine* 71, 1719–1727.

Campbell, O.M.R. and Graham, W.J. (2006) Strategies for reducing maternal mortality: Getting on with what works. *Lancet* 368, 1284–1299.

Castro-Leal, F., Dayton, J., Demery, L. and Mehra, K. (2000) Public spending on health care in Africa: Do the poor benefit? *Bulletin of the World Health Organization* 78(1), doi: 10.1590/S0042-96862000000100007.

Chapman, R.R. (2004) A nova vida: The commoditization of reproduction in Central Mozambique. *Medical Anthropology* 23, 229–261.

Chowdhury, R.I., Islam, M.A., Gulshan, J. and Chakraboty, M.S. (2007) Delivery complications and health-care-seeking behaviour: The Bangladesh Demographic Health Survey, 1999–2000. *Health and Social Care in the Community* 15(3), 254–264.

Department of Community Medicine and Family Health (2004) *Utilization of Emergency Obstetric Care in Selected Districts in Nepal.* Institute of Medicine, Kathmandu, Nepal.

DiStephano, C. (1990) Dilemmas of difference. In: Nicholson, L. (ed.) *Feminism/Postmodernism.* Routledge, London.

Donnan, H. (1988) *Marriage among Muslims: preference and choice in northern Pakistan.* Hindustan Publishing Corporation, Delhi.

Doyal, L. (1998) Gender and health technical paper. World Health Organization, Geneva. Available at: http://www.who.int/docstore/gender-and-health/pages/WHO%20-%20Gender%20and%20Health%20Technical%20Paper.htm (accessed 16 August 2011).

Dujardin, B., Clarysse, G., Criel, B., De Brouwere, V. and Wangata, N. (1995) The strategy of risk approach in antenatal care: Evaluation of the referral compliance. *Social Science and Medicine* 40(4), 529–535.

Dutta, M.J. (2010) The critical cultural turn in Health Communication: Reflexivity, solidarity and praxis. *Health Communication* 25(6), 534–539.

Ensor, T. and Cooper, S. (2004) Overcoming barriers to health service access: Influencing the demand side. *Health Policy and Planning* 19(2), 69–79.

Fonn, S. and Xaba, M. (2001) Health Workers for Change: Developing the initiative. *Health Policy and Planning* 16(S1), 13–18.

Freedman, L.P. (2005) Achieving the MDGs: Health systems as core social institutions. *Development* 48(1), 19–24.

Freedman, L.P., Waldman, R.J., de Pinho, H., Wirth, M.E., Chowdhury, A.M.R. and Rosenfield, A. (2005) *Who's Got the Power? Transforming health systems for women and children.* Earthscan, London.

Freire, P. (1970) *Pedagogy of the Oppressed.* Herder and Herder, New York.

Garikipati, S. (2008) The impact of lending to women on household vulnerability and women's empowerment: Evidence from India. *World Development* 36(12), 2620–2642.

Gilson, L. (2003) Trust and the development of health care as a social institution. *Social Science and Medicine* 56, 1453–1468.

Goetz, A.M. and Gupta, R.S. (1996) Who takes the credit? Gender, power, and control over loan use in rural credit programs in Bangladesh. *World Development* 24(1), 45–63.

Harrison, A. and Montgomery, E. (2001) Life histories, reproductive histories: Rural South African women's narratives of fertility, reproductive health and illness. *Journal of South African Studies* 27(2), 311–328.

Holford, J. (1995) Why social movements matter: Adult education theory, cognitive praxis, and the creation of knowledge. *Adult Education Quarterly* 45, 95–111.

Horton, R. (2010) Maternal mortality: Surprise, hope and urgent action. *Lancet* 375, 1581–1582.

Jewkes, R., Abrahams, N. and Mvo, Z. (1998) Why do nurses abuse patients? Reflections from South African obstetric services. *Social Science and Medicine* 47(11), 1781–1795.

Jewkes, R., Nduna, M., Levin, J., Dunkle, K., Khuzwayo, N., Koss, M., Puren, A., Wood, K. and Duvvury, N. (2006) A cluster randomized-controlled trial to determine the effectiveness of Stepping Stones in preventing HIV infections and promoting safer sexual behaviour amongst youth in the rural Eastern Cape, South Africa: Trial design, methods and baseline findings. *Tropical Medicine and International Health* 11(1), 3–16.

Kabeer, N. (1994) The structure of 'revealed' preference: Race, community and female labour supply in the London clothing industry. *Development and Change* 25(2), 307–331.

Kayongo, M., Esquiche, E., Luna, M.R., Frias, G., Vega-Centeno, L. and Bailey, P. (2006) Strengthening emergency obstetric care in Ayacucho, Peru. *International Journal of Gynecology and Obstetrics* 92, 299–307.

Khan, M., Matendo Mwaku, R., McClamroch, K., Kinkela, D.N. and Van Rie, A. (2005) Prenatal care in Kinshasa: Knowledge, beliefs, and barriers to timely care. *Cahiers d'Études et de Recherches Francophones/Santé* 15(2), 93–97.

Laverack, G. and Labonte, R. (2000) A planning framework for community empowerment goals within health promotion. *Health Policy and Planning* 15(3), 255–262.

Mabsout, R. and Van Staveren, I. (2010) Disentangling bargaining power from individual and household level institutions: Evidence on women's position in Ethiopia. *World Development* 38(5), 783–796.

Maine, D. and Larsen, M. (2004) *Blaming the Victim? The literature on utilization of health services.* Background paper prepared for the UN Millennium Project Task Force on Child Health and Maternal Health. United Nations, New York.

Manandhar, D.S., Osrin, D., Shrestha, B.P., Mesko, N., Morrison, J., Tumbahangphe, K.M., Tamang, S., Thappa, S., Shrestha, D., Thapa, B., Shrestha, J.R., Wade, A., Borghi, J., Standing, H., Manandhar, M., de La Costello, A.M. and members of the MIRA Makwanpur trial team (2004) Effect of a participatory intervention with women's groups on birth outcomes in Nepal: Cluster-randomized controlled trial. *Lancet* 364, 970–979.

Matsuyama, A. and Moji, K. (2008) Perception of bleeding as a danger sign during pregnancy, delivery, and the postpartum period in rural Nepal. *Qualitative Health Research* 18(2), 196–208.

Mayhew, M., Hansen, P.M., Peters, D., Edward, A., Singh, L.P., Dwivedi, V., Mashkoor, A. and Burnham, G. (2008) Determinants of skilled birth attendant utilization in Afghanistan: A cross-sectional study. *American Journal of Public Health* 98(10), 1849–1856.

McCray, T.M. (2004) An issue of culture: The effects of daily activities on prenatal care utilization patterns in rural South Africa. *Social Science and Medicine* 59, 1843–1855.

McPake, B., Asiimwe, D., Mwesigye, F., Ofumbi, M., Ortenblad, L., Streefland, P. and Turinade, A. (1999) Informal economic activities of public health workers in Uganda: Implications for quality and accessibility of care. *Social Science and Medicine* 49, 849–865.

Mezirow, J. (1991) *Transformative Dimensions of Adult Learning.* Jossey-Bass, San Francisco, California.

Minkler, M. (ed.) (1998) *Community Organizing and Community Building for Health.* Rutgers University Press, New Brunswick, New Jersey.

Mohana, N. (2005) Maternal mortality in Islamic and Arabic countries. *The Internet Journal of Health* 4(1).

Mullany, B.C., Lakhey, B., Shrestha, D., Hindin, M.J. and Becker, S. (2009) Impact of husband's participation in antenatal health education services on maternal health knowledge. *Journal of Nepal Medical Association* 48(173), 28–34.

Mumtaz, Z. (2002) Gender and reproductive health: a need for reconceptualization. Unpublished Doctoral Dissertation, University of London, London School of Hygiene and Tropical Medicine, London.

Mumtaz, Z. and Salway, S. (2005) 'I never go anywhere': Extricating the links between women's mobility and uptake of reproductive health services in Pakistan. *Social Science and Medicine* 60, 1751–1765.

Mumtaz, Z. and Salway, S. (2007) Gender, pregnancy and the uptake of antenatal services in Pakistan. *Sociology of Health and Illness* 29(1), 1–26.

Mumtaz, Z. and Salway, S. (2009) Understanding gendered influences on women's reproductive health in Pakistan: Moving beyond the autonomy paradigm. *Social Science and Medicine* 68, 1349–1356.

Mumtaz, Z., Salway, S., Waseem, M. and Umer, N. (2003) Gender-based barriers to primary health care provision in Pakistan: The experience of female providers. *Health Policy and Planning* 18(3), 261–269.

Myer, L. and Harrison, A. (2003) Why do women seek antenatal care late? Perspectives from rural South Africa. *The Journal of Midwifery and Women's Health* 48(4), 268–272.

NIPS National Institute of Population Studies (2008) Demographic and Health Survey 2006-07 Pakistan. Available at: http://www.measuredhs.com/pubs (accessed 16 August 2011).

Norris, M. (2009) Curing the blood and balancing life: Understanding, impact and health seeking behaviour following stroke in Central Aceh, Indonesia. Unpublished PhD thesis. Brunel University School of Health Sciences and Social Care, London.

Obermeyer, C. (2000) Risk, uncertainty, and agency: Culture and safe motherhood in Morocco. *Medical Anthropology: Cross-Cultural Studies in Health and Illness* 19(2), 173–201.

Okojie, C.E. (1994) Gender inequalities of health in the third world. *Social Science and Medicine* 39(9), 1237–1247.

Onyango-Ouma, W., Laisser, R., Mbilima, M., Araoye, M., Pittman, P., Agyepong, I., Zakari, M., Fonn, S., Tanner, M. and Vlassoff, C. (2001) An evaluation of Health Workers for Change in seven settings: A useful management and health system development tool. *Health Policy and Planning* 16(S1), 24–32.

Oppenheim Mason, K. (1987) The impact of women's social position on fertility in developing countries. *Sociological Forum* 2(4), 718–744.

Papanek, H. (1973) Purdah: Separate worlds and symbolic shelter. *Comparative Studies in Society and History* 15(3), 289–325.

Pigg, S.L. (1995) Acronyms and effacement: Traditional medical practitioners (TMP) in international development. *Social Science and Medicine* 41(1), 47–68.

Porter, G. (2002) Living in a walking world: Rural mobility and social equity issues in Sub-Saharan Africa. *World Development* 30(2), 285–300.

Price, N.L. and Hawkins, K. (2007) A conceptual framework for the social analysis of reproductive health. *Journal of Health, Population and Nutrition* 25(1), 24–36.

Raikes, A., Shoo, R. and Brabin, L. (1992) Gender-planned health services. *Annals of Tropical Medicine and Parasitology* 86(S1), 19–23.

Rosato, M., Laverack, G., Howard-Graham, L., Tripathy, P., Nair, N., Mwasamba, C., Azad, K., Morrison, J., Bhutta, Z., Perry, H., Rifkin, S. and Costello, A. (2008) Community participation: Lessons for maternal, newborn, and child health. *Lancet* 9642(372), 962–971.

Salam, S.S., Khan, M.A., Salahuddin, S., Choudhury, N., Nicholls, P. and Nasreen, H. (2009) Maternal, neonatal and child health in selected northern districts of Bangladesh: Findings from baseline survey 2008.

BRAC Research and Evaluation Division, Dhaka. Available at: http://www.bracresearch.org/reports/MNCH_baseline_2008_new.pdf (accessed 16 August 2011).

Shaheed, F. (1989) Women, Religion and Social Change in Pakistan: A Proposed Framework for Research – Draft. An International Centre for Ethnic Studies Project (1988–1989). Dossier 5-6, December 1988–May 1989. Women Living under Muslim Laws, London. Available at: http://www.wluml.org (accessed 11 August 2011).

Simawa, B., Theobold, S., Amakudzi, Y.P. and Tolhurst, R. (2005) Meeting millennium development goals 3 and 5. *British Medical Journal* 331, 708–709.

Smid, M., Campero, L., Cragin, L., Hernandez, D.G. and Walker, D. (2010) Bringing two worlds together: Exploring the integration of traditional midwives as Doulas in Mexican public hospitals. *Health Care for Women International* 31(6), 475–498.

Standing, H. (1991) *Dependence and Autonomy: Women's Employment and the Family in Calcutta.* Routledge, London.

Sundari, T.K. (1992) The untold story: How the health care systems in developing countries contribute to maternal mortality. *International Journal of Health Services* 22(3), 513–528.

Thaddeus, S. and Maine, D. (1994) Too far to walk: Maternal mortality in context. *Social Science and Medicine* 38(8), 1091–1110.

Thomas, P. (1994) Participatory development communication: Philosophical premises. In: White, S.A., Nair, K.S. and Ashcroft, J. (eds) *Participatory Communication: Working for change and development.* Sage, New Delhi, pp. 49–59.

Umoiyoho, A.J., Abasiattai, M. and Etuk, S.J. (2010) Perceptions among the Annang women of South-South Nigeria regarding antenatal healthcare information. *International Journal of Gynaecology and Obstetrics* 108(1), 77–78.

United Nations International Children's Emergency Fund (UNICEF) (2009) Maternal and newborn health. Available at: http://www.unicef.org/health/index_maternalhealth.html (accessed 13 April 2010).

Van Staveren, I. and Odebode, O. (2007) Gender norms as asymmetric institutions: A case study of Yoruba women in Nigeria. *Journal of Economic Issues* 61(4), 093–925.

Varley, E. (2010) Targeted doctors, missing patients: Obstetric health services and sectarian conflict in Northern Pakistan. *Social Science and Medicine* 70, 61–70.

Waisbord, S. (2001) *Family Tree Theories, Methodologies and Strategies in Development Communication: Convergences and Differences.* Rockefeller Foundation, New York.

Wall, L.L. (1998) Dead mothers and injured wives: The social context of maternal morbidity and mortality among the Hausa of Northern Nigeria. *Studies in Family Planning* 29(4), 341–359.

Weiss, M.G. (1988) Cultural models of diarrheal illness: Conceptual framework and review. *Social Science and Medicine* 27(1), 5–16.

West, C. and Zimmerman, D.H. (1987) Doing gender. *Gender and Society* 1(2), 125–151.

White, P.M. (2002) Crossing the river: Khmer women's perceptions of pregnancy and postpartum. *The Journal of Midwifery and Women's Health* 47(4), 239–246.

Whiteford, L.M. and Szelag, B.J. (2000) Access and utility as reflections of cultural constructions of pregnancy. *Primary Care Update for OBGYNS* 7(3), 98–104.

WHO (1997) *IEC Interventions for Reproductive Health: What do we know and where do we go?* Family Planning and Population Unit, Division for Reproductive Health, Geneva.

WHO (2010) Trends in maternal mortality: 1990 to 2008. Available at: http://www.who.int/reproductive-health/publications/monitoring/9789241500265/en/index.html (accessed 11 August 2011).

Wilkinson, S.E. and Callister, L.C. (2010) Giving birth: The voices of Ghanaian women. *Health Care for Women International* 31(3), 201–220.

Winkvist, A. and Akhtar, H.Z. (1997) Images of health and health care options among low income women in Punjab, Pakistan. *Social Science and Medicine* 45(10), 1483–1491.

Winkvist, A. and Akhtar, H.Z. (2000) God should give daughters to rich families only: Attitudes towards child-bearing among low income women in Punjab, Pakistan. *Social Science and Medicine* 51(1), 73–81.

Wreford, J. (2005) 'Sincedisa-we can help!' A literature review of current practice involving traditional African healers in biomedical HIV/AIDS interventions in South Africa. *Social Dynamics: A Journal of African Studies* 31(2), 90–117.

Yeha, N.A. and Dutta, M.J. (2010) Health, religion, and meaning: A culture-centered study of Druze women. *Qualitative Health Research* 20(6), 845–858.

13 Empowering the Community: BRAC's Approach in Bangladesh

Kaosar Afsana
BRAC, Dhaka, Bangladesh

Summary

- BRAC is an international development organization based in Bangladesh that is dedicated to alleviating poverty by empowering the poor.
- Empowerment can be viewed as a process of transformational change. Community participation is an empowering tool through which local communities can take action to resolve their health and development problems.
- A community empowerment framework of six elements, capacity building, human rights, organizational sustainability, institutional accountability, contribution and enabling environment (CHOICE), can be used as an underlying foundation to plan maternal health programmes.
- Strategies for community empowerment, which include building up skilled human resources for health and community resources, are meant to free the community from powerlessness, lack of choice and poverty.
- The community is a source of valuable resources, in particular, people with expertise and skills who can act as agents for change.
- The community health workers introduced by BRAC create demand, provide community services and are themselves members of the community whose capacity is being built to influence pathways to community empowerment.
- Other means to engage the community for social change include the establishment of structured community support networks and use of interactive communication methods that engage a broad and diverse base of people in maternity care interventions.

Introduction

Historically, there is no single, universally accepted definition of empowerment (World Bank, 2002; Rifkin, 2003). Its definition varies with context, culture, time and needs. It can apply to the individual's or the collective community's power and control over their resources, capacity, confidence and active participation (Rifkin, 2003).

Community participation has drawn attention for its cosmetic value (Chambers, 1995). It is deemed an essential element of community health and development because its approach is acceptable and desirable to donors and the international community. In paradigms for achieving health, community participation is envisaged as a magic bullet, elucidating the deep-rooted problems of health and political struggles (Rifkin, 1996).

©CAB International 2012. *Maternal and Perinatal Health in Developing Countries*
(eds J. Hussein, A. McCaw-Binns and R. Webber)

Empowerment and participation are sometimes used as reciprocal concepts, but empowerment is actually a process of transformational change whereas participation is not (Sen, 1997; Laverack and Wallerstein, 2001; Rifkin 2003). Community empowerment is a process where people can acquire more power in different forms (Labonté and Laverack, 2008). Community participation, on the other hand, is a tool through which local communities take responsibility for scrutinizing and resolving their health and development problems, thereby increasing their control over the factors that determine their wellbeing (WHO, 1989). Others see participation as the drive and motivation used to plan, design and implement a programme, pointing out that it is not necessarily a result of community consensus (Chambers, 1998; Morgan, 2001).

It is argued that 'struggles over power are not always destructive' but can create space for participation when it is accommodative and receptive to change for the betterment of people's lives (Chambers, 1998). Whatever the debates on definition and contextual meaning, it is widely agreed that community empowerment and participation are both essential. More importantly, empowerment is necessary to improve health care for long term sustainable development.

Amartya Sen (1999) views development as a process of expanding freedom. He points out that development requires removal of major sources of 'unfreedom', that is, poverty and the associated lack of economic opportunities, education and health care. In keeping with this broad perspective, the MDGs set out development to include poverty alleviation, education, health, gender equity and fostering of partnerships (UN General Assembly, 2000). Despite the strong messages and call for actions to translate the MDGs through holistic means, empowerment for health improvement is not yet fully integrated within conventional approaches.

Bangladesh has made remarkable achievements in improving maternal and child mortality and fertility, but still suffers a high burden of death and disease. This chapter describes how BRAC (http://www.brac.net) has been engaged in empowering the community for improving maternal and neonatal health.

BRAC is one of largest non-government organizations in the world and it originated in Bangladesh with a philosophy rooted in empowerment. It started in rural Bangladesh in 1972 as the 'Bangladesh Rehabilitation Assistance Committee', but its name has been changed simply to BRAC, which is no longer an acronym. A focus of BRAC is on women-initiated maternal, neonatal and child health interventions for disadvantaged populations in urban and rural areas. Experiences and evidence from BRAC's community-based interventions are described in this chapter to illustrate how community empowerment can be central to bringing about improvements in health.

About Bangladesh

Anindita is a young woman, born in a country that carries the insanity and melancholy of chronic deprivation of wealth, health and education. This is Bangladesh, once known as *sonar bangla* or Golden Bengal for its richness in wealth and productivity (Ahmed, 2001). However, ages of colonial and post-colonial exploitation, combined with the burden of a neo-colonial era, now place this nation state at a low rating of human development, ranking 129 out of 169 countries (Human Development Report, 2010). Sadly, Bangladesh also endures the unceasing agony of natural calamities due to its geographical location, affecting its growth and development (Ahmed, 2001). A multiplicity of factors complicates the situation, leading to a vicious cycle of poverty, malnutrition and ill health. As a result, the many 'Aninditas' and their children suffer the 'unfreedom' impinging on empowerment and health care (Sen, 1999).

The home of over 150 million people, Bangladesh is now the most densely populated country in the world. The per capita income is US$750 and increasing. Life expectancy is 65.1 years and the overall literacy rate is 56%, indicating that Bangladesh is slowly turning into a middle income country

(Bangladesh Bureau of Statistics, 2010). Yet 32% of the population live below the poverty line. MDG 4 is on track with the under-5 child mortality rate declining from 133 in 1990 to 65 per 1000 live births in 2007 (NIPORT, 2009). The MDG target for maternal mortality is also on track, with the maternal mortality ratio dropping from 574 to 194 per 100,000 live births since the 1990s (NIPORT, 2011). Nevertheless, the health system is not adequately responding to the demands of the increasing population, in spite of the existence of good and expanding infrastructure all over Bangladesh. Currently, 71% of pregnant women seek antenatal care, 77% of childbirths take place at home and 26% of births are attended by skilled personnel. Despite the stable economic growth, the country suffers from diverse disparity across wealth quintiles, geographical terrain, territoriality and culture (NIPORT, 2009). Understanding of birth, social and cultural norms, religion, education, poverty and access to functional health facilities pose challenges to effective use of maternal and newborn care (Afsana, 2005).

BRAC's Approach

As part of BRAC's approach to development, its health programmes are founded on a multi-sectoral platform. In a contribution to national efforts to achieve MDGs 4 and 5, BRAC launched its most recent maternal, newborn and child health programme in rural and urban areas of Bangladesh (IMNCS, 2010; Manoshi, 2010). Community empowerment and creating demand for maternal and newborn care are the prime components of the interventions, but, to fulfil the needs for health care, provision of services is equally vital and embedded within the approach.

A framework for community empowerment

It is critical to understand the pathways of community empowerment and how they influence behaviour change and practice for health. Laverack and Labonte (2000) framed approaches to community empowerment either as top down or bottom up. They stress the point that the programme design, regardless of content, is empowering when strategic and participatory planning processes are used – the principle being that choice enables people to improve their development and 'freedom' (Sen, 1999). Rifkin (2003) subsequently developed a framework for community empowerment called CHOICE – capacity building, human rights, organizational sustainability, institutional accountability, contribution and enabling environment. This framework captures the notion of empowerment relevant to a broad multi-sectoral perspective and matched BRAC's development ideology. Maternal health programme interventions were therefore based on consideration of the pathways leading to empowerment. BRAC begins with building up human resources for health at community level, then gradually moves towards developing capacity of women, men, families and communities. The ultimate objectives are to create awareness amongst the community of maternal and newborn health and act at both individual and collective levels to bring about change in people's practices.

Agents of change: community health workers

Given the shortages in the skilled health workforce and limitations of a low resource setting, the foundations of strengthening community participation and using community resources have resulted in the idea to develop and empower community health workers to extend health services to poor and underserved populations. Rebecca, Anowara and Monira are all BRAC's community health workers. These are the agents of change – women who are revolutionizing health behaviour and practices at community level. According to WHO (1989), community health workers are 'members of the communities where they work, selected by the communities, answerable to the communities for their activities, supported by the health system but not necessarily a part of its organization, and have shorter training than professional workers'. BRAC's community health workers are based in the community, selected by the community and meant to serve the community. *Shasthya Shebikas* are the first level frontline workers and *Shasthya Kormis* the second level frontline health workers. A third cadre of community health worker known as the Newborn Health Worker has recently been introduced. Within their targeted catchment areas, these workers enrol eligible populations to render maternal, newborn and under-5 child health services, make linkages with health facilities and social support services and engage community members in community development activities. These health workers are the community health resource and the 'change-makers' in rural areas of Bangladesh, engaged in empowering the community to improve health and create demand for health services.

Shasthya Shebikas act as the link to BRAC's Village Organization. The Village Organization is an existing community 'institution' comprising women members much involved in socio-economic empowerment and institutional building within their communities. The *Shasthya Shebika* is a member of the Village Organization selected according to a number of criteria. She should be married, preferably with reading and writing skills, aged 25–45 years, with the youngest child over 2 years old. The women should be willing to offer their time voluntarily and their selection has to be acceptable to other community members. *Shasthya Shebikas* work in neighbourhoods of 150 families, visiting seven or eight houses every day to cover all allocated households within a month. They provide simple preventive, promotive and curative services.

The second level frontline workers are the *Shasthya Kormis*. They were introduced as a result of lessons learned from past programmes and to meet demand. The *Shasthya Kormis* are educated women chosen from the local vicinity who are aged between 25 and 45 years, married, with at least 10 years' schooling. They should be willing to work in the community and their selection has to be acceptable to the community. They support

and supervise activities of ten *Shasthya Shebikas* each and five Newborn Health Workers, thus reaching 1500 families and covering populations of up to 7000 people. Their activities are overseen directly by BRAC staff, posted at local offices.

The Newborn Health Workers are a more recently introduced cadre of community health workers with similar characteristics to the *Shasthya Shebikas*. Their major focus is to provide physical and emotional support for birthing women and their newborn babies. They are trained to detect maternal complications, arrange the mothers' referral to hospitals and offer immediate newborn care. Having experience in attending birth, acceptability to the community and willingness to offer voluntary services are among the criteria for their selection.

Services provided

ANTENATAL CARE During household visits, the *Shasthya Shebikas* follow up couples of reproductive age and discuss their menstrual history and contraceptive use. Possible pregnancies are noted and communicated to the *Shasthya Kormis*, who confirm pregnancies with a pregnancy test. The confirmed pregnant women are registered and the *Shasthya Kormis* provide antenatal care for each pregnant woman every month. The antenatal check-up is provided jointly by the two health workers to include health education (danger signs, nutrition and hygiene), symptomatic detection of anaemia and oedema, measurement of blood pressure, abdominal examination, tetanus toxoid injections, provision of iron and folic acid tablets and birth planning and preparedness. The pregnant women are also encouraged to attend for comprehensive antenatal care in a health facility.

CHILDBIRTH When labour commences, the *Shasthya Shebika* and Newborn Health Worker are informed, so they can assist in delivery. Both have responsibility for attending the mother and baby during the birth. The mother is given a misoprostol tablet for prevention of postpartum haemorrhage and Vitamin A is provided. Advice on special care for low birth-weight babies is shared. If complications have arisen in the mother or baby, referral to health facilities is organized.

POSTNATAL CARE   The community health workers conduct postnatal visits to mothers and newborn babies, giving special attention to low birth weight and asphyxiated babies. As soon as the baby is born, the *Shasthya Kormis* are informed so that they can conduct a postnatal visit within 24 h of birth. The *Shasthya Kormis* subsequently offer visits on the 7th and 28th day to counsel on nutrition, hygiene and family planning, encourage exclusive breastfeeding and ensure special attention is given to low birth-weight babies and to mothers. In addition, the *Shasthya Shebikas* visit low birth-weight babies every alternate day from 0 to 28 days. Referral is organized if necessary. In the event that the mother has puerperal sepsis and refuses to seek treatment in a health facility, the *Shasthya Kormis* can initiate treatment following a protocol.

Training for competency

The competency and skills of community health workers are gradually built up within the BRAC programme, with the intent of extending improved quality of health services to the grass-roots level. The foundation training for *Shasthya Shebikas* and *Shasthya Kormis* began as 3 weeks' residential training, followed by continuing education for 2 years. The basic training is modular, allowing the training to be tailored alongside their community work. The *Shasthya Kormis* also receive training on health communication and supervision. The *Shasthya Shebikas* and *Shasthya Kormis* are provided refresher training every month. The Newborn Health Workers receive an initial six-day training followed by refresher training every alternate month.

As part of the continued capacity building, *Shasthya Kormis* with experience can be selected for further training to become government-accredited skilled birth attendants. For this, they attend designated training institutes and hospitals for 6 months.

Performance-based incentives

To enhance motivation, continue with the community activities, attract more capable women and compensate for opportunity costs, a performace-based incentive package has been introduced for the community health workers (Alam *et al.*, 2009; Afsana, 2011; Kinoti, 2011). The *Shasthya Shebikas* earn small amounts of money based on their activities of diagnosing and treating basic ailments and selling of health commodities. *Shasthya Shebikas* and Newborn Health Workers also receive performance-based incentives. The *Shasthya Kormis* are given a modest monthly honorarium, as well as receiving incentives for their performance. The incentives provided for the community health workers are summarized in Table 13.1.

Engaging the community for social change

Community participation and voice in health care are crucial for strengthening and enhancing the accountability of the health system and for improving access of poor and disadvantaged populations to quality health services, so engaging the community should be an essential ingredient to acheiving positive health outcomes (Rifkin, 2003). This concept is not new – for example, people's right to participate individually or collectively in planning and implementing health programmes was put forward in the Alma-Ata Declaration more than three decades ago (WHO, 1978). By developing longstanding partnerships within communities, BRAC has engaged people in community actvities and created public demand for their health-care needs.

Local health committees

A community support network locally known as the maternal, neonatal and child health committee addresses issues particularly to meet the matenity care needs of the poor living in the locality. BRAC personnel hold discussions with the local community first before forming the committee, to explore issues of engagement and participation. A general meeting is then organized, where the committee is formed. The committee usually comprises respected community members who are locally endorsed – but also considers representation of gender, adolescents and marginalized populations. The committee has a president (usually the female member of the local government council) and a secretary (usually the *Shasthya Kormi*). The committee has a broad mandate, which institutionalizes the importance of maternity care within the community and links pregnancy and childbirth with issues of rights and accountability (Box 13.1).

Health communications

Information on maternal and neonatal care is given to mothers, family members and the community through interactive communications such as performance of street folk music and theatre, broadcasting on radio and television, group discussions and advocacy workshops. Folk music shows produced by local folk groups are performed at village level and these are organized to reach the same audience twice a year. Television and radio are used periodically to air information about danger signs. The community health workers use pictorial messages during their service provision activities. For broader dissemination, posters, stickers and billboards are also used. Meetings with various stakeholders are conducted to raise their awareness and motivate them to take pro-active roles in maternity-related activities. These meetings bring local government council, government health workers and local influential people together to discuss interventions and expectations for improved service delivery.

Table 13.1. Incentives for community health workers, in Bangladeshi taka, 2010.[a]

Task-based indicator	Shasthya Shebika	Newborn Health Worker	Shasthya Kormi
Pregnancy identification in first trimester	30	–	–
Antenatal care 80%	–	–	100
Delivery attendance	100	100	–
Newborn care just after delivery	25	–	–
Birth asphyxia management	50	–	–
Referral of complications	50	50	–
Birth weight measure	30	–	–
First postnatal visit 80%	–	–	200
Second postnatal visit 80%	–	–	100
Postpartum contraception	20	–	–
Neonatal sepsis diagnosis and management	50	–	–

[a]Exchange rate 2011: US$1 = 75 taka.

Box 13.1. Functions of the BRAC maternal, neonatal and child health committee.

- Maintain an environment suitable for the *Shasthya Shebika*, Newborn Health Worker and *Shasthya Kormi* to work.
- Remain aware of maternal, newborn and child health in their areas, including identification and follow up of women who are pregnant, including those requiring hospital delivery or who have experienced complications.
- Facilitate referral of complications to hospitals.
- Manage community financing activities.
- Monitor activities of community health workers.
- Audit pregnancy, births, complications and deaths.
- Raise issues related to hospital care in relevant meetings.
- Stop malpractice and misuse of drugs in the community (for example, inappropriate use of uterotonics).

Safe motherhood day is celebrated each year with activities such as workshops, blood donation camps and other public events. A wide range of participants is engaged – local government administrative officials, health and family planning professionals, non-government organizations, media, religious leaders and social workers – to reinforce and create constant awareness about maternity services and status. Blood donation activities involve employees in the public and private sectors, students, scouts, community members and others. BRAC organizes blood donation camps with Shandhani and Friends (a charitable Medical Students Association), stores collected blood in its blood banks and arranges timely supply of fresh blood in acute maternal emergencies.

Community services

In addition to the services provided by the community health workers, BRAC has established a referral system that connects the community with the health facilities. Birth plans are maintained in a mother-baby card, which contains information on a pre-identified vehicle for transport, a named birth companion and mobile phone numbers of the responsible *Shasthya Kormi* and a responsible BRAC staff member. Husbands are asked to be prepared for potential unexpected problems and to make advance decisions for such events in case they are not immediately available. Memoranda of understanding with local owners of motor vehicles are made to ease the

process of transfer to hospitals. A designated BRAC staff member, known as the Referral Programme Organizer, is specifically placed in hospitals to support the referred patients and assist women and their families in communicating with doctors and nurses. In case of emergencies, women, families and the community health workers can contact BRAC personnel and ambulance services by calling a special number for urgent transfer to hospital. In remote communities, pre-selected referral pick-up spots have been identified which are close to households and, at the same time, easily accessible to emergency vehicles.

Effects of Interventions

In 2005, the BRAC maternal, neonatal and child health programme commenced in Nilphamari, a northern district of Bangladesh with a population of 1.5 million. Here, each intervention was gradually introduced and the experience used to learn lessons and adapt activities to fit the context. Key effects of the programme are summarized in Box 13.2. Funding from the Australian, UK and Dutch governments and collaboration with UNICEF and the government of Bangladesh allowed a phased expansion of programme activities into nine more districts by 2008, to reach a current figure of 19 million people.

Despite the positive trend observed in maternal mortality, the reduction of neonatal mortality rate has been slow, declining in

---

Box 13.2. Key effects of BRAC's maternal, neonatal and child health programme, Nilphamari district.

- The maternal mortality in the district (through collection of data from a census of the district population) dropped from 256 per 100,000 live births in 2007 to 156 in 2010, representing a decline of 39% with an annual reduction rate of 13%. This can be compared with the national reduction of maternal mortality ratio of 40% in 9 years (an annual reduction of 4.2%).
- Over 93% of women now receive more than four antenatal visits and 28% were referred to hospitals for maternal health problems.
- Of 38,000 total births, 75% occurred at home, but 87% of them were attended by the community health workers. All received misoprostol tablets for prevention of postpartum haemorrhage.
- 87% of women receive more than three postnatal visits.
- Referral of maternal complications to hospitals has increased deliveries in hospitals from 13.5% in 2007 to 25% in 2010.
- A group of community health workers is being equipped with a skill mix that addresses the crisis of human resources for health in rural areas.

Nilphamari from 31 in 2008 to 26 per 1000 live births in 2010. The national neonatal mortality rate is 37 per 1000 livebirths. Although deliveries with health professionals and in hospitals remained low, a proportion of this reduction in maternal mortality may be explained by the use of misoprostol: 87% of home births were provided misoprostol tablets by community health workers to prevent postpartum haemorrhage. On the other hand, it is suspected that management of birth asphyxia in the community is not optimal and referral levels to hospitals are low. This and the lack of trained hospital personnel and facilities to manage sick newborns in hospitals may be reasons for the slow progress in reducing neonatal mortality.

Capacity Building and Participation

The emancipation of women is regarded as an integral aspect of social development (Dereze and Sen, 1995). In the total of ten current intervention districts, 48,125 female community health workers have been trained to empower the community by raising awareness and providing maternity services. Frequent contact with mothers at domiciliary level, offering them continuity of care and providing women-centric services, has made women receptive to the community health worker. The community health workers' role in service provision is central, and this function highlights the observation that community health workers engaged only in demand creation for services cannot have credibility unless a strong connection with health service provision exists. By creating demand and providing services together, the community health worker is uniquely empowered to act effectively as an agent who brings about changes in behaviour and practice of women and their families. Community trust and confidence in the skills of the community health workers are motivating – bringing a sense of pride in their work and raising their social status. The impetus to bring about changes in women's behaviour and practices by empowering and engaging community health workers has led to women themselves being

changed and participating in influencing the pathways to empowerment.

Nevertheless, it is acknowledged that behaviour change is a gradual process. Maternity-related problems are likely to be only an occasional event in a person's life, so changing behaviour and practices cannot be expected to happen quickly. Interventions will be needed at individual and collective levels and indeed support across generations may be necessary.

A challenge in building capacity in a scaled up intervention is related to issues of quality. In this programme, recruitment and training of community health workers are conducted side by side. Once the training is completed, the community health workers immediately start working. Some supervisors are new and may only be recently trained. As standards are influenced by experience, competency and supervisory skills, quality may fluctuate until those skills are sufficient. Continuous refresher training and supportive supervision are provided to overcome such obstacles.

Voice and Accountability

Community empowerment is a transformational process which involves multiple stakeholders, whose engagement may vary. For the community health workers who are directly involved in the programme, the meaning and objectives of the programme are largely clearer to them, resulting in proactive participation. Although the contribution of other groups such as the community support network cannot be overlooked, their participation is less proactive. On the other hand, their role in referral of maternal complications is not negligible. Many members influenced family members, provided monetary support and informed hospital doctors about referred cases. However, a study assessing the effect of the BRAC programme found that many members of the committee were not aware of their responsibilities, nor did they regularly participate in meetings (Rashid et al., 2010). It is understood that the roles of the committees are insufficiently defined and not clear to the members. More importantly, the process of their inclusion has followed a top-down approach. Better understanding of the means through which ownership can be created and further efforts to enhance the participation of the community support network are required.

The Right to an Enabling Environment

To effectively improve health outcomes, the creation of demand for services and the provision of basic services in the community have to be paralleled by improvements in the availability, accessibility and quality of services in health facilities. In BRAC's programme, women are referred to public health facilities maintained by the government, with UNICEF providing support to enhance the quality of these services. The partnership between these organizations allows linkages between the various levels of the health system from community to referral level. Although programme assessments have revealed that gains have been made in improving facility-based care, as in many other developing country settings, impediments remain. They include absent health personnel, fear of the hospital environment and costs, and lack of 24 h emergency services in sub-district and district hospitals. Scarcity of medicines and blood is also experienced and services can be affected by poor interpersonal relationships and conflicting interests between health personnel in hospitals.

Sustainability

Various problems related to sustainability remain. Even though communities can be observed to have begun adopting recommended practices after 5 years in Nilphamari, long term interventions are required to instil behavioural change. Finding enough women who fit the criteria necessary to fulfil the designated functions of the community health worker is difficult, and the dropout rate is sometimes high. The community health workers may be offered better job opportunities as their incentive package is not priced at market rates. Strategies to overcome some of these barriers are being considered and include reassessments of the incentives, introducing career structures within the overall health system and providing other inducements such as advanced training and flexible working conditions.

Conclusion

Community empowerment is a process of transformational change. Strategies to achieve this change include building up skilled health human resources and employing community resources to free the community from the 'unfreedom' of powerlessness, lack of choice and poverty (Sen, 1999). The experiences of the large scaled up programme described in this chapter illustrate how various interventions, grounded in the priniciples of CHOICE – capacity building, human rights, organizational sustainability, institutional accountability, contribution and enabling environment (Rifkin, 2003) – can work together to change demand, behaviours and health outcomes in women and children.

The approach of empowerment described in this chapter has elements of both top down and bottom up approaches, yet engagement of the community basically happens at the grass roots. The argument in support of this mixed model is that an external driving force is a necessity to catalyse development and remove 'unfreedom', especially in developing country settings where chronic deprivation of health, wealth and literacy requires an accelerated form of freedom from this oppression. The question may be raised in this context as to whether the desired change can be sustained. To do so, unceasing efforts to create demand with concurrent provision of quality services to meet the needs of the community are imperative. Strategies for community empowerment should remain responsive to the needs of the community health workers, the community support network and, most importantly, women and the community beneficiaries.

References

Afsana, K. (2005) *Disciplining Birth. Power, Knowledge and Childbirth Practices in Bangladesh*. The University Press Limited, Bangladesh.

Afsana, K. (2011) Scaling up of BRAC's Maternal, Neonatal and Child Health Interventions in Bangladesh. In: Cash, R., Chowdhury, A.M.R., Smith, G.B. and Ahmed, F. (eds) *From One to Many: Scaling Health Programs in Low Income Countries*. The University Press Limited, Dhaka.

Ahmed, R. (2001) The emergence of the Bengal Muslims. In: Ahmed, R. (ed.) *Understanding Bengal Muslims. Interpretative essays*. The University Press Limited, Dhaka, pp. 1–25.

Alam, K., Oliveras, E. and Tasneem, S. (2009) *Retention of Female Volunteer Community Health Worker: A Case-Control Study in the Urban Slums of Dhaka*. Manoshi Working Paper 08. ICDDR,B and BRAC, Dhaka.

Bangladesh Bureau of Statistics (2010) *Statistical Yearbook of Bangladesh 2010*. Ministry of Planning, Government of the People's Republic of Bangladesh, Dhaka.

Chambers, R. (1995) Paradigms shifts and the practice of participatory research and development. In: Nelson, N. and Wrights, S. (eds) *Power and Participatory Development: Theory and practice*. Intermediate Technology Publications, London, pp. 30–42.

Chambers, R. (1998) Foreword. In: Guijt, I. and Shah, M.K. (eds) *The Myth of Community: Gender issues in participatory development: Theory and practice*. Intermediate Technology Publications, London, pp. xvii–xx.

Dereze, J. and Sen, A. (1995) *India: Economic Development and Social Opportunity*. Oxford University Press, New York, 178 pp.

Human Development Report (2010) *The Real Wealth of Nations: Pathways to Human Development, 20th Anniversary Edition*. UNDP, Palgrave Macmillan, New York.

IMNCS (2010) *Annual Report Improving Maternal, Neonatal and Child Health Survival. A Partnership Approach to Achieve MDGs 4 and 5*. BRAC, Dhaka.

Kinoti, S. (2011) Effects of Performance Based Financing on Maternal Care in Developing Countries: Access, Utilization, Coverage, and Health Impact. USAID. Available at: http://www.tractionproject.org/sites/default/files/upload/Reports/Effects (accessed 20 July 2011).

Labonté, R. and Laverack, G. (2008) *Health Promotion in Action: From local to global empowerment*. Palgrave Macmillan, London.

Laverack, G. and Labonte, R. (2000) A planning framework for community empowerment goals within health promotion. *Health Policy and Planning* 15(3), 255–262.

Laverack, G. and Wallerstein, N. (2001) Measuring community empowerment: a fresh look at organisational domains. *Health Promotion International* 16, 179–185.

Manoshi (2010) *Annual Report Community Health Solutions in Urban Slums*. BRAC, Dhaka.

Morgan, M.M. (2001) Community participation in health: Perpetual allure, persistent challenge. *Health Policy and Planning* 16(3), 221–230.

National Institute of Population Research and Training (NIPORT) (2009) *Bangladesh Demographic and Health Survey 2007*. Mitra and Associates and Macro International, Dhaka, Bangladesh and Calverton, Maryland.

National Institute for Population Research and Training (NIPORT) (2011) *Bangladesh Maternal Mortality and Health Care Survey 2010. Preliminary Results*. Measure Evaluation, UNC-CH, USA and ICDDR,B, Dhaka.

Rashid, S., Leppard, M., Nasreen, H.E. and Akhter, M. (2010) Voice and accountability: the role of maternal, neonatal and child health committee, working paper. BRAC Research and Evaluation Division, BRAC, Dhaka.

Rifkin, S.B. (1996) Paradigms lost: toward a new understanding of community participation in health programmes. *Acta Tropical* 61, 79–92.

Rifkin, S.B. (2003) A Framework Linking Community Empowerment and Health Equity: It Is a Matter of CHOICE. *Journal of Health, Population and Nutrition* 21(3),168–180.

Sen, A. (1999) *Development as Freedom*, 1st edn. Knopf, New York, 366 pp.

Sen, G. (1997) Empowerment as an approach to poverty. Background paper to the Human Development Report, 1997. Available at: http://www.hsph.harvard.edu/Organizations/healthnet/Hupapers/97_or.pdf (accessed 20 July 2011).

UN General Assembly (2000) United Nations Millennium Declaration, Millennium Summit, New York. Available at: http://www.un.org/millennium/declaration/ares552e.pdf (accessed 20 July 2011).

WHO (1978) *Primary Health Care: Report of the International Conference on Primary Health Care.* World Health Organization, Geneva, 79 pp.

WHO (1989) Strengthening the performance of community health workers in primary health care. Report of a WHO Study Group. *Technical Report Series, No. 780.* World Health Organization, Geneva.

World Bank (2002) Empowerment and poverty: a sources book (draft). Available at: http://www.worldbank.org/poverty/empowerment/index.htm (accessed 20 July 2011).

14   Quality of Care

Endang Achadi,[1] Emma Pitchforth[2] and Julia Hussein[3]
*[1]University of Indonesia, West Java, Indonesia; [2]RAND Europe, Cambridge, UK;
[3]University of Aberdeen, Scotland, UK*

Summary

- Definitions of quality of care vary, but all recognize the multidimensional nature of quality. Choosing a suitable quality of care framework should be driven by the purpose of assessing quality of care, the setting in which quality improvements are planned, the nature of the interventions and the target beneficiaries.
- Improving quality of care cannot be isolated from the function of the health system.
- Quality aspects permeate through all levels of the health system and at all stages of the reproductive life cycle, thus encompassing the concept of the continuum of care.
- Failure to maintain this 'continuum of quality' at any stage will result in death or severe disability, a failure occurring in too many maternity care services in countries where levels of maternal mortality are still high.
- Certain times of pregnancy are particularly risky. Most maternal and newborn deaths occur during childbirth and in the first few days after delivery. To save lives, quality of care during childbirth and in the immediate postpartum period is crucial, as well as attention to high quality care during complications.
- The person who provides maternity care, her/his knowledge, attitudes and practice are essential aspects of quality, but ensuring that a 'skilled attendant at delivery' is present is not a sufficient factor to ensure good quality care.
- The place where women seek maternity care (whether at home, en route or in a health facility) influences quality, and consideration of these different settings affects how quality is assessed.
- Studies indicate that quality of maternity care is poor in many developing country settings. Quality improvement strategies that are widely recommended include interactive educational events, reminders, use of opinion leaders and mass media to change provider practice, audit and combinations of interventions.

Introduction

The provision of good quality care cannot be isolated from the function of the overall health system. It is well recognized that three types of delays in receiving obstetric care contribute significantly to the prognosis of a woman's survival (Thaddeus and Maine, 1994). The first delay comprises recognition of complications and making decisions to refer. The second delay occurs in reaching emergency care. The third delay is the delay experienced in receiving appropriate treatment for an obstetric complication. To overcome these delays, pregnant women must have access to obstetric care including four key elements, namely: a skilled attendant at delivery; emergency care in case of a complication; a referral system to ensure that those women who experience complications can reach life-saving emergency obstetric care (EmOC) in time; and finally, having reached a point of care, the service provided should be of the highest quality (Chowdhury and Rosenfield, 2004). All of these elements have links to the various health system components such as the workforce, availability of equipment and supplies or health services such as clinic and hospital infrastructure and referral systems.

This chapter highlights the importance of focusing on improving quality of care during childbirth as part of national and international efforts to improve maternal and neonatal outcomes. Various concepts and definitions for quality of care are discussed, as knowledge of these different frameworks may help in the selection of the most appropriate ones to use in the implementation of maternal health programmes and interventions. Quality of care around the time of childbirth is a focus of the next section, as this is a time of particular risk for achievement of maternal and perinatal health goals. Quality improvement interventions in obstetric care are reviewed in the final part of this chapter.

Definitions and Frameworks

There is no universally accepted definition of quality of care, but it is recognized that any definition needs to account for the composite nature of quality and the purpose for which the definition is used (van den Broek and Graham, 2009; Creel *et al.*, 2011). Several frameworks have been recommended in maternity care and related reproductive health fields. Bruce (1990) addressed six elements of quality for family planning: choice of method (for example, inventory and control system, logistics, times of service); technical competence of the provider; contraceptive method and delivery of key messages to clients; interpersonal interaction between client and provider; follow-up care; and appropriateness of services. Emphasis has been placed on the internal enabling environment with policy, leadership, core values and resources as structures upon which quality objectives should be based (Silimperi *et al.*, 2002). Other core elements that quality definitions encompass include follow-up care, continuity of care, gender interactions, formalized standards of care and access (Bertrand *et al.*, 1995; Vlassoff *et al.*, 1996; Brown *et al.*, 2000; Creel *et al.*, 2011).

The concept of quality of care can be described for an individual or for populations, at community and household level, in health facilities and for national or programme use, depending on the context and purpose. From the perspective of community-level maternity care, factors related to knowledge, accessibility and community readiness to respond in the event of emergencies are likely to be important. Quality in health facilities is usually defined based on certain clinical standards, and also in terms of user acceptability and meeting client needs. For national and programme use, quality concepts can be put into two main categories: standards for performance of services and standards for qualification to provide services, for example through certification, licensure or other professional regulation (USAID, 2007).

At individual level, quality can be viewed from the basis of whether individuals can access the health structures and processes of care which they need; and whether the care received is effective. A definition of quality of care for populations has been suggested as 'the ability of the community to access effective care on an efficient and equitable basis for the optimisation of health benefit/wellbeing for the whole population' (Campbell *et al.*, 2000). Campbell's definition highlights two principal dimensions of quality of care: access and effectiveness. Within these dimensions, two key components of effectiveness are differentiated: effectiveness of clinical care and effectiveness of interpersonal care. These various components of access, clinical effectiveness and interpersonal care are interrelated. The quality of interpersonal care in health facilities may affect women's willingness to access and use the facility. It is also an essential factor that motivates women to seek professional care when they choose to deliver in their homes. The effectiveness of clinical care depends on the application of knowledge, which may be evidence based (Sackett *et al.*, 1996) or widely accepted as legitimate (Donabedian, 1990).

Donabedian's 'Structure-process-outcome' framework (Donabedian, 1966) has withstood the test of time, being influential as a quality concept for over four decades. Structure refers to organizational factors that define the health system under which care is provided. Process involves the interactions between users and health-care providers and can be thought of as the actual delivery and receipt of care. Outcomes refer to the consequences of care, commonly health outcomes (such as maternal death) or satisfaction. More recently, the Institute of Medicine's quality framework has become influential in developed and developing countries. The framework uses a systems perspective and the definition of quality is deliberately broad so that it can encompass all elements and levels of care. Its underlying premise is that, if a health-care system achieves major gains in relation to six dimensions (safe, effective, patient-centred, timely, efficient and equitable), then the system will be far better at meeting users' needs. In turn, such a system would also benefit health-care providers, who experience satisfaction from giving care that is more reliable, more responsive to patients and more coordinated in nature (IOM, 2001).

As attention is increasingly brought to quality improvements in developing countries, the elements of the various approaches have been adopted within global development initiatives (Box 14.1).

Emerging from the broader frameworks of quality discussed above, paradigms specific to maternity care in developing countries have resulted. In a review of the various definitions of quality, it was concluded that high quality maternity services necessitated all the following criteria (Pittroff and Campbell, 2000):

- A minimum level of care for all pregnant women and their newborn babies.
- A higher level of care for those who need it.
- Care provision with the best possible medical outcome.
- Satisfaction of women and their families and providers with care provided.
- Maintenance of managerial and financial performance.
- Development of existing services to raise the standards of care.

Hulton *et al.* (2000) proposed two distinct streams of quality in maternity care: the provision of care and the experience of care. Unsurprisingly, the provision of care stream contains elements akin to those of the building blocks of the health system (see Mavalankar and Sankara Raman, Chapter 6 this volume), including human and physical resources, technologies and information and referral systems. The facets included in the 'experience of care' category aid in highlighting women's perspectives, choices and exposure

---

Box 14.1. Nine dimensions of quality of care from a health systems perspective (USAID, 2007).

USAID sets out nine important dimensions of quality important to a health-care delivery system's stakeholders (service users, communities, providers, managers and payers). The nine dimensions are:

- The compliance of performance with technical standards.
- Access to services in terms of geographical, economic, social, organizational or linguistic barriers to services.
- Effectiveness of care and the degree to which desired results or outcomes are achieved.
- Efficiency of service delivery, i.e. the appropriate use of resources to produce effective services.
- Effective interpersonal relations.
- Continuity of services.
- Safety – the degree to which the risks of injury, infection or other harmful side effects are minimized.
- Physical infrastructure and comfort.
- Client choice.

to quality-related factors. Another framework, used to assess quality of delivery care provided by Indonesian midwives in the community, presents quality as the interaction between the user and the health service (D'Ambruoso *et al.*, 2009).

The concept of quality encompasses that of 'skilled care' or 'skilled attendance' at delivery, defined as the 'process by which a woman is provided with adequate care during labour, delivery and the postpartum period' (Family Care International, 2000). Various frameworks are available to describe skilled care (Graham *et al.*, 2001; Adegoke *et al.*, 2011). The term 'skilled attendance' (the process) should be distinguished from 'skilled attendant' (the person) defined as 'an accredited health professional – such as a midwife, doctor or nurse – who has been educated and trained to proficiency in the skills needed to manage normal (uncomplicated) pregnancies, childbirth and the immediate postnatal period, and in the identification, management and referral of complications in women and newborns' (WHO, 2004a).

Overall, the frameworks available are complementary and contain similar elements. They lead to the conclusion that it is imperative that providers have sufficient skills to provide clinical care, with an approach that is humane and interpersonal. The care can be provided in the community or in a health facility, but the policies, regulations and physical environment should be conducive for the provision of adequate care. When referral from household and primary health facilities to higher level facilities is needed, standards of care pertinent to each level should be met. It should be noted that some frameworks of quality have focused on the risky period around childbirth and the immediate days after delivery (D'Ambruoso *et al.*, 2009) while others cover maternity care more broadly (Hulton *et al.*, 2000; Pittroff and Campbell, 2000). It can thus be seen that concepts of quality are indeed multicomponent and multifaceted and deal with the various elements within the idea of the 'continuum of care' with its two dimensions of place (different levels of the health system, from household to facility and with referral linking them) and time (comprising the reproductive life cycle from before pregnancy, through to pregnancy and after, including the neonate, infant and child) (PMNCH, 2011).

The Care Provider: a Skilled Attendant

It is widely accepted that a skilled attendant present during childbirth reduces the risk of maternal mortality (WHO, 2004a). In the early 20th century, it was observed that maternal mortality in industrialized countries halved in association with the provision of professional midwifery care at childbirth. Such successes were repeated in the 1950s and 1960s in Malaysia, Sri Lanka and Thailand, where increasing numbers of midwives attended deliveries (Pathmanathan *et al.*, 2003). In Egypt, maternal mortality was also reduced by 50% between 1983 and 2000, when the proportion of deliveries assisted by skilled birth attendants doubled (Campbell *et al.*, 2005). Without a trained health professional attending childbirth, many women who are at risk of having complications may not be identified, may be referred late for adequate care and may not receive life-saving first aid.

Globally, levels of professional assistance at birth are rising and currently stand at 64% in developing countries, although progress is slow or stagnant in rural areas of sub-Saharan Africa and parts of Asia (Koblinsky *et al.*, 2006; UNICEF, 2011). In many countries, few births are attended by skilled attendants. Taking a few examples from Asia (Table 14.1), the proportion of deliveries with health professionals is as low as 18% in Bangladesh and 19% in Nepal (UN, 2010), although exact levels vary depending on the source of data (see, for example, Afsana, Chapter 13 this volume). Birth attendants other than health professionals usually comprise traditional birth attendants, family welfare visitors, auxiliary midwives, relatives or friends; and some women deliver alone (Bell *et al.*, 2003). In Indonesia, the increase in deliveries with health professionals has been remarkable, with a rise of about 12% per year between 1991 and 1997 (UN, 2010), although differences between rich and poor and urban and rural women remain large (Hatt *et al.*, 2007).

Table 14.1. Births attended by skilled health personnel in a selection of Asian countries (UN, 2010).

Country	Total (%)		By wealth and residence (%)				
	Earliest (year)	Latest (year)	Poorest quintile	Richest quintile	Rural	Urban	Latest year
Bangladesh	10 (1994)	18 (2007)	3	40	9	30	2004
Cambodia		44 (2005)	21	90	39	70	2005
India	34 (1993)	47 (2006)	19	89	38	74	2006
Indonesia	41 (1990)	73 (2007)	40	94	55	79	2003
Myanmar	46 (1991)	57 (2001)	–	–	–	–	–
Nepal	7 (1991)	19 (2006)	5	58	19	52	2006
Pakistan	19 (1991)	39 (2007)	5	55	8	42	1991
The Philippines	53 (1993)	60 (2003)	25	92	41	79	2003
Vietnam		88 (2006)	58	100	82	99	2002

It should be noted that, despite low levels of health professionals present during childbirth, some countries such as Bangladesh and Nepal have nevertheless seen reductions in maternal and perinatal mortality. Many other factors play a part. In Bangladesh, abortion-related services and better access to emergency care have been noted (Chowdhury *et al.*, 2007; Ronsmans *et al.*, 2008), while, in Nepal, factors related to general improvement in women's health, female education and gender empowerment have been postulated as reasons for the observed falls in mortality (Hussein *et al.*, 2011). Disparities in wealth are likely to play a part in patterns of mortality reduction. Even in countries with high levels of health professional attendance overall, gaps between urban and rural or poorer and richer populations are considerable (Table 14.1), with evidence indicating that the disadvantaged are also the groups that suffer higher maternal mortality (Graham *et al.*, 2004; Ronsmans *et al.*, 2009).

Yet levels of maternal mortality can be surprisingly high even among groups of richer women who received professional care, as was found in Banten province, Indonesia (Ronsmans *et al.*, 2009). Independently of wealth, the risk of maternal death was not necessarily lower if a delivery was attended by a health professional. The study by Ronsmans *et al.* (2009) showed that 43.4% of the 355 women who died had been managed by a health professional during the birth; and that the odds of having a health professional present during delivery or around the time of

death was 1.9 times higher (95% CI: 1.4–2.5) among women who died than among those who survived. Various explanations are possible. Women may have sought care too late, health professionals may not have had access to the necessary equipment or supplies or their skills in managing complications may not have been sufficient – underscoring another important concept related to quality and skill – that simply being a health professional may not necessarily imply that a person possesses adequate or appropriate skills or the necessary resources. The presence of a health professional, even if he or she is skilled, is a necessary but not a sufficient factor to ensure good quality care (Graham *et al.*, 2001; Ronsmans *et al.*, 2009).

The Continuum of Quality

High quality care should guarantee that appropriate care is available wherever and whenever it is needed (Kerber *et al.*, 2007). An effective 'continuum of quality care' implies that the continuum of dimensions both of place and of time has to be considered (PMNCH, 2011).

Place of delivery and levels of health-care provision

Most professional assistance for childbirth is provided in health facilities, so the rate of deliveries in health facilities globally follows the same change as has been observed for deliveries with health professionals (Stanton *et al.*, 2007). In developing countries, 58% of deliveries occur in health facilities, although in the poorest countries only 35% of deliveries are institutional (UNICEF, 2011). Utilization patterns between urban and rural populations and the richer and poorer women are similar across countries (Montagu *et al.*, 2011).

Most deliveries outside health facilities take place at home, usually in a woman's own home, a relative's or friend's house or the home of the birth attendant. A small percentage may take place en route to a facility – in Indonesia, 3% of births happened in this way (Ronsmans *et al.*, 2009), clearly an undesirable outcome. Many home deliveries are not attended by health professionals, raising questions of quality on the assumption that the presence of a health professional is a necessary component for good quality care. Nevertheless, women may prefer to deliver at home, with a perception that the quality is better for various reasons that include comfort, familiarity of environment and lower costs. Many women and their families see a facility delivery as unnecessary (Montagu *et al.*, 2011).

In Indonesia, a considerable proportion of the population is located in remote and rural areas, far from health centres and hospitals. The Indonesia national village midwife strategy was a large scale programme set up in 1989 to post professional midwives and enable them to attend deliveries at community level. The initiative has resulted in a situation where 44.6% of the deliveries assisted by a health professional occur in a professional midwife's home, 7.2% in a health centre and 13.5% in hospital (Ronsmans *et al.*, 2009). Although seen as an improvement in the quality of care available for childbirth, various barriers remain that hinder access to adequate care, especially when complications occur. Response times by the midwife could be slow and referral delays were common. Women did not always choose to call the midwife first, and the competency and standards of care provided by the midwife were not considered optimal (D'Ambruoso *et al.*, 2009).

Within health facilities, a number of studies from developing countries show that the quality of maternity care is poor. Health professionals' knowledge and skills are inadequate, while the ability to meet specified clinical criteria at various levels of health facilities have been shown to be deficient (Wagaarachchi and Fernando, 2002; Gbangbade *et al.*, 2003; Hussein *et al.*, 2004; McCaw-Binns *et al.*, 2004; Koblinsky *et al.*, 2006; van den Broek and Graham, 2009). The standards of quality expected at different levels of health facilities have not been clearly defined, except in terms of levels of expected function (see Phoya *et al.*, Chapter 10 this volume). There have been some attempts to disaggregate quality assessments by level of maternity facility, for example in Ghana, showing that health centres perform less well than hospitals and that mission hospitals perform better than public facilities, although the findings may be subject to bias due to the reliance on availability of medical records (Hussein *et al.*, 2004).

From the perspective of reducing maternal and perinatal mortality, good quality care in dealing with the complications of childbirth, with access to and utilization of high quality EmOC, is central to saving lives (Paxton *et al.*, 2005). Most births are normal and the expected outcome is a healthy mother and baby. Major obstetric complications are expected in 15% of births (WHO *et al.*, 2009) and death can be averted in the majority of these events, but only if the complication is identified early, prevented from progressing, supported by timely and effective referral and managed adequately at an emergency care facility. This series of actions echoes the need to consider quality within the context of a continuum of care. Three scenarios illustrate its importance. The first represents a situation commonly found, where there is lack of a continuum between levels of care. In this case, few complications will be prevented or detected early, because of poor access, poor provision of care or both. Of the women with complications, only a few may receive adequate first aid and appropriate referral. The ones that reach an EmOC facility may not receive appropriate high quality care (Pitchforth *et al.*, 2006). The outcome is a low proportion of survival in the mother and the fetus or newborn. The second scenario represents a situation where the quality of care is adequate at lower levels of the health service but with inadequate support at referral level. Complications are detected and referred but casualties occur at the high levels of the system. The last scenario is what health systems aspire to reach, where complications are identified and referred early at primary level and adequately managed in higher level health facilities. If coverage levels are high, decreased levels of mortality can be expected. This last scenario also highlights the principle that coverage (see Phoya *et al.*, Chapter 10 this volume) and quality need to be improved alongside each other for effective realization of MDGs 4 and 5.

The dimension of time: when is quality crucial?

Childbirth and obstetric complications have been a focus of much of the discussion thus far and there are good reasons for this. Obstetric complications are the direct causes of maternal and perinatal death. Childbirth and the immediate few days after delivery appear to be the most risky times of pregnancy. A meta-analysis showed that over two-thirds of maternal deaths occurred in the postpartum period and, of these, 45% occurred within 1 day of childbirth (Li *et al.*, 1996). More recently, data from Bangladesh demonstrated that the highest mortality levels occurred on the first day after childbirth, fell by one-third on the second day and continued to fall thereafter (Ronsmans and Graham, 2006). At least 30% of stillbirths also occur during childbirth (Kerber *et al.*, 2007) and up to 45% of neonatal deaths in the first 24h after birth (Lawn *et al.*, 2005). Globally recommended and evidence-based interventions for the management of complications in pregnancy and childbirth and for managing newborn problems are available from a number of sources, including the WHO-led series 'Integrated Management of Pregnancy and Childbirth' (IMPAC) (WHO, 2011) and the Cochrane Library (2010) and are also reviewed elsewhere in this book (see Langer *et al.*, Chapter 8 this volume).

Taking the broader perspective of maternal and perinatal health (in contrast to mortality reduction), the quality of care provided during antenatal and postnatal care are of importance. These services are usually of a non-urgent routine nature. Evidence-based interventions that should be provided as part of antenatal and postnatal care are recommended (Cochrane Library, 2010; WHO, 2011). Apart from the early detection of complications in the mother, antenatal care is believed to be protective for the unborn fetus and neonate in particular. In Indonesia, data from a study of 52,917 singleton infants showed that the risk of early neonatal deaths was reduced by half or more in women who received antenatal care (Titaley *et al.*, 2011) The quality of antenatal care in developing countries has been investigated from the viewpoint of numbers of visits with the conclusion that there may be an increased perinatal mortality and lower levels of satisfaction among women who used a reduced, four-visit programme (Dowswell *et al.*, 2010; see Phoya *et al.*, Chapter 10 this volume). Calls to focus attention on postnatal care are growing, especially in the light of the commitments to newborn health (Lawn *et al.*, 2005; Sines *et al.*, 2007; Seims, 2008). Studies of postnatal care in some developing countries have revealed poor use, low awareness of importance and dissatisfaction amongst women (Kabakian-Khasholian *et al.*, 2000; Lomoro *et al.*, 2002; Mrisho *et al.*, 2009).

Quality Improvement

Strategies to improve the quality of maternity care have been implemented in many countries (Raven *et al.*, 2011). The majority of quality improvement initiatives may be classified as educational, organizational and financial. A systematic review relevant to maternal and child health identified at least five specific quality improvement strategies with sufficient evidence to support their implementation in developing countries. Combinations of more than one intervention also appear to have positive effects, while a number of other interventions merit further study (Table 14.2) (Althabe *et al.*, 2008).

Table 14.2. Quality improvement strategies in maternal and child health (Althabe *et al.*, 2008).

Type of intervention	Summary of effects
Education and feedback	
Passive distribution of materials	No improvement in provider practice unless combined with other strategies
Audit	Small to moderate improvements in provider practice
Reminders to providers to perform an action[a]	Improved provider practice
Meetings (workshops, seminars, conferences, training courses)	Improved provider practice if active and interactive in nature (workshops, small group sessions).[a] Passive processes such as conferences and lectures not effective
Developing consensus	No evidence of effectiveness
Tutor-facilitated problem-based learning	Inconclusive
Outreach visits by educator	Improved prescribing practices, otherwise unclear
Opinion leaders[a]	Small positive changes in provider practice
Patient-mediated (information sought from or given to patients)	Inconclusive
Mass media[a]	Improved provider practice
Tailored interventions to address specific barriers	Inconclusive
Organization of care	
Integration of primary health-care services	Inconclusive
Improving office procedures[a] (appointment-based systems, provision of screening by nurses)	Increased use of services
Changing medical record systems	Inconclusive
Others	
Financial incentives to providers	Inconclusive
Combinations of above[a]	Improved provider practice

[a]Sufficient evidence to implement intervention in developing countries.

Innovative initiatives to train community health workers and family members to administer first aid to mothers and their new-borns, while also assessing their care provision, are being tried out in countries such as Ethiopia (URC, 2010). Standards-based management and recognition systems have been used to improve quality of maternity services and other essential health-care services in Ethiopia and Afghanistan (Necochia and Bossemeyer, 2010), using a quality improvement tool called the balanced scorecard, which is based on the principles of strategic planning tools like the logical framework (see Hounton *et al.*, Chapter 15 this volume). A quality improvement initiative to improve EmOC specifically in rural hospitals was used in Nepal to improve health staff motivation and function of the hospital system (Clapham *et al.*, 2004), while quality improvement in a community-based setting was implemented in Indonesia (Box 14.2).

Audit and feedback in particular have been used extensively in maternity care as a quality improvement intervention, for example, confidential enquiries on maternal death, maternal and perinatal death audits and criterion-based clinical audit (Wagaarachchi *et al.*, 2001; WHO, 2004b; Hussein, 2007; Adisasmita *et al.*, 2009; Kongnyuy and Uthman, 2009; van den Broek and Graham, 2009). Overall, the evidence on audit and feedback suggests a positive effect (Jamtvedt *et al.*, 2006; Althabe *et al.*, 2008; Kongnyuy and Uthman, 2009), although some limitations include their reliance on adequate routine record and data collection systems and difficulties in scaling up and maintaining the rigour of the process in health systems that are not functioning well (Althabe *et al.*, 2008). Audit and feedback are likely to have greater effect in situations where baseline adherence to recommended practice is low and when feedback is delivered intensively (Jamtvedt *et al.*, 2006).

Box 14.2. A combination quality improvement strategy, Indonesia.

The USAID MotherCare project, working with the Indonesian Ministry of Health, provincial health office, three district health offices in South Kalimantan, the Indonesian Midwifery Association and the American College of Nurse Midwives, provides an example of a combination quality improvement strategy for maternal and neonatal health. Specific interventions comprised training courses, audit and feedback activities and organizational improvements. Recognizing the fact that the pathway to maternal survival needs a continuum of care, the quality improvement strategy was directed at all levels of care.

Training courses were conducted for midwives in life-saving skills, interpersonal communication and counselling. Training, supervision and support were provided within the existing service structure through the community health centres, district hospitals and provincial hospitals. Policy formulation, improved referral systems and equipment and drug supplies were also strengthened or made coherent with the training and expected practice of the midwives. After the training was completed, midwives continued to participate in educational workshops and interactive peer-review sessions.

Throughout the project period, 130 maternal deaths were reported in the project area and assessed through maternal and perinatal audit activities, at community level and in facilities, which resulted in the generation of recommendations to improve quality, including the need for additional training of midwives, a blood bank and specific drugs and for standardized treatment guidelines. Many of these recommendations led to concrete improvements in aspects of the district health system, while a formal end of project evaluation indicated significant improvement in both clinical and communication skills of the midwives (Achadi *et al.*, 2000).

Conclusion

The multidimensional nature of quality, even in a field as specific as maternal and perinatal health, is clear from the frameworks discussed. Quality assessments have to take into account broad perspectives and recognize the need to move beyond the clinical encounter to incorporate health systems and organizational perspectives, user experiences and the choice preferences of women and their families.

Improving the quality of obstetric care, not least in developing country settings, is nevertheless crucial, but is challenged by the diverse array of the factors linked to quality and the need to be comprehensive in defining quality and to address all dimensions of the continuum of care, at all levels of care provision and at the various stages of the reproductive life cycle. New methods to improve approaches to quality improvement and to capture the complexity of quality continue to be pioneered and tested, but many gaps in knowledge remain, with future work warranted on indicators of quality, incorporation of data on user experiences, standardization of measures and evaluations of quality improvement.

References

Achadi, E., Beck, D., Zazri, A., Supratikto, G., Zizic, L., Cohen, S., Jus'at, I., Ronsmans, C. and McDermott, J. (2000) *The Mothercare Experience in Indonesia*. Final Report, John Snow Inc. MotherCare Project and USAID, Washington, DC.

Adegoke, A.A., Hofman, J.J., Kongnyuy, E.J. and van den Broek, N. (2011) Monitoring and evaluation of skilled birth attendance: a proposed new framework. *Midwifery* 27(3), 350–359.

Adisasmita, A., Respatiasih, J. and Izzati, Y. (2009) *Report on Confidential Enquiries into Maternal Deaths Implementation Pilot in West Nusa Tenggara*. Report to WHO Indonesia University of Indonesia, Jakarta.

Althabe, F., Bergelb, E., Cafferatac, M.L., Gibbonsa, L., Ciapponia, A., Colantonioa, A.A.L. and Palaciosa, A.R. (2008) Strategies for improving the quality of health care in maternal and child health in low- and middle-income countries: an overview of systematic reviews. *Paediatric and Perinatal Epidemiology* 22 (Suppl. 1), 42–60.

Bell, J., Curtis, S.L. and Alayón, S. (2003) Trends in delivery care in six countries. *DHS Analytical Studies No.7.* International Research Partnership for Skilled Attendance for Everyone (SAFE) and ORC Macro, Calverton, Maryland.

Bertrand, J.T., Hardee, K., Magnani, R.J. and Angleet, M.A. (1995) Access, quality of care, and medical barriers in family planning programs. *International Family Planning Perspectives* 21(2), 64–69.

Brown, L.D., Franco, L.M., Rafeh, N. and Hatzell, T. (2000) *Quality Assurance of Health Care in Developing Countries.* Quality Assurance Methodology Refinement Series, Quality Assurance Project, Bethesda, Maryland.

Bruce, J. (1990) Fundamental elements of quality of care: a simple framework. *Studies in Family Planning* 21(2), 61–91.

Campbell, O., Gipson, R., Issa, A.H., Matta, N., El Deeb, B., El Mohandes, A., Alwen, A. and Mansour, E. (2005) National maternal mortality ratio in Egypt halved between 1992–93 and 2000. *Bulletin of the World Health Organization* 83(6), 462–471.

Campbell, S.M., Roland, M.O. and Buetow, S.A. (2000) Defining quality of care. *Social Science and Medicine* 51, 1611–1625.

Chowdhury, M. and Rosenfield, A. (2004) Interim Report of Task Force 4 on Child Health and Maternal Health. Millennium Project. Available at: http://www.unmillenniumproject.org/documents/tf4interim. pdf (accessed 23 August 2011).

Chowdhury, M.E., Botlero, R., Koblinsky, M., Saha, S.K., Dieltiens, G. and Ronsmans, C. (2007) Determinants of reduction in maternal mortality in Matlab, Bangladesh: a 30-year cohort study. *Lancet* 370(9595), 1320–1328.

Clapham, S., Basnet, I., Pathak, L.R. and McCall, M. (2004) The evolution of a quality of care approach for improving emergency obstetric care in rural hospitals in Nepal. *International Journal of Gynecology and Obstetrics* 86(1), 86–97.

Cochrane Library (2010) Available at: http://www.thecochranelibrary.com/view/0/index.html (accessed 25 August 2011).

Creel, L.C., Sass, J.C. and Yinger, N.V. (2011) Overview of Quality of Care in Reproductive Health: Definitions and Measurements of Quality, Population Reference Bureau. Available at: http://www.prb.org/Publications/PolicyBriefs/OverviewofQualityofCareinReproductiveHealthDefinitionsandMeasurements.aspx (accessed 23 August 2011).

D'Ambruoso, L., Achadi, E., Adisasmita, A., Izati, Y., Makowiecka, K. and Hussein, J. (2009) Assessing quality of care provided by Indonesian village midwives with a confidential enquiry. *Midwifery* 25, 528–539.

Donabedian, A. (1966) Evaluating the quality of medical care. *Milbank Quarterly* 44, 166–203.

Donabedian, A. (1990) The seven pillars of quality. *Archives of Pathology and Laboratory Medicine* 114, 1115–1118.

Dowswell, T., Carroli, G., Duley, L., Gates, S., Gülmezoglu, A.M., Khan-Neelofur, D. and Piaggio, G.G.P. (2010) Alternative versus standard packages of antenatal care for low-risk pregnancy. *Cochrane Database of Systematic Reviews* 2010, Issue 10. Art. No.: CD000934. DOI:10.1002/14651858. CD000934.pub2.

Family Care International (2000) *Skilled Attendance at Delivery: a review of the evidence.* Safe Motherhood Inter-Agency Group, New York.

Gbangbade, S., Harvey, S.A., Edson, W., Burkhalter, B. and Antonakos, C. (2003) *Safe Motherhood Studies: results from Benin.* Quality Assurance Project, Bethesda, Maryland.

Graham, W.J., Bell, J.S. and Bullough, C.H.W. (2001) Can skilled attendance at delivery reduce maternal mortality in developing countries? *Studies in Health Services Organisation and Policy* 17, 97–130.

Graham, W.J., Fitzmaurice, A.E., Bell, J.S. and Cairns, J.A. (2004) The familial technique for linking maternal death with poverty. *Lancet* 363, 23–27.

Hatt, L., Stanton, C., Makowiecka, K., Adisasmita, A., Achadi, E. and Ronsmans, C. (2007) Did the strategy of skilled attendance at birth reach the poor in Indonesia? *Bulletin of the World Health Organization* 85(10), 774–782.

Hulton, L.A., Matthews, Z. and Stones, R.W. (2000) A Framework for the Evaluation of Quality Maternity Services. University of Southampton, Southampton. Available at: http://www.socstats.soton.ac.uk/choices (accessed 20 August 2011).

Hussein, J. (2007) Improving the use of confidential enquiries into maternal deaths in developing countries. *Bulletin of the World Health Organization* 85(1), 68–69.

Hussein, J., Bell, J., Nazzar, A., Abbey, M., Adjei, S. and Graham, W.J. (2004) The skilled attendance index (SAI): proposal for a new measure of skilled attendance at delivery. *Reproductive Health Matters* 12, 160–170.

Hussein, J., Bell, J., Dar Iang, M., Mesko, N., Amery, J. and Graham, W. (2011) An appraisal of the maternal mortality decline in Nepal. *PLoS ONE* 6(5), e19898. doi:10.1371/journal.pone.0019898.

Institute of Medicine (IOM) (2001) *Crossing the Quality Chasm*. National Academy Press, Washington, DC.

Jamtvedt, G., Young, J.M., Kristoffersen, D.T., O'Brien, M.A. and Oxman, A.D. (2006) Audit and feedback: effects on professional practice and health care outcomes. *Cochrane Database of Systematic Reviews 2006*, Issue 2. Art. No.: CD000259. DOI: 10.1002/14651858.CD000259.pub2.

Kabakian-Khasholian, T., Campbell, O., Shediac-Rizkallah, M. and Ghorayeb, F. (2000) Women's experiences of maternity care: satisfaction or passivity? *Social Science and Medicine* 51(1), 103–113.

Kerber, K.J., de Graft-Johnson, J.E., Bhutta, Z., Okong, P., Starrs, A. and Lawn, J.E. (2007) Continuum of care for maternal, newborn, and child health: from slogan to service delivery. *Lancet* 370, 1358–1369.

Koblinsky, M., Matthews, Z., Hussein, J., Mavalankar, D., Mridha, M.K., Anwar, I., Achadi, E., Adjei, S., Padmanabhan, P. and van Leberghe, W. (2006) Going to scale with professional skilled care. *Lancet* 368(9544), 1377–1386.

Kongnyuy, E.J. and Uthman, O.A. (2009) Use of criterion-based clinical audit to improve the quality of obstetric care: A systematic review. *Acta Obstetricia et Gynecologica Scandinavica* 88(8), 873–881.

Lawn, J.E., Cousens, S., Zupan, J. and Lancet Neonatal Survival Steering Team (2005) 4 million neonatal deaths: When? Where? Why? *Lancet* 365, 891–900.

Li, X.F., Fortney, J.A., Kotelchuck, M. and Glover, L.H. (1996) The postpartum period: the key to maternal mortality. *International Journal of Gynecology and Obstetrics* 54(1), 1–10.

Lomoro, O.A., Ehiri, J.E., Qian, X. and Tang, S.L. (2002) Mothers' perspectives on the quality of postpartum care in Central Shanghai, China. *International Journal of Quality in Health Care* 14(5), 393–402.

McCaw-Binns, A., Burkhalter, B., Edson, W., Harvey, S.A. and Antonakos, C. (2004) *Safe Motherhood Studies: Results from Jamaica*. Quality Assurance Project, Bethesda, Maryland.

Montagu, D., Yamey, G., Visconti, A., Harding, A. and Yoong, J. (2011) Where do poor women in developing countries give birth? A multi-country analysis of demographic and health survey data. *PLoS One* 28, 6(2), e17155.

Mrisho, M., Obrist, B., Schellenberg, J.A., Haws, R.A., Mushi, A.K., Mshinda, H., Tanner, M. and Schellenberg, D. (2009) The use of antenatal and postnatal care: perspectives and experiences of women and health care providers in rural southern Tanzania. *BMC Pregnancy Childbirth* 9(10), doi: 10.1186/1471-2393-9-10.

Necochia, E. and Bossemeyer, D. (2010) Standards based management and recognition. USAID and JHPIEGO, Baltimore. Available at: http://www.jhpiego.org/files/SBMR%20FieldGuide.pdf (accessed 20 August 2011).

Pathmanathan, I., Liljestrand, J., Martins, J.M., Rajapaksa, L.C., Lissner, C., de Silva, A., Selvaraju, S. and Singh, P.J. (2003) Sri Lanka. In: *Investing in Maternal Health: Learning from Malaysia and Sri Lanka*. Health Population and Nutrition Series, World Bank, Washington, DC.

Paxton, A., Maine, D., Freedman, L., Fry, D. and Lobis, S. (2005) The evidence for emergency obstetric care. *International Journal of Gynaecology and Obstetrics* 88(2), 181–193.

Pitchforth, E., van Teijlingen, E., Graham, W., Dixon-Woods, M. and Chowdhury, M. (2006) Getting women to hospital is not enough: a qualitative study of access to emergency obstetric care in Bangladesh. *Quality and Safety in Health Care* 15, 214–219.

Pittroff, R. and Campbell, O. (2000) Quality of Maternity Care: Silver Bullet or Red Herring? London School of Hygiene and Tropical Medicine, London. Available at: http://www.dfid.gov.uk/r4d/SearchResearch DatabaseWord.asp?OutputID=50072 (accessed 20 August 2011).

Partnership for Maternal, Newborn and Child Health (PMNCH) (2011) The continuum of care. Available at: http://www.who.int/pmnch/about/continuum_of_care/en/index.html (accessed 23 August 2011).

Raven, J., Hofman, J., Adegoke, A. and van den Broek, N. (2011) Methodology and tools for quality improvement in maternal and newborn health care. *International Journal of Gynecology and Obstetrics* 114(1), 4–9.

Ronsmans, C. and Graham, W.J. (2006) Maternal mortality: who, when, where and why. *Lancet* 368(9542), 1189–1200.

Ronsmans, C., Chowdhury, M.E., Alam, N., Koblinsky, M. and El Arifeen, S. (2008) Trends in stillbirths, early and late neonatal mortality in rural Bangladesh: the role of public health interventions. *Paediatric and Perinatal Epidemiology* 22(3), 269–279.

Ronsmans, C., Scott, S., Qomariyah, S.N., Achadi, E., Braunholtz, D., Marshall, T., Pambudi, E., Witten, K.H. and Graham, W.J. (2009) Professional assistance during birth and maternal mortality in two Indonesian districts. *Bulletin of the World Health Organization* 87, 416–423.

Sackett, D.L., Rosenberg, W.M.C., Gray, J.A.M., Haynes, R.B. and Richardson, W.S. (1996) Evidence based medicine: what it is and what it isn't. *British Medical Journal* 312, 71–72.

Seims, L.K. (2008) Postnatal care of newborns and mothers in developing countries. *Journal of Health, Population and Nutrition* 26(1), 110–111.

Silimperi, D.R., Franco, L.M., Van Zanten, T.V. and Macaulay, C. (2002) A framework for institutionalizing quality assurance. *International Journal for Quality in Health Care* 14(Suppl. 1), 67–73.

Sines, E., Syed, U., Wall, S. and Worley, H. (2007) Postnatal Care: A Critical Opportunity to Save Mothers and Newborns. Save the Children and Population Reference Bureau, Washington, DC. Available at: http://www.prb.org/pdf07/SNL_PNCBriefFinal.pdf (accessed 10 August 2011).

Stanton, C., Blanc, A.K., Croft, T. and Choi, Y. (2007) Skilled care at birth in the developing world: progress to date and strategies for expanding coverage. *Journal of Biosocial Science* 39(1), 109–120.

Thaddeus, S. and Maine, D. (1994) Too far to walk: maternal mortality in context. *Social Science and Medicine* 38, 1091–1110.

Titaley, C.R., Dibley, M.J. and Roberts, C.L. (2011) Type of delivery attendant, place of delivery and risk of early neonatal mortality: analyses of the 1994–2007 Indonesia Demographic and Health Surveys. *Health Policy and Planning* [Epub ahead of print].

UN (2010) Economic and Social Commission for Asia and the Pacific Statistical Yearbook for Asia and the Pacific 2009. Available at: http://www.unescap.org/stat/data/syb2009/index.asp (accessed 24 August 2011).

UNICEF (2011) *State of the World's Children 2011*. UNICEF, New York.

University Research Corporation (URC) (2010) Available at: http://www.urc-chs.com/quality_improvement (accessed 24 August 2011).

USAID (2007) *Child Survival and Health Grants Program Technical Reference Materials: Quality Assurance*. USAID, Washington, DC.

van den Broek, N.R. and Graham, W.J. (2009) Quality of care for maternal and newborn health: the neglected agenda. *BJOG* 116(Suppl.1), 18–21.

Vlassoff, C., Abou-Zahr, C. and Kumar, A. (1996) Quality health care for women: a global challenge. *Health Care for Women International* 17, 449–467.

Wagaarachchi, P.T. and Fernando, L. (2002) Trends in maternal mortality and assessment of substandard care in a tertiary care hospital. *European Journal of Obstetrics, Gynecology and Reproductive Biology* 101(1), 36–40.

Wagaarachchi, P.T., Graham, W.J., Penney, G.C., McCaw-Binns, A., Yeboah Antwi, K. and Hall, M.H. (2001) Holding up a mirror: changing obstetric practice through criterion-based clinical audit in developing countries. *International Journal of Gynaecology and Obstetrics* 74(2), 119–130.

WHO (2004a) Making pregnancy safer: the critical role of the skilled attendant. A joint statement by WHO, ICM and FIGO WHO, Geneva. Available at: http://www.who.int/making_pregnancy_safer/documents/92415916692/en/index.html (accessed 14 August 2008).

WHO (2004b) *Beyond the Numbers: Reviewing Maternal Deaths and Complications to Make Pregnancy Safer*. WHO, Geneva.

WHO (2011) Making Pregnancy Safer. IMPAC. Available at: http://www.who.int/making_pregnancy_safer/documents/impac/en/index.html (accessed 23 August 2011).

WHO, UNFPA, UNICEF and AMDD (2009) *Monitoring Emergency Obstetric Care: A Handbook*. WHO, Geneva.

15 Monitoring and Evaluation

Sennen Hounton,[1] David Newlands,[2] Nicolas Meda[3] and Julia Hussein[2]
[1]UNFPA, New York, USA; [2]University of Aberdeen, Scotland, UK;
[3]Centre MURAZ, Bobo-Dioulasso, Burkina Faso

Summary

- Monitoring and evaluation are essential components of all programmes to improve maternal and perinatal health and to ensure that programme effects and value can be documented.
- A plan for monitoring and evaluation should be done when programmes are being designed and at the start of implementation, not after implementation has commenced.
- Monitoring and evaluation are two distinct, essential programme activities, which are linked, but have different purposes. Monitoring is the routine and continuous tracking of performance to provide information on ongoing progress, while evaluation is an objective assessment that determines achievement of objectives.
- A wide range of indicators has been formulated to measure the effect of programme interventions on maternal and perinatal health. Selection of indicators should take into account the programme activities, existence of current data collection systems, human resources and cost. The indicators selected should include a mix of process and outcome measures.
- Four essential tools that can be used as a basis for monitoring and evaluation of programmes are discussed: theory of change, logical frameworks, evaluation criteria and a framework for evaluation.
- Managing an evaluation is a complex process and requires allocation of adequate time, funding and expertise.
- Country level investment is required for vital registration and health information systems with real-time monitoring to improve accountability and provide locally relevant information for action.

Introduction

A goal which is not monitored cannot be met or missed (Johansson and Stewart, 2002). As obvious as this statement might seem, it is worth a pause for reflection. Without the information provided by monitoring and evaluation activities, it will not be possible to document whether a programme has been implemented as planned, whether there are intended or unintended effects or whether targets set at the beginning are achieved or not. The value of any investment made in the programme will not be known. Questions on whether the activities should be supported again or replicated would remain unanswered.

There is general acceptance that development activities should be implemented efficiently, responsibly and with a high degree of accountability. This has heightened the importance of demonstrating value for money and effort, underscoring the need to monitor and document effectiveness and cost-effectiveness. At a practical level, such needs are translated as activities involving development of results frameworks, mid-term assessments and final evaluations of programmes.

There are numerous resources for monitoring and evaluation available. Despite this, programme managers and public health practitioners continue to be faced with many challenges – technical and resource related – when planning, designing and implementing monitoring and evaluation activities. Maternal and newborn health programmes are not an exception. This chapter will provide guidance on good practices in monitoring and evaluation, with specific reference to maternal and perinatal health. We draw from our field experiences and focus on programme monitoring and evaluation in support of national processes, national ownership and national accountability, rather than on global monitoring mechanisms of maternal and newborn indicators such as of the Millennium Development Goals (MDGs) or the Countdown reports, which are discussed in earlier chapters.

The Purposes and Characteristics of Monitoring and Evaluation

Monitoring is the routine and continuous tracking of performance against planned activities. Data are collected and analysed on specified indicators. An effective monitoring system will provide programme managers with timely information on progress – or lack of it – towards achieving results, which are expressed in terms of outputs, outcomes and goals. Through regular record keeping and analysis, programme managers can assess performance of a programme in a systematic manner. Strengths and weaknesses of the implementation activities are identified early and corrective action taken if necessary, without waiting for the completion of the programme. In this way, the monitoring system provides constant feedback on programme implementation, enhances the ongoing learning experience of programme implementers, improves subsequent planning processes

and guides implementation towards achievement of desired goals.

Evaluation is a 'systematic and objective assessment' of a programme (Kuseck and Rist, 2004). In general, the term refers to a periodic time-bound exercise, usually conducted by external evaluators (independent evaluation), with the aim of answering questions on why and how programme results were achieved (or not achieved). Evaluations may rely on data generated through monitoring activities, can use existing data to conduct new in-depth analysis or can gather primary data obtained from a range of sources such as research studies, in-depth interviews, focus group discussions and surveys.

External evaluations in particular can be viewed as threatening, especially by programme managers, who may feel blamed or intimidated during evaluation activities. Those involved in implementing programme activities may feel that an external evaluator visiting their programme for a short time may not understand the full realities and challenges posed during implementation. However, evaluation should be valued by all – donor agencies and external stakeholders as well as programme staff – as it allows learning from past experiences to improve service delivery, planning and allocation of resources, ultimately ensuring that target beneficiaries' health is improved through programme interventions. Tensions between evaluators and programme implementers/managers can be managed through clear identification of a monitoring and evaluation framework from the earliest stages of programme planning, with specified and appropriate indicators, data sources and data collection tools. Programme staff should be involved in specifying the terms of reference for the evaluation. Interpretation and use of monitoring data as part of the evaluation are important to instil ownership of the evaluation findings by the programme staff. Evaluations should be designed to be objective and evidence-based rather than being opinion-based.

Monitoring and evaluation are thus two distinct activities (Table 15.1) but also intrinsically linked. Evaluation is not a substitute for monitoring nor is monitoring a substitute for

Table 15.1. Characteristics of monitoring and evaluation (adapted from UNFPA, 2004).

Criteria	Monitoring	Evaluation
Frequency	Continuous	Periodic: at important milestones such as the inception and the mid-term of programme implementation; at the end of the programme/project
Main actions	Keeps track; oversight; analyses and documents progress	Assessment, in-depth and comparative analysis
Scope	Focuses on inputs, activities, outputs, implementation processes	Focuses on: outcomes in relation to inputs; results in relation to cost (value for money); processes used to achieve results; overall effectiveness and relevance; impact and sustainability
Objectives and usefulness	Answers what activities were implemented and results achieved Alerts managers to problems and provides options for corrective actions	Answers why and how results were achieved Contributes to building theories and models for change Provides managers with strategy and policy options
Information sources	Routine systems, field observations, progress reports, rapid assessments	Same as monitoring plus surveys/studies
Internal versus external team	Self-assessment by programme managers, supervisors, community stakeholders and funders	Internal and/or external analysis by programme managers, supervisors, community stakeholders, funders and/or external evaluators

evaluation. Both are an essential part of the complete programme cycle. They comprise similar activities and processes but produce different kinds of information. Both are necessary management tools to inform decision making and to demonstrate accountability.

Tools for Monitoring and Evaluation

Indicators

At the core of any monitoring results framework and any evaluation are the indicators. An indicator is defined as 'a quantitative or qualitative factor or variable that provides a simple and reliable means to measure achievement, to reflect changes connected to an intervention, or to help assess the performance of a development actor' (OECD,

2002). In practice, indicators often describe quantity (how many, how much), time (when), place (where), target groups (who) and sometimes quality. A commonly used mnemonic used to ascertain important criteria for indicators is 'SMART', i.e. indicators should be Specific, Measurable, Achievable (or applicable, appropriate), Relevant and Time bound (a specified change over time, implying the need for a baseline and target). 'SMART' provides an objective approach to indicator criteria, although there are other considerations that are important, including ensuring that indicators should be empowering, diverse, relatively easy to collect and credible and have potential for influencing change (Roche, 1999).

Indicators can be categorized as input, output, outcome and impact indicators, although the terms are not always consistently used in the literature (Kuseck and Rist, 2004; AusAID, 2005; Immpact, 2007):

- Input indicators measure the resources that are employed in the implementation of the programme. Examples of inputs are funds, time, equipment, supplies or personnel.
- Outputs are the immediate results of the programme activities, examples being improved service utilization (number of new contraceptive acceptors, number of deliveries by health personnel) and availability of health facilities and quality of care. What are commonly known as 'process indicators' in maternal health are usually output measures.
- Outcome indicators are the intermediate (medium term) results, usually measured in terms of benefits to the target groups or at the population level. Examples of such indicators include contraceptive prevalence rate and proportion of births by skilled health personnel.
- Impact indicators (sometimes confusingly referred to as health outcomes) are measures of the long-term goals of programmes, such as maternal mortality ratio and stillbirth rates. It is not usually feasible to use impact indicators to monitor typical programmes, although evaluation of large-scale programmes can involve the use of impact indicators.

Data sources

To monitor and evaluate programmes, a specific data source must be identified for each indicator selected and consistently used, because different sources may give different data for the same indicator. There are several sources of data for tracking maternal and newborn indicators. They include the use of national health management information systems, health facility data including medical registers and clinical case notes, population-based surveys and existing administrative records – a unique source of data for information on inputs and costs.

Routine health management information data are the source of data for most output indicators and many outcome indicators. Civil registration systems record vital events (births, deaths, migrations) and can be reliable data sources for maternal and child deaths as well as births. Such systems can provide disaggregated data at the regional/provincial, district and health facility levels for the monitoring of programmes and services. The international community, donors and externally funded programmes in developing countries have traditionally relied on independent household surveys for assessing progress in maternal, newborn and child health. This was mainly due to the weakness of the national health information systems, with quality, coverage and reliability issues.

Population-based surveys such as demographic and health surveys and the Multiple Indicator Cluster Survey (UNICEF, 2011) are sources of data for outcome and impact indicators. The drawback of these surveys is that they do not provide annual estimates for continuous monitoring. These surveys also do not provide district and health facility data to inform the planning and management of programmes at these levels. Health facility surveys are another source of data. Many independent health facility surveys are conducted (MEASURE DHS, 2011) although the recommendation is that they support national health information systems to contribute to their completeness, timeliness and accuracy.

Selecting indicators

It is a common mistake within programmes to invent indicators, often with no clear mechanisms to produce, collect and analyse data. In selecting indicators, programme managers should ensure there is a clear definition for the indicator, defined methods to calculate the indicators by specification of the numerator and denominator, identified sources of data and frequencies of monitoring. There is a large body of literature recommending indicators to measure the effects of maternity care and programme interventions (examples are provided in Table 15.2), so it will be rare that new indicators will have to be created. The decision to create a new indicator should take into account programme activities, existence of current data collection systems, human resources and cost.

Table 15.2. Examples of indicators used in maternal health programmes.

Reference	Indicator
WHO Mother Baby Package (WHO, 1994)	Antenatal care uptake Contraceptive prevalence rate Average age at first birth for women under 25 years Percentage of births attended by trained health personnel Percentage of population living within 1 h travel time of health facility offering obstetric care Prevalence of anaemia by gestation Percentage of women screened for syphilis
UN process indicators (WHO *et al.*, 2009)	Availability of emergency obstetric care Geographical distribution of emergency obstetric care facilities Proportion of all births in emergency obstetric care facilities Proportion of women with major direct obstetric complications treated in emergency obstetric care facilities Caesarean sections as a proportion of all births Direct obstetric case fatality rate Intrapartum and very early neonatal death rate Proportion of maternal deaths due to indirect causes in emergency obstetric care facilities
Unmet Obstetric Need (UON, 1999)	An indicator which compares the need for obstetric care with the ability of the health service to provide the care, expressed in terms of women who should have benefited from an intervention but for whom the intervention did not take place
Skilled Attendance Index (Hussein *et al.*, 2004)	Composite measure of skilled care based on summarizing scores on over 40 clinical criteria
Gabrysch *et al.*, 2011	Health professionals Density of health facilities Geographical access Birth density
Criterion-based clinical audit (Wagaarachchi *et al.*, 2001)	Clinical indicators of quality of care for obstetric complications

Frameworks

The key foundation for monitoring and evaluation is the underlying conceptual framework. A variety of tools and frameworks exist. Four basic tools are discussed here: theory of change, logical frameworks, evaluation criteria and a framework for evaluation.

Theory of change

A theory of change is a way to describe the pathway through which a programme objective or goal might be achieved (Pawson and Tilley, 2003). It is an essential step required to design programmes and to formulate a coherent monitoring and evaluation plan yet is often not conducted well and even more often is poorly documented.

Programme interventions and activities that depict the intended pathway of change can be simply mapped out using a programme logic chain (Leeuw, 2003). This process helps to identify the way in which a programme is expected to work. The logic chain is created by identifying elements that would need to be achieved for the expected result to occur. If a theory of change or logic chain is not available, even if a programme is already being implemented, it is advisable to formulate one. To inform the development of this logic chain, the following activities could be conducted (Immpact, 2007):

- Hold discussions with people who are familiar with the programme, such as programme staff, as well as ministry officials and representatives of development partners external to the programme.

- Observe programme activities as they are being implemented.
- Review and retrieve historical and current programme documents.

An intervention conceptual framework is a type of logic chain which describes a programme and the postulated rationale through which it will achieve change. It helps clarify objectives and aids in the identification of the expected causal links, the 'programme logic' and the sequence of anticipated results. Figure 15.1 is an example of a conceptual framework of an intervention developed and implemented in Burkina Faso by Family Care International, called the Skilled Care Initiative (see: http://www.familycareintl.org/en/issues/30) (Family Care International, 2007; Hounton *et al.*, 2008). The programme aimed to reduce maternal and perinatal mortality by developing a comprehensive set of interventions to target service delivery, quality of care and demand for quality maternity care. The figure conceptually represents what the programme was trying to achieve and how. It was used to identify indicators to measure performance and impact. It is useful to note

that such representation of programme interventions may evolve over time as programmes are adjusted and modified according to barriers encountered, shifting contexts, new evidence or/and policy change. Having the original framework and a record of its evolution will assist in assessment and aid understanding of the effects of the programme.

Other general examples of logic chains and additional information on the theory and practice of developing logic chains can be found in McLaughlin and Jordan (1999) and Frechtling (2007). Adegoke *et al.* (2011) describe a framework for monitoring skilled attendance at delivery using a theory of change approach.

The logical framework

A logical framework is a widely employed management tool used to establish a hierarchy of means through which the programme goals will be reached (AusAID, 2005). It is often represented as a matrix which describes a programme according to the desired impact of the programme, its intermediate outputs

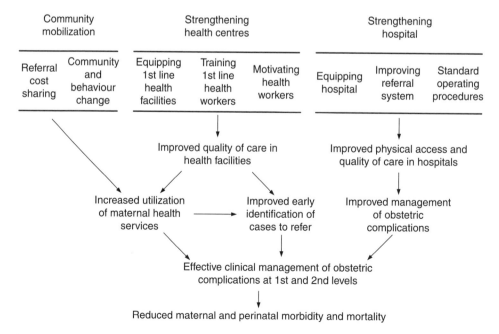

Fig. 15.1. Skilled Care Initiative impact model, Burkina Faso (Family Care International, 2007).

and outcomes, the inputs and activities that the programme will undertake and the environment in which it operates. Activities are carried out by programmes when inputs in the form of funds and resources such as know-how and skills are available. For a programme to achieve its expected outputs and outcomes, activities must be relevant and appropriate to the setting within which the programme operates. Hence, the activities must address factors such as culturally relevant needs, political instability or conflict and identified needs within the target population. At the same time, the activities must be congruent with expected outputs, outcomes and goals: for example, if a project goal were to reduce neonatal mortality, an activity involving immunization of a 6-month-old child is unlikely to be relevant to the attainment of the goal. Activities are closely related to outputs, which are the tangible products or deliverables of completed activities. Examples of logical frameworks are widely available (AusAID, 2005; DFID, 2011). SAFE (2003) provides an example of a maternal health programme logical framework which has been developed through a situation analysis and analysis of root problems.

Based on the logical framework, a simplified results-based table can be used to monitor the progress of a programme (Fig. 15.2). The results framework for the programme should include: the goal, outcome (purpose) and output indicators and also activities or inputs. For each indicator the definition (including numerator and denominator), baseline, targets, sources of data and how the data will be collected should be included. A more detailed calendar (days, weeks and months) could be used, depending on the nature, the frequency and the changeability of the activities being carried out. The template should be seen not as a mechanical activity of filling out the cells, but as a tool for analysis and reiterative planning of activities. It is also crucial to ensure that factors outside the programme activities are taken into account. An example is the provision of reproductive health commodities, which requires several conditions to execute, including effective procurement, shipping, storage and waste management, logistics and supply chain management, timely monitoring and responses for stock-outs. To enable access to and use of reproductive health commodities, all the factors that affect the route of

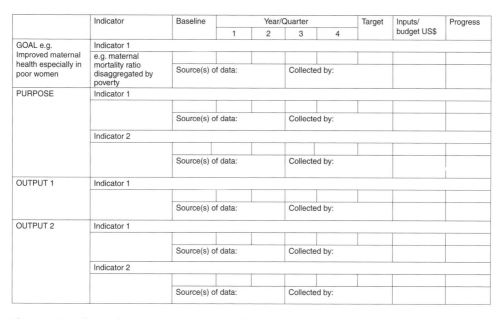

Fig. 15.2. Sample template for monitoring results (adapted from DFID, 2011).

the product from manufacturing to the client's hand and use need to be monitored. A programme may not undertake all areas of logistics and supply chain management, but should have a system for monitoring major factors that affect the programming of the activities.

Evaluation criteria

The Development Assistance Committee (DAC) has drawn upon results and logical frameworks to assess the inputs, activities, expected outcomes and goals of a project or programme and identified five key criteria (Table 15.3) to be considered when conducting an evaluation (OECD, 2011).

The relevance of activities to the programme goals has been discussed earlier. Expected outcomes may be achieved within the programme: these are measured by effectiveness. Attainment of effectiveness may be efficient or not, depending on whether the activities have been implemented in a timely manner and whether the intensity and quality of implementation are optimal. Programmes that are not effective cannot be efficient. If it can be shown that the minimum resources possible have been used to reach the expected outcomes, efficiency can be measured, although this is not always easy to do unless specific, measurable and time-bound targets are set on expected outcomes and comparisons with alternative modes of implementation

are available. One measure of efficiency is cost-effectiveness, which requires the comparison of alternative approaches to achieving the same or comparable results (Box 15.1).

Although impact is generally thought of only in terms of positive change, a programme may also result in unexpected or unintended consequences. The size of population affected by either positive or negative changes is important and usually measured in terms of coverage of the programme. Finally, programmes may have effects or influences that extend beyond its life, so factors of sustainability will need to be accounted for as part of the evaluation.

The likelihood of the goal being achieved will be constrained or increased depending on factors of relevance, effectiveness, efficiency, impact and sustainability. Goals are not always measured within programmes, so implementation of many of the projects and programmes reviewed assumes contributions to the goal if expected outcomes are achieved.

An evaluation framework

Figure 15.3 provides a diagram of six key steps to take when conducting an evaluation. It will be noted that the steps are cyclical. Once the final step of documentation is completed, the stakeholder should be re-engaged and her/his feedback and inputs will help to inform the other steps for the next planned evaluation.

Table 15.3. Five key evaluation criteria.

	Evaluation criteria	Explanation
Activities/outputs	Relevance	Relevance and appropriateness of activities and outputs to reach expected outcomes and goals
Expected outcomes	Effectiveness	Attainment of expected outcomes
		Factors contributing to and impeding achievement of outcomes
	Efficiency	Intensity and quality of implementation of activities, including cost-effectiveness
	Impact	Positive and negative changes resulting from activities that would affect attainment of the goal, including coverage
	Sustainability	Activities or benefits continuing beyond the project or programme and factors influencing these
Goals		Likelihood of reaching goals

Box 15.1. Designing an economic evaluation.

Resources – people, time, financial, facilities, equipment and knowledge – are scarce. Choices must be made concerning their deployment. Systematic consideration of the decision to commit resources to one use instead of another is important. If some maternal and newborn health programmes cost more in terms of women's deaths or complications averted than others, then the reallocation of resources from the less to the more cost-effective programmes will result in an increase in the number of women's and newborn's lives saved and complications averted – with overall expenditure unchanged.

Economic evaluation can be defined as: the comparative analysis of alternative courses of action in terms of their costs and consequences. The basic tasks of any economic evaluation are to identify, measure, value and compare the costs and consequences of the alternatives being considered. There are various types of economic evaluation. In order of increasing complexity, the most common types are: cost–consequences analysis, cost-minimization analysis, cost-effectiveness analysis and cost–benefit analysis (Drummond *et al.*, 2005). The majority of economic evaluations consist of some form of cost-effectiveness analysis to provide better value for money.

Economic evaluation is not an exact science and some critical steps in planning a cost-effectiveness analysis of a maternal health programme include the identification of relevant costs and consequences, the perspective taken for the analysis and the magnitude and the accuracy of the costing exercise.

Resources are consumed by any health-care programme in the health-care sector, in other sectors and by the woman concerned and her family. The resources consumed in the health-care sector are relatively easy to identify, measure and value. They include drugs and other medical supplies, equipment, health workers, buildings and vehicles. The resources used by women and their families in seeking maternal care include out-of-pocket expenses in travelling to hospital and various co-payments and expenditure in the home, but often one of the most important resources consumed in health care is time. As a consequence, the resources consumed by women and their families are often difficult to identify, measure and value.

The main consequence of a maternal and newborn health programme is that the woman's health status will be changed (improved). This can be measured in terms of effects, such as deaths averted, complications averted, life-years gained or disability days reduced. It can also be valued in monetary terms, for example using the willingness-to-pay approach (Drummond *et al.*, 2005). There are common indicators in assessing effectiveness of a maternal and newborn health programme including the UN process indicators.

Another critical step is the specification of viewpoint or perspective, since an item may be a cost from one point of view but not a cost from another. For example, patients' travel costs are a cost from the patients' point of view and from the point of view of society, but not a cost from the Ministry of Health's point of view.

Regarding the accuracy and magnitude of the costing exercise, an important rule of thumb or mantra is: 'Costing can take considerable time and effort and it is important not to make the perfect the enemy of the merely good' (Drummond *et al.*, 2005). Analysts need to decide how accurate or precise cost estimates need to be within a given study.

Sensitivity analysis can and should be employed to consider the impact which different values for the main uncertain factors have upon the overall results. Some costs are so small that even a large variation in their magnitude will make little significant difference to the result of the study. It is not worth investing a great deal of time and effort considering such costs. Some costs are merely likely to confirm a result that would be obtained by consideration of a narrower range of costs. For example, the consideration of patients' costs may simply confirm a result that might be obtained from consideration of health sector operating costs alone. If analysis of patients' costs requires extra effort and the choice of programme is unlikely to be changed it may not be worthwhile to complicate the analysis unnecessarily. There are some existing resources for costing packages, which are valuable aids in economic evaluation of maternal and newborn health programmes. These costing packages differ according to which costing, financing, demographic and epidemiological components are incorporated. They include the Mother-Baby Package (WHO), Marginal Budgeting for Bottlenecks (UNICEF/World Bank), CHOICE (WHO), the Reproductive Health Costing Tool (UNFPA) and Making Pregnancy Safer (Integrated Healthcare Technology Package).

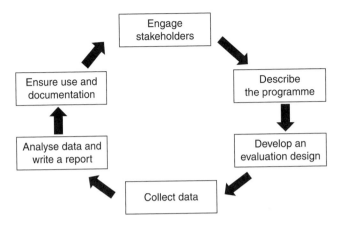

Fig. 15.3. An evaluation framework (adapted from CDC, 1999).

ENGAGE STAKEHOLDERS   Here the aim is to ensure that all stakeholders are engaged and support the evaluation from the beginning of the process. The range of perspectives and viewpoints in judging success of the programme can be taken into account by this step. It may be conducted through one-to-one interviews, focus-group discussions, surveys, workshops or even using electronic media.

DESCRIBE THE PROGRAMME   Some tools to assist in describing programmes have been discussed, such as the theory of change and logical framework. Key factors to include in a programme description are the context, stakeholders and priorities of the programme (the situation); its objectives, interventions, corresponding activities and implementation mechanisms (the programme); and monitoring and evaluation processes, human resources and budget (supporting components).

DEVELOP AN EVALUATION DESIGN   Evaluations should be designed to include inputs from a multidisciplinary technical team (epidemiologist, economist, socio-anthropologist, etc.). The design will usually need to ascertain to what extent results can be associated with or attributed to the programme (Box 15.2) but will also depend on the resources available and the requirements of decision makers regarding issues such as plausibility and probability levels. The availability of comparisons can add a crucial dimension to evaluations. Readers are referred to the numerous

resources available on evaluation designs (Habicht, 2006; Hounton *et al.*, 2008; Victora *et al.*, 2011).

COLLECT DATA   Credible data sources are required to inform the evaluation and this may be achieved by triangulating different sources. Data collection instruments, tools and methods need to be developed accordingly, avoiding unnecessary data collection or duplication by careful design of tools and advance planning of how data will be analysed.

ANALYSE DATA AND WRITE A REPORT   The evaluation team should develop an analysis plan and structure for the report before the evaluation starts. Sufficient time should be provided for this stage and the analysis will usually assess most, if not all, of the evaluation criteria discussed earlier.

ENSURE USE AND DOCUMENTATION   This last step emphasizes the need for transfer and application of the learning and evidence generated through the evaluation. The minimum requirement is to ensure the report is widely disseminated to local, regional and national stakeholders, including the international scientific and technical community where appropriate. Ideally, dissemination activities should be interactive and are more likely to be successful when stakeholders are engaged in the evaluation process and possess ownership of the findings.

Box 15.2. The need for comparisons in evaluation.

One of the common problems faced when assessing the effectiveness of programme interventions is the lack of comparison data from non-intervention facilities or areas. Without these comparisons, it will not be known whether the observed changes were due to other, non-programme activities or to background factors (such as a nationwide change in policy of fees for delivery care or closure of a nearby non-project health facility). This case study illustrates how improvements in utilization of maternity services could be inadvertently attributed to programme interventions without comparisons.

Projects 1, 2 and 3 were maternal health projects which aimed to improve availability, quality and utilization of obstetric care services. Data on delivery care utilization in 'project' and 'non-project' districts were obtained from routine health information systems from 1998 to 2006, during the time the projects were implemented. Deliveries with health professionals as a percentage of expected pregnancies are shown in Fig. 15.4.

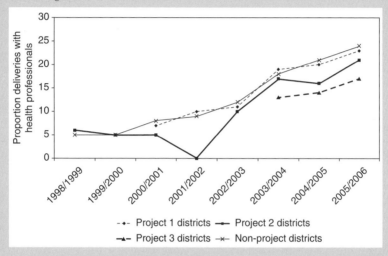

Fig. 15.4. Comparison of deliveries with health professionals in project and non-project districts (Hussein *et al.*, 2008).

If data from only the project districts were looked at, it would appear that all three projects improved the rate of deliveries with health professionals. However, by including data from the non-project districts in the analysis, it can be seen that the levels and the rate of increase of delivery attendance with health professionals in project districts and non-project districts are similar. The pattern suggests that the three projects may not have affected the proportion of births attended. Background increases in birth attendance are occurring irrespective of project interventions. Although it would be expected that project interventions would have accelerated improvements in birth attendance, the rate of change is no different in project and non-project districts.

One of the lessons learned from this analysis is that comparisons with non-intervention areas are important to include in the design of monitoring and evaluation activities. It should also be recognized that a 'non-intervention' area does not mean that nothing is happening there and that, although therefore not a true 'control', it can nevertheless be used to compare with other similar areas (Victora *et al.*, 2011).

Good Practices in Monitoring and Evaluation

Managing an evaluation

Adequate time, funding and staff should be available and allocated when a programme is designed and should be reassessed at the commencement of a programme. Evaluations should be planned early in a programme, preferably before any interventions are implemented. Too often, planning for an evaluation only happens when a mid-term review approaches or at the end of a programme.

A checklist for the main points to consider when managing an evaluation is provided in Table 15.4.

Alignment and country ownership

It is not unusual to have several monitoring results frameworks and parallel information systems for each programme in countries, often with no connection to the national health information system. Programme activities, including monitoring and evaluation efforts, should be aligned and be supportive of national processes and systems to contribute to efforts for sustainable development through, for example, use of vital registration systems and health information systems.

There has been steady progress in improving national health information systems, with advancements in data quality, development of innovations (for example, in data storage and communications technology) and integration of community data collection activities. Continued investment in and strengthening of these systems are essential to improve the efficiency of monitoring processes and to minimize duplication of effort, although there have been constraints experienced in doing so (Box 15.3).

Capacity building

When planning and implementing maternal and newborn programmes, building national capacity is often a necessity. It is currently common practice to implement donor-funded programmes with technical assistance from a northern university or research institute. We recommend support is instead obtained from national institutions whenever possible, to enable continuity, improve the follow up of implementation activities and enable timely corrections to be made based on local knowledge. National statistical or public health institutes or universities can be identified and supported to increase the likelihood of sustainability in capacity building.

Real-time monitoring of health outcomes for accountability

Recent technological advances such as mobile communication systems have provided a way forward for monitoring health outcomes now and in the future. Real-time surveillance has been made possible due to better communication systems and innovations. Countries such as Bangladesh, Cambodia, India, Madagascar and Rwanda have spearheaded efforts to make maternal mortality more visible (Box 15.4).

Conclusion

Monitoring and evaluation give feedback on whether planned interventions have been implemented. They promote accountability and provide information for planning (WHO, 2006). They require careful reflection and advance planning, as well as adequate resources in terms of technical skills, funding and time. They are not often done well, and standards can be raised by supporting commitment to the process and engendering cultural change when planning maternal and newborn health programmes. Their value as a learning exercise has been undermined by a fear of their potential threats. Without effective monitoring and evaluation, we cannot increase self reliance, know-how and accountability for effective programme implementation. Investment is required to develop innovative strategies such as real-time surveillance.

Acknowledgement

We would like to acknowledge the contributions of Samuel Mills, who reviewed this chapter and provided valuable comments and insights.

Table 15.4. Guidance for managing an evaluation.

Checklist	Description
Timing	The time from the development of the terms of reference to the finalization of the report irrespective of the size and scope of the evaluation usually requires a minimum of 12–24 months. It is therefore important to start planning early, working backwards from when the evaluation results are needed so as not to rush through the process
Terms of reference	Detailed terms of reference should be developed through a participatory process, involving all stakeholders and under the leadership of technical monitoring and evaluation advisers
Selection of evaluation team	The selection of the evaluation team is critical as team members lacking the requisite skills may cause the evaluation to fail or be unsatisfactory. Previous experience with maternal and newborn health programme evaluations in related settings and feedback from clients will assist in selecting appropriate individuals for the evaluation
Reference group	A technical reference group can advise, steer and guide the evaluation team. Individuals on the reference group should possess a mix of skills, competencies and experience. The reference group can help to refine the terms of reference
Preparatory phase	Required to arrange meetings with key stakeholders, identify focal points, ensure an inter-office memorandum for the evaluation (so that all stakeholders are kept up to date) and gather relevant programme documents
The evaluation inception phase	The evaluation team should be required to produce an evaluation inception report during this phase. This report will describe the final evaluation questions, methods and tools, elaborate on the analysis and provide a detailed work plan and timeline for the evaluation process
The evaluation desk phase	In this phase, existing literature, past reports and other programme-relevant documents will be gathered and analysed. An assessment of the feasibility of the evaluation design will be made, the hypothesis refined and the methodology for data collection, data analysis and data inference refined
The evaluation field phase	The field missions will collect primary data and assist in verifying programme deliverables as well as judge progress from target beneficiaries' perspectives
Analysis and report writing	The analysis and preliminary report should have clear, useful and practical recommendations with a timeline for implementation. They should be accompanied by alternatives with benefits and risks associated with each alternative
Feedback on preliminary findings	The reference group and other key stakeholders should reflect on preliminary findings and conclusions to provide the evaluation team with perspectives, further information or insights that may affect the interpretation and conclusions
Management response	A formal management response to the final report should be produced
Dissemination phase	This could include policy briefs, pamphlets, scientific publications and workshops for local, regional and national stakeholders
Completion and archiving	Rating of the evaluation team: a standardized rating form should be used for assessing the performance of the evaluation team Archiving: all documents relevant to the evaluation should be filed, including assessments of evaluation bids, awarding of the evaluation exercise, rating forms of the evaluation team and the final management response

Box 15.3. Vital registration in Jamaica (McCaw-Binns, Kingston, 2011, personal communication).

Use of vital registration to monitor maternal mortality should be validated in countries with civil registration systems to ensure that these relatively rare events are accurately and consistently reported. Misclassification can result in significant under-reporting. In Jamaica, some of the constraints encountered have included:

- Inadequate training and quality assurance of the practices of doctors who complete medical certificates of cause of death.
- Need to improve layout of the medical certificate of cause of death to better identify maternal deaths (for example, the check box for deaths among reproductive-age women is rarely used; the font on the certificate is too small to read, the wording is ambiguous).
- One of four health regions was treating maternal deaths as a Coroner's case, resulting in delays of up to 2 years to register these deaths and defeating the use of the system to provide reliable, up-to-date data.
- Need for WHO coding guidelines to improve identification of maternal deaths from vital records, especially indirect deaths (see Pattinson *et al.*, 2009).
- Lack of decision rules in software programmes to correctly code maternal deaths. When chronic disease rules are applied, maternal deaths are misclassified to the chronic condition, instead of the alternative pregnancy-related codes.
- Registrars not trained to look for maternal deaths among women of reproductive age by cross-referencing with registered births and fetal deaths.
- Lack of training of coders to manually code pregnancy-related deaths.

Box 15.4. Real-time surveillance.

Figures 15.5 and 15.6 illustrate the results of an active surveillance of maternal mortality in Cambodia (UNFPA, 2010), demonstrating the feasibility of timely notification of events and confirmation of cases; and the opportunities for awareness raising, advocacy and, most importantly, accountability for health service provision by monitoring. This active surveillance of pregnancy-related deaths has been made possible through technological advances in mobile and electronic communications, used to report events as they occur, thus paving the way for timely detection of changes in trends, outbreaks or recrudescence of adverse events or complications. Such information may also stimulate operational research to identify context specific determinants and improve quality of care.

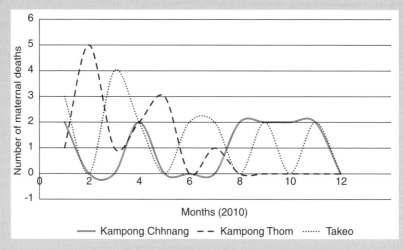

Fig. 15.5. Real-time surveillance of maternal deaths in three provinces in Cambodia (UNFPA, 2010).

Box 15.4. Continued.

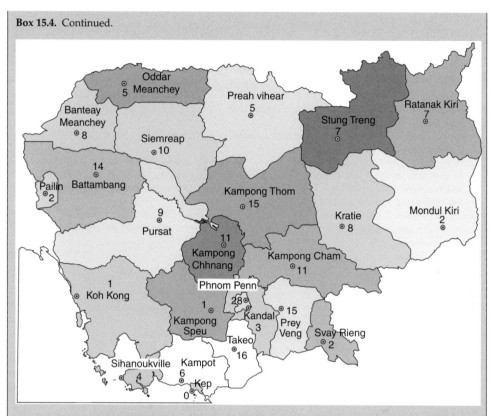

Fig. 15.6. Map of maternal deaths in Cambodia (UNFPA, 2010).

Most importantly, real-time surveillance provides the means to create accountability by generating data that can be owned by countries, is meaningful and relevant at sub-national and district levels and allows a timely and rapid response. It is currently unusual to be able to provide real-time estimates of the magnitude of mortality and morbidity. The availability of these techniques is a significant advance to the current situation. Up until now, there has been reliance either on globally modelled estimates of maternal mortality or on large scale community surveys. The modelled estimates do not engender country ownership, and they provide data often contested by policy makers in countries for lack of accuracy (McCaw-Binns and Lewis-Bell, 2010; Meda *et al.*, 2010). Large scale community surveys are expensive and require large teams of interviewers and considerable logistic support, so are usually completed only once every 5 to 10 years. In addition, estimates derived have wide confidence intervals due to the relative rarity of maternal mortality and constraints of sample sizes. Long delays are experienced in obtaining a result because data entry and cleaning take time.

We cannot continue to promote efforts that only provide information every 5 or 10 years. To monitor effectively and use monitoring to enhance accountability, data are needed to be monitored on a weekly, monthly or quarterly basis. Surveys and modelling efforts have their place, but these have to be invested in concurrently with efforts to improve systems such as real-time surveillance.

References

Adegoke, A.A., Hofman, J.J., Kongnyuy, E.J. and van den Broek, N. (2011) Monitoring and evaluation of skilled birth attendance: a proposed new framework. *Midwifery* 27(3), 350–359.

AusAID (2005) The logical framework approach. Available at: http://www.ausaid.gov.au/ausguide/pdf/ausguideline3.3.pdf (accessed 11 August 2011).

Centers for Disease Control and Prevention (CDC) (1999) Framework for program evaluation in public health. Mortality and Morbidity Weekly Report 48, No. RR–11. Available at: http://www.cdc.gov/mmwr/indrr_1999.html (accessed 11 August 2011).

DFID (2011) Guidance on using the revised logical framework. Available at: http://www.dfid.gov.uk/Documents/publications1/how-to-guid-rev-log-fmwk.pdf (accessed 11 August 2011).

Drummond, M.F., Sculpher, M.J., Torrance, G.W., O'Brien, B.J. and Stoddart, G.L. (2005) *Methods for the Economic Evaluation of Health Care Programmes*, 3rd edn. Oxford University Press, Oxford, UK.

Family Care International (2007) *The Skilled Care Initiative: Overview and Key Findings. Technical Brief.* FCI, New York.

Frechtling, J.A. (2007) *Logic Modeling Methods in Program Evaluation.* Wiley, Jossey-Bass, San Francisco, California.

Gabrysch, S., Zanger, P., Seneviratne, H.R., Mbewe, R. and Campbell, O.M.R. (2011) Tracking progress towards safe motherhood: meeting the benchmark yet missing the goal? An appeal for better use of health-system output indicators with evidence from Zambia and Sri Lanka. *Tropical Medicine and International Health* 16(5), 627–639.

Habicht, J.P., Victora, C.G. and Vaughan, J.P. (1999) Evaluation designs for adequacy, plausibility and probability of public health programme performance and impact. *International Journal of Epidemiology* 28, 10–18.

Hounton, S., Sombié, I., Meda, N., Bassane, B., Byass, P., Stanton, C. and De Brouwere, V. (2008) Methods for evaluating effectiveness and cost-effectiveness of a Skilled Care Initiative in rural Burkina Faso. *Tropical Medicine and International Health* 13, 14–24.

Hussein, J., Bell, J., Nazzar, A., Abbey, M., Adjei, S. and Graham, W.J. (2004) The Skilled Attendance Index (SAI): Proposal for a new measure of skilled attendance at delivery. *Reproductive Health Matters* 12(24), 160–170.

Hussein, J., Newlands, D., Makowiecka, K. and D'Ambruoso, L. (2008) Maternal and neonatal health review in the South Asia region. Unpublished report to the UNICEF/UNFPA/WHO steering committee for review of programmes for maternal and neonatal mortality reduction in South Asia. Ipact at University of Aberdeen, Scotland.

Immpact (2007) Immpact Toolkit: A Guide and Tools for Maternal Mortality Programme Assessment. Module 3 Designing and managing an evaluation. University of Aberdeen, Scotland. Available at: http://www.immpact-international.org/toolkit/module3/index.html (accessed 11 August 2011).

Johansson, C. and Stewart, D. (2002) *The Millennium Development Goals: Commitments and Prospects.* Human Development Report Office Working Papers and Notes: Working Paper No 1. UNDP, New York.

Kuseck, J.Z. and Rist, R.C. (2004) *Ten Steps to a Results Based Monitoring and Evaluation System: A Handbook for Development Practitioners.* World Bank, Washington, DC.

Leeuw, F.L. (2003) Reconstructing program theories: Methods available and problems to be solved. *American Journal of Evaluation* 24(1), 5–20.

McCaw-Binns, A. and Lewis-Bell, K. (2010) New modelled estimates of maternal mortality. *Lancet* 375, 1967–1968.

McLaughlin, J. and Jordan, G. (1999) Logic models: A tool for telling your program's performance story. *Evaluating and Program Planning* 22, 65–72.

MEASURE DHS (2011) Service Provision Assessments. Available at: http://www.measuredhs.com/aboutsurveys/spa/start.cfm (accessed 11 August 2011).

Meda, N., Ouedraogo, M. and Ouedraogo, L. (2010) New modelled estimates of maternal mortality. *Lancet* 375, 1965–1966.

OECD (2002) Glossary of key terms in evaluation and results based management. Available at: http://www.oecd.org/dataoecd/29/21/2754804.pdf (accessed 11 August 2011).

OECD (2011) DAC criteria for evaluating development assistance. Available at: http://www.oecd.org/document/22/0,2340,en_2649_34435_2086550_1_1_1_1,00.html (accessed 11 August 2011).

Pattinson, R., Say, L., Souza, J.P., van den Broek, N. and Rooney, C. on behalf of the Working Group on Maternal Mortality and Morbidity Classifications (2009) WHO maternal death and near-miss classifications (editorial). *Bulletin of the World Health Organanization* 87, 734.

Pawson, R. and Tilley, N. (2003) *Realistic Evaluation.* Sage Publications, London.

Roche, C. (1999) *Impact Assessment for Development Agencies: Learning to Value Change.* Oxfam, Oxford, UK.

SAFE International Research Partnership (2003) SAFE Strategy Development Tool: A guide for developing strategies to improve skilled attendance at delivery. Module 5 P 176. The Dugald Baird Centre for

Research on Women's Health, University of Aberdeen, Scotland. Available at: http://www.abdn.ac.uk/dugaldbairdcentre/safe/pdfs/sdt_manual.pdf (accessed 12 August 2011).

UNFPA (2004) The programme managers planning, monitoring and evaluation toolkit. Available at: http://www.unfpa.org/monitoring/toolkit.htm (accessed 11 August 2011).

UNFPA (2010) *Maternal Health Thematic Fund Annual Report, 2009.* UNFPA, New York.

UNICEF (2011) Multiple Indicator Cluster Surveys. Available at: http://www.unicef.org/statistics/index_24302.html (accessed 11 August 2011).

Unmet Obstetric Need Network (UON) (1999) Guide 2: Tackling Unmet Obstetric Needs Part 2: Establishment of the protocol on the collection of data. Available at: http://www.uonn.org/uonn/eng/home2.html (accessed 11 August 2011).

Victora, C.G., Black, R.E., Boerma, J.T. and Bryce, J. (2011) Measuring impact in the Millennium Development Goal era and beyond: a new approach to large-scale effectiveness evaluations. *Lancet* 377, 85–95.

Wagaarachchi, P.T., Graham, W.J., Penney, G.C., McCaw-Binns, A., Yeboah Antwi, K. and Hall, M.H. (2001) Holding up a mirror: changing obstetric practice through criterion-based clinical audit in developing countries. *International Journal of Gynaecology and Obstetrics* 74(2), 119–130.

WHO (1994) *The Mother Baby Package. Implementing Safe Motherhood in Countries. A Practical Guide.* WHO, Geneva.

WHO (2006) *Monitoring and Evaluation of Maternal and Newborn Health and Services at the District Level.* Technical consultation report, WHO, Geneva.

WHO, UNFPA, UNICEF and AMDD (2009) *Monitoring Emergency Obstetric Care: A Handbook.* WHO, Geneva.

16 Addressing Maternal Health in Emergency Settings

Linda Bartlett,[1] Iain Aitken,[2] Jeffrey Michael Smith,[3] Lisa J. Thomas,[4] Heather E. Rosen,[1] Hannah Tappis[1] and Gilbert Burnham[1]
[1]*Johns Hopkins Bloomberg School of Public Health, Baltimore, USA;* [2]*Management Sciences for Health, Cambridge, USA;* [3]*Jhpiego, Baltimore, USA;* [4]*World Health Organization, Geneva, Switzerland*

Summary

- Emergency and crises situations are special circumstances in which maternal and perinatal health programmes are required.
- Countries that have just gone through a conflict or civil war typically have among the highest maternal and newborn mortality in the world, along with other poor reproductive health indicators.
- In acute emergencies, globally endorsed best practice guidelines for response focus on urgent life-saving interventions, largely implemented by humanitarian relief agencies. Essential core services in these settings include family planning, care for labour and delivery, newborn care and emergency obstetric care to handle complications, within a 'Minimal Initial Service Package' of reproductive health interventions.
- After the acute phase, in protracted emergencies or during recovery, the priority is to strengthen the health system, with early and long-term inputs needed especially for effective leadership, health service delivery, performance monitoring and improvement and health workforce development.
- A 'Basic Package of Health Services' is being adopted in many post-conflict countries as a framework for reconstruction of the health system. Components of the package typically include the essential core services provided in the acute phase, but including a broader range of promotive, preventive and curative services.
- Although the government health system may undertake to provide health services in the post-crisis phase, the priority is to strengthen government's stewardship over health care. The delivery of services may be contracted out to non-state actors such as non-government organizations, at least until the government's human resource, supply chain and financial management capacities are built.
- Depending on the type of emergency and the extent of the destruction or development, there may also be the opportunity to introduce new health priorities and evidence-based interventions and approaches into what is left of the previous system.

Introduction

Emergency situations include natural or technological disasters, conflict, forced migration, lack of government capacity to meet basic population needs and vulnerable populations living in very poor or remote areas or under great political pressure (Nabarro, 2004; O'Heir, 2004; Bostoen *et al.*, 2007). Fragile states lack the capacity or are so overwhelmed by emergency situations that they cannot perform the basic functions of the state – maintaining security across their terrain, enabling economic development and ensuring that the essential needs of the population are met. A crisis is a humanitarian situation characterized by damage to infrastructure or the environment, loss of human life and deterioration of basic services on a scale sufficient to warrant an extraordinary response from outside the affected community, or where populations such as refugees or internally displaced persons face extreme vulnerabilities and challenges in meeting basic needs for survival (Relief Web Project, 2008).

Reproductive health in emergency settings has gained recognition as a public health issue (O'Heir, 2004; Anderlini, 2010). Approaches and frameworks in emergency settings address reproductive health holistically, but in this chapter specific issues related to maternal health service response in emergencies are highlighted. An overview of the challenges related to maternal health is provided with discussion on the information, resources and strategies needed for planning and delivering maternal health services. Two main phases of emergencies are used as a framework, the acute phase and a protracted/recovery phase.

Trends in Emergency Situations

The number of acute and protracted emergencies requiring humanitarian assistance has doubled in the past 30 years (Noji, 2005; WHO, 2008a; CRED, 2009; Guha-Sapir *et al.*, 2011). Figure 16.1 shows trends in natural and technological disasters and armed conflicts since 1945, alongside global population growth. The increase in frequency of disasters is due to several factors, including: population growth and urbanization resulting in more people living in geographically or politically vulnerable areas; increasing hazardous technology; environmental degradation; and climate change.

The frequency of these types of emergencies is projected to increase (Noji, 2005; CRED, 2009). Although the number of active armed conflicts has remained relatively stable over the same time period, the number of people living in conflict and disaster affected settings with increased health risks and limited access to essential services continues to grow. The 2011 World Development Report focused on 'Conflict, Security and Development', reporting that 1.5 billion people were subjected to conflict or were living in fragile states: a staggering 'one in four persons on the planet'.

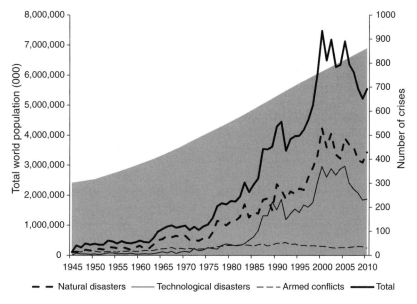

Fig. 16.1. Trends in numbers of crises and world population, 1945–2010 (CRED, 2009; UNESA 2010).

Forty two million people are refugees or internally displaced (World Bank, 2011). UNHCR reports an equivalent figure of people forcibly displaced around the world, the highest number of people uprooted by conflict and persecution since the mid-1990s (UNHCR, 2011a). Millions of those affected by humanitarian disasters and conflict have been living in protracted emergency situations with no option of return, reintegration or recovery for more than 10 years.

Maternal and Perinatal Health in Emergencies

Although the impact of humanitarian situations on health may vary by the type, phase and duration of the disaster (WHO, 2000a), generally the populations most affected are poor, with high fertility, low general health and poor nutrition status, alongside high burdens of morbidity and mortality, including maternal mortality. The populations face higher risk of injury, death and, commonly, enormous socio-economic pressures as homes, livelihoods and families are lost. Typically, they live in environments with insufficient access to quality preventive and curative health-care services. Women, particularly pregnant and postpartum women, are an especially vulnerable group.

Afghanistan, Chad, Somalia and Guinea-Bissau, with an extremely high maternal mortality ratio of greater than 1000 maternal deaths per 100,000 live births, are on the World Bank's list of fragile situations (World Bank, 2010), as are eight of the ten countries in sub-Saharan Africa with the highest maternal mortality (WHO, 2010). An ecologic analysis comparing 21 countries that had recently experienced conflict and 21 that had not indicated significantly higher maternal and neonatal mortality rates in the conflict-affected countries (O'Hare and Southall, 2007). Apart from higher maternal and neonatal mortality, other reported maternity-related effects of emergency situations include preterm birth, low birth weight, spontaneous abortions and congenital defects in the fetus such as orofacial and neural tube defects associated with inadequate nutrition during pregnancy or exposure to noxious substances (Cordero, 1993; Ahuka *et al.*, 2004, 2006; Kelsey *et al.*, 2011).

Given the clear vulnerability of pregnant women, heightened risk of maternal and perinatal mortality during the emergency phases of disasters is very likely (McGinn, 2000; RAISE, 2007). Research shows that some displaced populations that have crossed borders and settled in stable refugee camps with dedicated health-care services provided by aid agencies have lower risks of maternal and newborn mortality than those of host populations, indicating that the provision of adequate maternity services in emergencies not only is possible but also ameliorates excess mortality (Bartlett, 2000; Hynes, 2000; McGinn, 2000). Access to services may be straightforward in a well-established refugee-camp setting. However, less than half of current refugees live in camps. A small proportion live among rural host communities and most are integrated among urban host-country populations (Spiegel *et al.*, 2010). Self-settled or scattered refugees often live at the legal and social margins of society and fear that if they seek services they will expose uncertain or even illegal residence status, subjecting themselves and their families to actions by local authorities. Access to services may be even more challenging for internally displaced people who do not cross international borders.

Emergency management includes elements of: disaster risk reduction and emergency preparedness (before a crisis); emergency response/relief (at the onset of a crisis); recovery (after the acute phase); and transition to development. More recently, 'protracted emergencies' have been recognized, defined as countries requiring assistance for more than 8 years or where refugees have lived in exile for more than 5 years (Relief Web Project, 2008). Frequently, there is no clear-cut boundary between the relief and recovery periods. In many settings, such as protracted emergencies, the phases do not necessarily occur linearly in time and may either overlap or cycle between phases.

Figure 16.2 depicts the overall impact of an emergency, which affects context, health

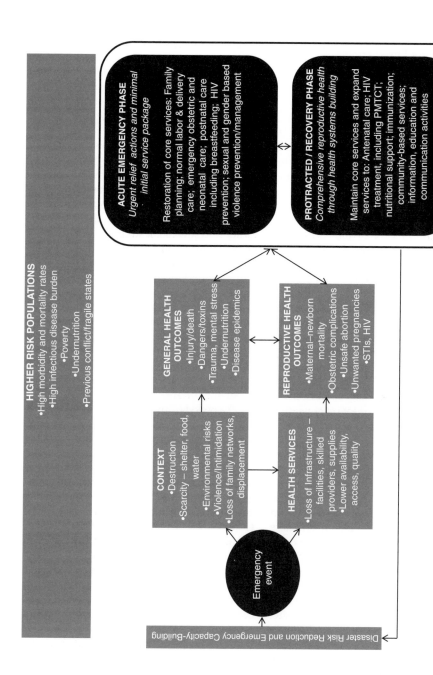

Fig. 16.2. Impact of emergency on maternal health and responses in differing phases.

services and health outcomes. Responses in the two phases of acute emergencies and protracted/recovery settings are outlined.

Acute Emergencies

Needs and challenges

In the acute phase of an emergency, health services and other infrastructure necessary for survival such as water, food distribution, shelter and sanitation may be destroyed. Deaths from injuries due directly to the event and morbidity ensue rapidly, as do exposure to environmental risks and potential violence, intimidation or displacement. Fewer health facilities may be functional due to physical destruction or isolation, whether due to conflict or natural disasters such as floods or earthquakes. Within the facilities, fewer health-care providers may be available due to factors such as: the possibility of their own injury or death; the need to care for their own families or flee the site; and inability to reach the health facility due to insecurity or destruction of infrastructure. Medical supplies and equipment for services such as EmOC may be unavailable due to destruction of facilities during the disaster or because they have been used for other medical and surgical emergencies. A review of EmOC in 31 facilities in nine conflict-affected countries found important shortcomings at most sites from both structural and human resource perspectives (Krause *et al.*, 2006).

Identifying the most vulnerable populations and providing services are difficult in both rural and urban situations and where there is insecurity, human rights abuses or restrictive cultures. For example, the civil war in Sri Lanka (1983–2009) resulted in understaffing and inability to provide emergency obstetric care at many hospitals (Kottegoda *et al.*, 2008). Available staff often lacked adequate technical capacity (Nagai *et al.*, 2007). As a consequence, the number of home deliveries increased in areas affected by fighting compared with unaffected areas. Even where services are available, persons displaced by conflict or natural disaster may not know about them, either because maternal health

services were not readily available where they previously lived or because they have low expectations of services in the new location. Consequently, displaced women may not actively seek health care. Among traditional households in Afghanistan, especially under the Taliban, women often lacked the knowledge to make appropriate decisions about seeking obstetric care (Williams and McCarthy, 2005).

Planning maternity services

The first step in planning for programme response to deliver essential maternal health services is to obtain information on the magnitude and severity of the crisis and the needs of the target population. Basic data required include the number of people affected, geographical distribution, physical access issues, health status and risk, number of women of reproductive age, estimated number of pregnant and postpartum women and their newborns and the availability of functioning obstetric health services (see Phoya *et al.*, Chapter 10 this volume). An interagency working group has developed a field manual for such assessments (IAWG, 2010).

Knowledge of pre-crisis reproductive health indicators such as the maternal mortality ratio, crude birth rate, abortion rate, contraceptive prevalence rate and percentage of births at health facilities can help guide programmatic response. Sources for pre-emergency data include health surveillance and health facility and survey data (see Hounton *et al.*, Chapter 15 this volume). Listings of health facilities by type are often available from the ministry of health, UN and non-government organizations working in the area. Much of the information on the extent of a crisis and population affected is compiled into situation reports, published online by the UN Office for the Coordination of Humanitarian Affairs (UN, undated) and WHO's Health Action for Emergencies programme (WHO, 2011). Other tools and resources to support rapid assessment in the acute emergency phase are available (IASC, 2007; WHO, 2009; UNHCR, 2011b).

Delivering services

Focus should be on relief efforts to provide essential life-saving assistance. Core services must be made available as rapidly as possible. These include family planning to prevent mistimed or unwanted pregnancies, normal labour, delivery and immediate postpartum and newborn care and EmOC to handle complications when they arise. To implement services, facilities where surgical procedures can be performed and health services can be provided must be identified and supported by assigning appropriate personnel and ensuring that adequate medical supplies and equipment are available. Community outreach can be implemented to identify pregnant and postpartum women and inform them of services. An effective referral system should reflect awareness of the area's current security and geographical, transport and communication constraints. Additional beds, equipment, supplies, medicines and human resources should also be provided to support the referral facility as necessary. Linkages with other sectors or clusters such as protection,

shelter, water and sanitation, nutrition and education and psychosocial support for women and girls should also be encouraged as much as possible. Several best practice guidance documents to help guide the delivery and management of maternity and reproductive health services in acute emergencies are available (Box 16.1).

A case study of the Haitian earthquake in 2010 demonstrates the services delivered as a result of recently improved awareness of reproductive health needs in emergency situations (Box 16.2).

Protracted Emergencies and Post-Crisis Recovery

Needs and challenges

In protracted emergencies and periods of transition and recovery from acute crisis situations, needs and challenges turn from providing essential life-saving assistance to rebuilding or establishing national capacity

---

Box 16.1. Guides for delivering reproductive health services in emergencies.

1. WHO's Health Cluster Guide has fully integrated reproductive health in its guidelines for situation mapping, immediate impact activities, key indicators, checklists and references: http://www.who.int/hac/network/global_health_cluster/guide/en/index.html
2. The Inter-agency Working Group for Reproductive Health in Emergencies provides a manual with information on the elements of a standard 'Minimal Initial Service Package' of reproductive health interventions that should be provided in all emergency settings to reduce excess maternal and newborn morbidity and mortality, prevent and manage the consequences of sexual violence and reduce HIV transmission: http://www.iawg.net/resources/field_manual.html
3. UNFPA and Save the Children have produced a companion volume to the above, an Adolescent Sexual and Reproductive Health Toolkit in Humanitarian Settings: http://www.unfpa.org/public/publications/pid/4169
4. A reproductive Health Kit for Emergency Situations is available as a standardized, affordable and quickly available list of essential medicines and medical devices that are urgently needed during emergencies. The kit contains approximately 170 different products in sufficient quantities to meet the initial primary health-care needs of approximately 10,000 crisis-affected people for 3 months: http://www.rhrc.org/resources/general_fieldtools/unfpa_rhkit.htm
5. The Women's Commission for Refugee Women and Children has developed a field guide on how to integrate emergency obstetric care within emergency programmes: http://www.rhrc.org/resources/emoc/EmOC_ffg.pdf
6. WHO's document entitled 'Key steps for maternal and newborn health care in humanitarian crises' outlines programme responses and includes a needs assessment planning tool where indicators to estimate the number of pregnant women and newborns are identified, plus a checklist for facility and service availability: http://www.who.int/making_pregnancy_safer/documents/keysteps.pdf

Box 16.2. Reproductive health services and the 2010 Haitian earthquake.

The Haitian earthquake of 12 January 2010 caused widespread death, injury and displacement. Like many disasters it created major reproductive health needs. But unlike many instances there was early and consistent attention paid to reproductive health needs by donors, responders and the media. Provision of the Minimal Initial Service Package for reproductive services began early, with the Interagency Reproductive Health Kits being available within days (see Box 16.1). Eventually these kits supported the provision of the minimal package to a population of 1.5 million concentrated in Port-au-Prince and surrounding areas.

Within the overall response, coordination of reproductive health issues was carried out by UNFPA as part of the health cluster activities. This worked well at the national level but less well at sub-national levels. Among problems seen were a failure to adequately involve Haitian non-government organizations and difficulties coordinating with other clusters. A surveillance system to track key reproductive health indicators was set up by the Centers for Disease Control. Participation was sporadic by some non-government organizations, yet with data from the sentinel surveillance system useful data were available to monitor needs.

Sexual violence became a considerable public health problem (Women's Refugee Commission, 2011). Centres were established shortly after the surveillance system reported it as a problem, enabling organizations to provide clinical and psychological support for victims. Widespread distribution of referral cards to clinical services built a high level of awareness among health providers. However, knowledge about where to receive services did not seem to diffuse well into the community. Even where established, these services had to compete for space with orthopaedic services and sometimes had limited privacy.

Preventing HIV transmission post-earthquake was an important activity in Haiti. These efforts built on an extensive pre-existing HIV programme. Starting within the first few weeks, 7 million male condoms were distributed, which met demands in Port-au-Prince, but did not fully reach areas that were more distant. Disposal of medical waste, a key element in universal precautions, proved difficult for smaller temporary health units. Antiretroviral therapy distribution started early and was sustained post-disaster.

Provision of free emergency obstetrical and newborn care was a priority, being established within days of the earthquake. In Port-au-Prince, 24-h services were provided, but the mobile clinics that provided maternal care for other areas could not provide this consistently. Further, the difficulty with transport made it difficult for many women to access those services that were available. Large numbers of clean delivery kits were distributed to support home deliveries, beginning within weeks after the earthquake. Keeping contraceptive methods readily available to all areas at times proved difficult.

As time passed, the initial levels of coordination and ready availability of supplies began to wane. As in many other relief services, there was poor utilization of local, non-government capacities. The rapid turnover among relief staff made it difficult to sustain initial efforts. However, most observers felt that reproductive health services were available within 1 or 2 weeks after the earthquake in some locations, eventually reaching many, but not all, affected populations (CARE *et al.*, 2011).

and systems for delivering health services and achieving development goals. Core services must still be maintained: family planning, normal labour, delivery and immediate postpartum and newborn care and EmOC. In addition, services should be expanded to include a fuller array of clinical and public health services such as antenatal care, HIV treatment and prevention, nutritional support and information and education interventions. Building the health system's capacity to establish functional and comprehensive obstetric care must begin early in the protracted or

recovery phase of an emergency (WHO and World Bank, 2005).

Humanitarian actors in protracted situations must recognize the long term nature of displacement and strive to provide more than the Minimal Initial Service Package. Programme design should ensure that populations affected can gain knowledge and skills to address maternal health issues as recovery from the emergency ensues or after repatriation and resettlement in the case of refugees.

A careful analysis of the political, economic and social situation is the first step in establishing effective maternal health services as the emergency stabilizes and reconstruction begins. The next step is to determine the most appropriate way to ensure that both immediate and longer term maternal health needs are considered in health-system strengthening and service delivery strategies (Burnham *et al.*, 2003). The transition from the relief phase to the recovery phase is a complex process and is often accompanied by a hiatus in effective support to health services. Figure 16.3 illustrates some of the key features. The relief phase during the conflict focuses on service delivery to save lives and is often led by international actors – independent of state – because of either limited capacity of the government or its being overwhelmed such that it cannot provide services. Funding is generally short term and precludes expenditures on long-term development activities. In the recovery phase, priorities turn to development goals, systems strengthening and increasing partnerships with establishing governments and local partners. Funding comes from different sources or allocations and development assistance is supplied by development agencies.

The immediate post-crisis period may be a time of opportunity for both state-building and the development of health services. There are renewed energy and enthusiasm and the return of exiles with skills and resources. Favourable international relationships result in expanded aid and direct investment. Depending on the type of emergency and the extent of the destruction or development,

there may also be the opportunity to introduce new priorities, interventions and approaches into what is left of the previous system. In places where emergencies have left little to no infrastructure, substantial or complete rebuilding may be necessary. The prospect to refresh considerations of equity, gender mainstreaming and evidence-based decision making into policy-making processes also exist (WHO and World Bank, 2005; Waldman, 2006; Gruber, 2009).

Planning services

In protracted emergencies and recovery phases, there is an opportunity to build on the information gathered during the acute phase using a greater variety of data collection methods. Health facility data are rich sources of information, for example, by using the UN process indicators (see Hounton *et al.*, Chapter 15 this volume). Many other standard tools for general use can be exploited, including those to assess the health management information systems (WHO, 2008b), facility reviews of maternal deaths or severe maternal morbidities and various quality improvement toolkits (see also Achadi *et al.*, Chapter 14 this volume) and some have been applied in recovery settings (Massoud *et al.*, 2001; WHO, 2008b; JHPIEGO, 2011).

In protracted emergencies, data may be available from humanitarian agency health information systems. UNHCR and its partners have developed and implemented a standardized system to support health facility data management in refugee camps and national governments that host them. It is now used to monitor refugee health programmes in both new and long-established refugee camps in at least 17 countries across Africa, Asia and the Middle East (Haskew *et al.*, 2010).

Qualitative research methods such as interviews and focus groups can also be used to understand better the knowledge, attitudes, beliefs and health-care-seeking practices of women, their families and communities. These provide information on how women, their husbands and families and community

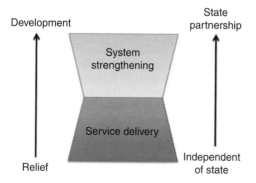

Fig. 16.3. The transition from relief to development (Vergeer *et al.*, 2009).

leaders perceive maternal health and the barriers that contribute to women dying, in order to guide rapid improvements to health programmes (UNFPA, 2010). Guides on methods for collecting data by rapid assessment and through surveys in communities affected by conflict are available (RHRC, 2004; CDC, 2007; ACAPS, 2011).

Delivering services

Establishing effective reproductive health services requires much more than just reconstituting pre-crisis services, which may have been inadequate. Building health services cannot be thought of as a merely technical exercise: it is a political and social process whose success depends upon the quality of governance and social justice. Reconstituting basic health services is a necessary condition for overcoming fragility and should be an early target for donors, but it is not a sufficient condition. The process of reconstructing health services needs to contribute to the legitimacy and strengthening of the state, for example, by improving the capacity and credibility of government or the ministry of health (WHO and World Bank, 2005). Each situation has its own special features, but several important generalizations will apply to the development of an appropriate approach. Key principles have been articulated by the Granada Consensus on Sexual and Reproductive Health in Protracted Emergencies and Recovery (UNFPA *et al.*, 2009) as follows:

1. Mainstream sexual and reproductive health in all health policies and strategies that aim to revitalize the health system during the recovery period and/or a protracted crisis.
2. Achieve sustainable consolidation and expansion of sexual and reproductive health services in protracted crises and recovery.
3. Secure the commitment of humanitarian and development actors to bridge the current service delivery and funding gaps.
4. Recognize and support the leadership role of national and local authorities, communities and beneficiaries in ensuring sexual and reproductive health.

One fundamental objective highlighted during the Granada consultation was to work towards quick, equitable and sustainable scaling up of sexual and reproductive health services. This can only be achieved through health systems strengthening, occurring within the framework of harmonized and coherent cross-sectoral policy, planning and action (WHO and World Bank, 2005; WHO, 2008a). The establishment of maternal and other priority health services in any country requires functionality of all aspects of the health system: effective leadership, the design and implementation of health services, information systems for initial assessment as well as ongoing monitoring and evaluation, human resources development and management and the supply of medical products and financing (see Mavalankar and Sankara Raman, Chapter 6 this volume). Some of these components are discussed here with specific reference to post-crisis recovery.

Building the health system

There are two main roles to play in management of a health system: stewardship and health-care delivery. The beginning of the recovery period is the time to decide which of these two roles the government will take responsibility for, especially as resources must be targeted carefully.

Typically, in fragile states that deteriorate into civil war, the voice of citizens gets heard less and less by those in government. Stewardship, support, incentives and supervision within the health system become increasingly weak (Roberts *et al.*, 2008). Services deteriorate from lack of supplies and staff motivation, and citizens seek health care from traditional sources or private providers. At the beginning of the recovery and development phase, service provision might have to rely on non-government mechanisms for finance, technical assistance and oversight. But over 5–10 year periods post crises reassumption of the stewardship role by government is important for long term health systems development.

Leadership and management

Stewardship comprises a set of functions concerned with policy, strategy and standards, the supply and allocation of resources and the monitoring and evaluation of services (WHO, 2000b). Even though the new administration may not have all the skills required to fulfil this role, stewardship of health care is recognized as a clear mandate of government.

Although the government health system may undertake to provide health services, priority is often on strengthening government's stewardship over health care, with delivery of services contracted out to non-state actors such as non-government organizations, at least until the government's human resources, supply chain and financial management capacities are built (Loevinsohn and Harding, 2004; Palmer, 2006). This makes good use of the experience and staff of the organizations that have been providing care during the conflict. This approach was tried nationwide in Afghanistan and on a limited scale in Cambodia and is now being used in other humanitarian settings such as Haiti, Rwanda, Liberia and southern Sudan (Roberts et al., 2008; Abramson, 2009).

Health services

Increasingly, a 'Basic Package of Health Services' is being adopted in post-conflict countries as both a framework for reconstruction of the health system and a policy to guide donors and implementers (Roberts et al., 2008). Such a policy document should be the result of a consensus process. The package specifies what activities are to be performed by each level of the health services and what staffing, equipment, drugs and supplies are required for their effective implementation. Essential components of the package typically include: maternal, newborn and child health; family planning; control of major infectious diseases; and management of common medical and surgical problems.

Community-based delivery of services is promoted, especially in countries where women's access to health facilities is constrained by distance, insecurity, culture or a combination of these. Interventions include provision of birth spacing methods, prevention of anaemia and malaria in pregnancy with micronutrients, haematinics, vaccination, intermittent preventive treatment for malaria, distribution of insecticide-treated bed nets and clean delivery kits, health promotion (information, education) and assisting women to access skilled care. Other community-based interventions currently being assessed include calcium supplementation and low dose aspirin to reduce incidence of severe pre-eclampsia and eclampsia (Campbell and Graham, 2006; Bhutta et al., 2008; see also Langer et al., Chapter 8 this volume). Misoprostol for the prevention and treatment of postpartum haemorrhage has shown promise in settings where skilled providers or the recommended injectable uterotonics such as oxytocin are not available (IAWG, 2010).

Delivery in a health facility by a midwife with referral capacity for comprehensive EmOC when needed is the ideal model (Baqui et al., 2008). Many of the fragile states that suffer from emergencies are countries with strong cultural traditions of traditional birth attendants and, typically, any earlier gains in the use of health professionals are lost with the onset of a humanitarian crisis. Creating a network of complementary first-referral hospitals with appropriately trained staff to provide EmOC (see Phoya et al., Chapter 10 this volume) is challenging due to resource limitations but programmes are in place. For example, the UK-based charity Merlin has established a midwifery training programme with the Ministry of Health and Social Welfare in Liberia (Keith, 2011). The Afghanistan Midwifery Education Programme has established 34 schools in 31 provinces serving women from all 34 provinces (Box 16.3). Education standards were developed and endorsed by the ministry of public health and a rigorous peer-reviewed school accreditation process put into place (Smith et al., 2008).

In situations of protracted crisis or the transition and recovery period, alternative service delivery models may be required. In eastern Burma, civil war and human rights violations were a major factor discouraging women and families from seeking antenatal

---

Box 16.3. The midwifery education programme in Afghanistan.

After 23 years of war and isolation, maternal health services in Afghanistan in 2002 were among the worst in the world. An early strategic focus of the Afghan Ministry of Public Health for expanding maternal health services was the education and deployment of large numbers of midwives. The major donors for Afghanistan supported two pre-service education programmes to train and graduate new midwives. The first programme aimed to strengthen existing institutes of health sciences for the placement of graduates in provincial, regional and national or speciality hospitals. The second programme established community midwifery education for community-based providers. Technical support was provided to lead the technical and quality components of the midwifery education programme.

The desire to rapidly open large numbers of midwifery schools created the potential for non-standardized educational approaches, which could have deepened the human resource crisis by deploying new but unskilled midwives, undermining the public's confidence in the concept of skilled care at birth. Therefore, a standards-based accreditation system was put in place to structure the process of establishing midwifery schools and to give the government a regulatory system through which to judge and mandate the quality of education.

Since 2004, when the first graduates were deployed, 34 education programmes (five within the institutes of health sciences and 29 as part of the community midwifery education initiative) were established in 31 provinces, serving all 34 provinces. As of the end of 2011, more than 2700 women will have graduated as midwives – an increase of five times the 467 midwives available in 2002. Assessments have shown that the rates of antenatal care and births with midwives increased substantially in provinces with midwifery schools, compared to those without. Focus groups among women in communities indicated that women were uniformly positive about the services that the midwives provided and their professionalism.

---

care and family planning services. The Back-Pack Health Worker Team, an independent community-based organization, used mobile workers to reach these communities with these services on a regular basis (Mullany *et al.*, 2008). Another successful alternative delivery model comes from northern Pakistan, where ethnic tensions prevented Sunni Islam women from seeking obstetric care and resulted in an increased maternal mortality. A Sunni Civil Hospital was established as a community initiative to cater to the excluded population (Varley, 2010).

Performance monitoring and improvement

Performance improvement under contracts has been achieved in four main ways: monitoring and evaluation, quality improvement mechanisms, technical assistance and performance-based incentives (Waldman, 2006; Sondorp *et al.*, 2009). Monitoring and evaluation are achieved through the health management information system, periodic household surveys and facility surveys. Standards-based quality improvement approaches have been applied in both state and contracted out

health systems. If provided, technical assistance may be in financial and organizational management, leadership and management of public health programmes, the implementation of specific training programmes, quality improvement activities, the provision of behaviour change communication materials and training in interpersonal communication skills.

Performance-based contracting is a variation on contracting out of services, which incorporates financial bonuses as incentives for reaching specific performance targets for priority programmes (Sondorp *et al.*, 2009). Rwanda has been cited as having long experience of performance-based contracts, with performance indicators measuring quality as well as quantity (Meessen *et al.*, 2006; Soeters *et al.*, 2006; Basinga *et al.*, 2010).

Health workforce development and management

During times of crisis human resource structures break down and mechanisms for preparing, maintaining and regulating the performance of health workers lose priority.

Access to training and professional development is typically restricted during times of conflict and hardship and health workers may go many years without updating their knowledge and skills. The need to improvise during times of crisis can result in the emergence of new, unofficial cadres of health workers without a globally recognized set of competencies.

A post-crisis approach to health systems reconstruction must include: a census of types, numbers and distribution of health workers; an analysis of health worker roles, qualifications and performance; an expansion of worker capacity to provide clearly defined sets of family planning and maternal and newborn health services; and a rebuilding of the institutions that educate and license health workers and regulate their performance (WHO, 2005). An early priority is to 'normalize' the maternal and newborn health workforce to determine how to regroup these cadres and where training is needed. This process of normalization rests upon the presence of a clearly defined package of maternal health services and a clear definition of who should provide those services.

As the roles of specific health worker cadres and the packages of health services they should deliver are clearly defined, the institutions and systems that support those health workers should also be supported to reemerge. Human resource policies and standards of practice for maternal health care providers should be prepared. Pre-service education institutions should be supported to revise curricula and be re-equipped to teach new clinical skills that may not have been included in prior curricula. Pre-service faculty must be brought up to date so they have the current knowledge as well as the clinical and pedagogic skills needed to prepare students. Processes for recruitment and selection of students must be modified and at times relaxed to allow for the admission of students from isolated, insecure and remote areas. Accreditation systems should be put in place to ensure that when schools reopen or new schools are established they meet a minimum set of educational standards (Box 16.3).

This process of institution building in post-conflict situations is also necessary to reestablish the credibility and accountability of health workers. In order to stimulate the demand for maternal and newborn health services among a potentially reluctant or cautious population, it is important to publicly and transparently clarify and declare that the chosen cadre, be they midwives, nurses, doctors or a combination, are the appropriate health workers to provide maternal health services and that the system is ensuring their readiness to work and their capacity to function. At the same time, these re-emerging professions must be held accountable to both the community and the system to provide high quality services according to a nationally defined set of standards or guidelines.

Conclusion

An acute emergency requires rapid deployment of resources to provide the core services to provide contraception, normal labour, delivery and essential newborn care and EmOC to manage complications. Organization of the response among relief organizations is important to ensure that no gaps in service or major overlaps occur. Community-based activities to refer women for skilled care during childbirth and for distribution of evidence-based interventions will help reach the majority of women of reproductive age, pregnant and postpartum women and their newborns.

In protracted emergencies and the recovery phase, a systematic rebuilding of the health system is necessary. Coordination and communication among actors, agencies and the local government are essential as is early consideration of a long term sustainable programme. Core services must continue to be maintained and expanded into a broader array of reproductive health services.

Several best practice standards exist that provide clear guidance on detailed implementation, although further understanding of the best practices for response in emergencies is needed. Retrospective evaluations can provide lessons learned but prospective evaluation is required to best inform future response efforts.

References

Abramson, W.B. (2009) Chapter 1 Lessons from Cambodia, Guatemala and Liberia. In: *Contracting out Health Services in Post-Conflict and Fragile Situations*. OECD, Paris, pp. 17–43. DOI: 10.1787/9789264066212-2-en. Available at: http://www.oecd-ilibrary.org/development/contracting-out-government-functions-and-services/contracting-out-health-services-in-post-conflict-and-fragile-situations_9789264066212-2-en (accessed 30 August 2011).

Ahuka, O.L., Chabikuli, N. and Ogunbanjo, G.A. (2004) The effects of armed conflict on pregnancy outcomes in the Congo. *International Journal of Gynecology and Obstetrics* 84(1), 91–92.

Ahuka, O.L., Toko, R.M., Omanga, F.U. and Tshimpanga, B.J. (2006) Congenital malformations in the north-eastern Democratic Republic of Congo during civil war. *East African Medical Journal* 83(2), 95–99.

Anderlini, S. (2010) Gender Background Paper. International Civil Society Action Network, Washington, DC and Center for International Studies, Massachusetts Institute of Technology, Cambridge, Massachusetts. In: *World development Report 2011. Conflict, Security and Development*. World Bank 2011, p. 6. Available at: http://wdr2011.worldbank.org/fulltext (accessed 27 July 2011).

Assessment Capacities Project (ACAPS) (2011) Technical brief: Direct observation and key informant techniques for primary data collection in rapid assessments. Available at: http://www.acaps.org/img/documents/direct-observation-and-key-informant-interview-techniques-direct-observation-and-key-informant-interview-techniques.pdf (accessed 30 August 2011).

Baqui, A.H., El-Arifeen, S., Darmstadt, G.L., Ahmed, S., Williams, E.K., Seraji, H.R., Mannan, I., Rahman, S.M., Shah, R., Saha, S.K., Syed, U., Winch, P.J., Lefevre, A., Santosham, M. and Black, R.E. for the Projahnmo Study Group (2008) Effect of community-based newborn-care intervention package implemented through two service-delivery strategies in Sylhet district, Bangladesh: a cluster-randomised controlled trial. *Lancet* 371(9628), 1936–1944.

Bartlett, L. (2000) The burden of mortality due to reproductive health-related causes among Afghan refugees in Pakistan. In: *Conference Proceedings: Findings on Reproductive Health of Refugees and Displaced Populations*, 5–6 December 2000. InterAction and the Global Health Council, Washington, DC.

Basinga, P., Gertler, P.J., Binagwaho, A., Soucat, A.L.B., Sturdy, J.R. and Vermeersch, C.M.J. (2010) *Policy Research Working Paper 5190 Paying Primary Health Care Centers for Performance in Rwanda*. The World Bank, Washington, DC.

Bhutta, Z.A., Ali, S., Cousens, S., Ali, T.M., Haider, B.A., Rizvi, A., Okong, P., Bhutta, S.Z. and Black, R.E. (2008) Alma Ata: Interventions to address MNC survivals: what difference can integrated primary health care strategies make? *Lancet* 372(9642), 972–989.

Bostoen, K., Bilukha, O.O., Fenn, B., Morgan, O.W., Tam, C.C., ter Veen, A. and Checchi, F. (2007) Methods for health surveys in difficult settings: charting progress, moving forward. *Emerging Themes in Epidemiology* 4, 13.

Burnham, G.M., Rowley, E.A. and Ovberedjo, M.O. (2003) Quality design: a planning methodology for the integration of refugee and local health services, West Nile, Uganda. *Disasters* 27, 54–71.

Campbell, O.M. and Graham, W.J. for the Lancet Maternal Survival Series steering group (2006) Strategies for reducing maternal mortality: Getting on with what works. *Lancet* 368(9543), 1284–1299.

CARE, International Planned Parenthood Federation, Save the Children and the Women's Refugee Commission (2011) Priority Reproductive Health Activities in Haiti. Available at: http://www.iawg.net/resources/Priority%20RH%20in%20Haiti_comprehensive%20report_2.21.2011.pdf (accessed 30 August 2011).

Centers for Disease Control and Prevention (CDC) (2007) *Reproductive Health Assessment Toolkit for Conflict-Affected Women Division of Reproductive Health*. National Center for Chronic Disease Prevention and Health Promotion, Coordinating Center for Health, Atlanta, Georgia.

Centre for Research on the Epidemiology of Disasters (CRED) (2009) Complex emergency database. Available at: http://www.cedat.be (accessed 20 August 2011).

Cordero, J.F. (1993) The epidemiology of disasters and adverse reproductive outcomes: lessons learned. *Environmental Health Perspectives* 101(Suppl. 2), 131–136.

Gruber, J. (2009) Technical assistance for health in non-conflict fragile states: challenges and opportunities. *International Journal of Health Planning and Management* 24, S4–S20.

Guha-Sapir, D., Vos, F., Below, R. and Ponserre, S. (2011) *Annual Disaster Statistical Review 2010: The Numbers and Trends*. Centre for Research on the Epidemiology of Disasters, Brussels.

Haskew, C., Spiegel, P., Tomczyk, B., Cornier, N. and Hering, H. (2010) A standardized health information system for refugee settings: rationale, challenges and the way forward. *Bulletin of the World Health Organization* 88, 792–794.

Hynes, M. (2000) Reproductive health indicators of displaced persons in post-emergency phase camps of humanitarian emergencies. In: *Conference Proceedings: Findings on Reproductive Health of Refugees and Displaced Populations*, 5–6 December 2000. InterAction and the Global Health Council, Washington, DC.

Inter-Agency Standing Committee (IASC) (2007) Initial Rapid Assessment Tool. Available at: http://www.humanitarianreform.org/humanitarianreform/Default.aspx?tabid=153 (accessed 30 August 2011).

Inter-Agency Working Group (IAWG) (2010) Field manual on reproductive health in humanitarian settings: 2010 version for field testing, Inter Agency Working Group on Reproductive Health in Crises. Available at: http://www.iawg.net/resources/field_manual.html (accessed 31 August 2011).

JHPIEGO (2011) Standards based management and recognition – a field guide. Available at: http://www.jhpiego.jhu.edu/resources/pubs/sbmr/sbmr_manual_dist.pdf (accessed 6 April 2011).

Keith, R. (2011) All mothers matter: investing in health workers to save lives in fragile states. Merlin, London. Available at: http://www.merlin.org.uk/sites/default/files/All_Mothers_Matter_1010_lowres(2).pdf (accessed 30 August 2011).

Kelsey, N., Dancause, D.P., Laplante, C.O., Fraser, S., Brunet, A. and King, S. (2011) Disaster-related prenatal maternal stress influences birth outcomes: Project Ice Storm. *Early Human Development*, In Press, Corrected Proof, Available online 23 July 2011.

Kottegoda, S., Samuel, K. and Emmanuel, S. (2008) Reproductive health concerns in six conflict-affected areas of Sri Lanka. *Reproductive Health Matters* 16, 75–82.

Krause, S.K., Meyers, J.L. and Friedlander, E. (2006) Improving the availability of emergency obstetric care in conflict-affected settings. *Global Public Health* 1, 205–228.

Loevinsohn, B. and Harding, A. (2004) *Contracting for the Delivery of Community Health Services: A Review of Global Experience*. World Bank Human Development Network, World Bank, Washington, DC.

Massoud, R., Askov, K., Reinke, J., Franco, L.M., Bornstein, T., Knebel, E. and MacAulay, C. (2001) *A Modern Paradigm for Improving Healthcare Quality*. QA Monograph Series 1(1). USAID and QAP/URC, Bethesda, Maryland.

McGinn, T. (2000) Reproductive Health of War-Affected Populations: What Do We Know? *International Family Planning Perspectives* 26(4), DOI: 10.1363/2617400.

Meessen, B., Musango, L., Kashala, J.P. and Lemlin, J. (2006) Reviewing institutions of rural health centers: the Performance Initiative in Butare, Rwanda. *Tropical Medicine and International Health* 11(8), 1303–1317.

Mullany, L.C., Lee, C.I., Yone, L., Paw, P., Oo, E.K.S., Maung, C., Lee, T.J. and Beyrer, C. (2008) Access to essential maternal health interventions and human rights violations among vulnerable communities in Eastern Burma. *PLoS Medicine* 5(12), e242 doi:10.1371/journal.pmed.0050242.

Nabarro, D. (2004) The Ultimate Challenge: Sustaining Life in Fragile States Presentation at HLF meeting in Abuja. In: *Rebuilding Health Systems and Providing Health Services in Fragile States*. Management Sciences for Health, Cambridge, Massachusetts.

Nagai, M., Abraham, S., Okamoto, M., Kita, E. and Aoyama, A. (2007) Reconstruction of health service systems in post-conflict Northern Province of Sri Lanka. *Health Policy and Planning* 83, 84–93.

Noji, E.K. (2005) Public health issues in disasters. *Critical Care Medicine* 33(1), S29–S33.

O'Hare, B.A. and Southall, D.P. (2007) First do no harm: the impact of recent armed conflict on maternal and child health in Sub-Saharan Africa. *Journal of the Royal Society of Medicine* 100(12), 564–570.

O'Heir, J. (2004) Pregnancy and childbirth care following conflict and displacement: care for refugee women in low-resource settings. *Journal of Midwifery and Women's Health* 49(4)(Suppl. 1), 14–18.

Palmer, N. (2006) An awkward threesome – donors, governments and non-state providers of health in low income countries. *Public Administration and Development* 26, 231–240.

RAISE (2007) Emergency Obstetric Care Fact Sheet. Available at: http://www.mariestopes.org/documents/Emergency%20obstectric%20care.pdf (accessed 30 August 2011).

Relief Web Project (2008) Glossary of Humanitarian terms. Available at: http://www.who.int/hac/about/reliefweb-aug2008.pdf (accessed 30 August 2011).

Reproductive Health Response in Conflict (RHRC) (2004) Consortium Monitoring and Evaluation ToolKit Combination Methods – Rapid Assessment Protocol, p. 2. Available at: http://www.rhrc.org/resources/general_fieldtools/toolkit/65%20Rapid%20Assessment%20Protocol.pdf (accessed 30 August 2011).

Roberts, B., Guy, S., Sondorp, E. and Lee-Jones, L. (2008) A basic package of health services for post-conflict countries: implications for sexual and reproductive health services. *Reproductive Health Matters* 16(31), 57–64.

Smith, J.M., Currie, S., Azfar, P. and Rahmanzai, A.J. (2008) Establishment of an accreditation system for midwifery education in Afghanistan: Maintaining quality during national expansion. *Public Health* 122(6), 558–567.

Soeters, R., Habineza, C. and Peerenboom, P.B. (2006) Performance-based financing and changing the district health system: experience from Rwanda. *Bulletin of the World Health Organization* 84(11), 884–889.

Sondorp, E., Palmer, N., Strong, L. and Wali, A. (2009) *Afghanistan: Paying NGOs for Performance in a Postconflict Setting.* Center for Global Development, Washington, DC.

Spiegel, P., Checchi, F., Colombo, S. and Pail, E. (2010) Health-care needs of people affected by conflict: future trends and changing frameworks. *Lancet* 375, 341–345.

UN (undated) United Nations Office for the Coordination of Humanitarian affairs. Available at: http://www.unocha.org (accessed 29 March 2011).

UN Department of Economic and Social Affairs (UNESA) (2010) Available at: http://www.esa.un.org/wpp (accessed 27 July 2011).

UNFPA (2010) Guidelines on Data Issues in Humanitarian Crisis Situations. Available at: http://www.unfpa.org/public/cache/offonce/home/publications/pid/6253;jsessionid=5A6402 (accessed 30 August 2011).

UNFPA, WHO and Andalusian School of Public Health (2009) Granada Consensus on Sexual and Reproductive Health in Protracted Crises and Recovery. Available at: http://www.rhrc.org/resources/index.cfm?sector=rh#207 (accessed 30 August 2011).

UNHCR (2011a) Figures at a glance. Available at: http://www.unhcr.org/pages/49c3646c11.html (accessed 30 August 2011).

UNHCR (2011b) Health information system. Available at: http://www.unhcr.org/pages/49c3646ce0.html (accessed 30 August 2011).

Varley, E. (2010) Targeted doctors, missing patients: obstetrical health services and sectarian conflict in Northern Pakistan. *Social Science and Medicine* 70, 61–70.

Vergeer, P., Canavan, A. and Rothmann, I. (2009) A rethink on the use of aid mechanisms in health sector early recovery. Development Policy and Practice, Royal Tropical Institute, Amsterdam. Available at: http://www.kit.nl/net/KIT_Publicaties_output/ShowFile2.aspx?e=1508 (accessed 31 August 2011).

Waldman, R. (2006) *Health Programming in Post-Conflict Fragile States.* Basic Support for Institutionalizing Child Survival (BASICS) for the United States Agency for International Development (USAID), Arlington, Virginia.

WHO (2000a) *Reproductive Health During Conflict and Displacement. A Guide for Programme Managers.* WHO, Geneva.

WHO (2000b) *The World Health Report 2000: Health Systems Improving Performance.* WHO, Geneva.

WHO (2005) *Guide to Health Workforce Development in Post Conflict Situations.* WHO, Geneva.

WHO (2008a) *Global Assessment of National Health Sector Emergency Preparedness and Response.* WHO, Geneva.

WHO (2008b) Assessing the national health information system: An assessment tool version 4.00. Available at: http://www.who.int/entity/healthmetrics/tools/Version_4.00_Assessment_Tool3.pdf (accessed 30 August 2011).

WHO (2009) HeRAMS Health Resources Availability Mapping System. Approach & Roles and Responsibilities of the Cluster. Global Health Cluster/Health Actions in Crisis/World Health Organization. Available at: http://www.who.int/entity/hac/network/global…/herams_users_guide.pdf (accessed 15 November 2011).

WHO (2010) Trends in Maternal Mortality: 1990 to 2008. World Health Organization, Geneva. Available at: http://whqlibdoc.who.int/publications/2010/9789241500265_eng.pdf (accessed 15 November 2011).

WHO (2011) Health Action in Crises Cluster Countries. Available at: http://www.who.int/hac/global_health_cluster/countries/en/index.html (accessed 20 March 2011).

WHO and World Bank (2005) High-Level Forum on the Health MDGs – Health Service delivery in post-conflict states, Paris 14–15 November 2005. Available at: http://www.hlfhealthmdgs.org/Documents/HealthServiceDelivery.pdf (accessed 30 September 2011).

Williams, J.L. and McCarthy, B. (2005) Observations from a maternal and infant hospital in Kabul Afghanistan, 2003. *Journal of Midwifery and Women's Health* 50, 31–35.

Women's Refugee Commission (2011) Four Months On: A Snapshot of Priority Reproductive Health Activities in Haiti. Available at: http://womensrefugeecommission.org/blog/1003-six-months-later-reproductive-health-needs-still-critical-in-haiti?q=four+months (accessed 30 August 2011).

World Bank (2010) Harmonized list of fragile situations. Available at: http://siteresources.worldbank.org/EXTLICUS/Resources/511777-1269623894864/Fragile_Situations_List_FY11_(Oct_19_2010).pdf (accessed 30 August 2011).

World Bank (2011) The World Development Report 2011. Available at: http://wdr2011.worldbank.org/ (accessed 30 August 2011).

Index

Page numbers in **bold** refer to illustrations and tables